Proceedings of the
TRACE ELEMENTS in DIET, NUTRITION, and HEALTH:
ESSENTIALITY and TOXICITY

Proceedings

of the

TRACE ELEMENTS in DIET, NUTRITION, and HEALTH: ESSENTIALITY and TOXICITY

A Joint Conference Constituting the

VIIIth Conference of the
International Society for Trace Element Research in Humans
(ISTERH)

IXth Conference of the
Nordic Trace Element Society
(NTES)

VIth Conference of the
Hellenic Trace Element Society
(HTES)

Hersonissos
CRETE-GREECE

October 21–26, 2007

Creta Maris Conference Center

Members of Planning Committee

Curtiss Hunt, Ph.D., Chair, Planning Committee; President, ISTERH
Sophie Ermidou-Pollet, Ph.D., President, HTES
Ole Andersen, Ph.D., Representative, NTES
Dorothy Klimis-Zacas, Ph.D., Chair, Local Organizing Committee; Member, ISTERH
Jeanne Freeland-Graves, Ph.D., Chair, Fundraising Committee; Council Member, ISTERH
Monica Nordberg, Ph.D., Chair, Abstract Committee; Vice-President, ISTERH
Hiroko Kodama, Ph.D., Chair, Publicity Committee; Secretary, ISTERH
Serge Pollet, Ph.D., Member at Large; Vice-President, HTES
George Brewer, M.D., Member at Large; Council Member, ISTERH
Harold Sandstead, M.D., Member at Large; Immediate Past-President, ISTERH

Reprinted from Cell Biology and Toxicology, Volume 24 Issues 4 & 5, 2008.

Editor
Curtiss Hunt
United States Department of Agriculture,
Agricultural Research Service,
Grand Forks ND 58202-9034
USA

ISBN: 978-1-4020-9068-4   e-ISBN: 978-1-4020-9056-1

DOI: 10.1007/978-1-4020-9056-1

Library of Congress Control Number: 2009920770

Printed on acid-free paper

springer.com

Cell Biology and Toxicology

An International Journal devoted to research at the cellular level

Official Journal of the Société Pharmaco-Toxicologie Cellulaire

Volume 24 · Numbers 4–5 · 2009

Indexed in *Current Contents*, *Index Medicus*, and *EMBASE*.

Instructions for authors for *Cell Biol Toxicol* are available at http://www.springer.com/10565.

ACKNOWLEDGEMENTS

Funding for this conference was made possible in part by 1 R13 DK080637-01 from the National Institutes of Health. The views expressed in written conference materials or publications and by speakers and moderators do not necessarily reflect the official policies of the Department of Health and Human Services; nor does mention of trade names, commercial practices, or organizations imply endorsement by the U.S. Government.

The project was supported by the National Research Initiative of the USDA Cooperative State Research, Education and Extension Service Grant number 2007-35200-18235.

Dimerumic acid protected oxidative stress-induced cytotoxicity in isolated rat hepatocytes

Jun-ichi Yamashiro · Sumihiro Shiraishi ·
Toru Fuwa · Toshiharu Horie

Originally published in the journal Cell Biology and Toxicology, Volume 24, Nos 4–5, 3–10.
DOI: 10.1007/s10565-007-9037-7 © Springer Science + Business Media B.V. 2007

Abstract Dimerumic acid (DMA) is contained in *Monascus anka* and *Monascus pilosus* fermented products. The purpose of this study was to evaluate the effect of DMA against salicylic acid (SA)- and tert-butylhydroperoxide (t-BHP)-induced oxidative stress and cytotoxicity in the liver, using rat liver microsomes and isolated rat hepatocytes. DMA was extracted from monascus-garlic-fermented extract using *M. pilosus*. In rat liver microsomes, 1 μM DMA decreased SA-induced lipid peroxidation but did not affect the production of the oxidative metabolite of SA via CYP. In isolated rat hepatocytes, 1 μM DMA decreased SA-induced lipid peroxidation and chemiluminescence (CL) generation and the intracellular glutathione-reduced form/oxidized form (GSH/GSSG) ratio in the presence of 1 μM DMA was higher than that without DMA; however, 100 μM DMA suppressed the leakage of lactate dehydrogenase (LDH). On the other hand, t-BHP-induced lipid peroxidation, CL generation, and LDH leakage were prevented by 100 μM DMA. Thus, DMA showed an antioxidative effect in hepatocytes and protected against hepatotoxicity by suppressing oxidative stress without affecting CYP enzymes.

Keywords Antioxidant · Dimerumic acid · Isolated rat hepatocyte · Oxidative stress

Abbreviations

CL	chemiluminescence
DHB	dihydroxybenzoic acid
DMA	dimerumic acid
GSH	glutathione
GSSG	glutathione oxidized form
LDH	lactate dehydrogenase
ROS	reactive oxygen species
SA	salicylic acid
TBARS	thiobarbituric acid reactive substances
t-BHP	tert-butylhydroperoxide

J.-i. Yamashiro · T. Horie (✉)
Department of Biopharmaceutics,
Graduate School of Pharmaceutical Sciences,
Chiba University,
1-8-1, Inohana, Chuo-ku,
Chiba 260-8675, Japan
e-mail: horieto@p.chiba-u.ac.jp

S. Shiraishi · T. Fuwa
Research and Development Division,
Wakunaga Pharmaceutical Company,
Osaka, Japan

Introduction

It is well known that reactive oxygen species (ROS) are one of the triggers of various disorders of biological systems (Kehrer 1993), aging (Barja 2004), and apoptosis (Haddad 2004) because of their high reactivity with lipids, proteins, and DNA. ROS are suggested to play an important role in cytochrome c release from mitochondria followed by apoptotic response. In addition, not only ROS but also products of lipid peroxidation are reported to be related to cellular signaling as shown by the example of 4-hydroxy-2-nonenal, which is an aldehyde (Forman and Dickinson 2004).

Dimerumic acid (DMA) of which structure was shown in Fig. 1 was reported as a breakdown product of Coprogen B, which was secreted as siderophore from microorganisms (Burt 1982) and obtained from fermented products by *Monascus anka* and *Monascus pilosus*. The genus *Monascus* was traditionally used for the preparation of fermented foods and food additives in Asia; moreover, it is utilized as Chinese herbal medicine. Recent studies suggest that DMA has an antioxidative effect in vitro (Taira et al. 2002) and a protective effect on carbon tetrachloride-induced liver injury in mice (Aniya et al. 2000); however, there is little evidence showing a direct correlation between the antioxidative effect and cytoprotective effect. It is uncertain whether the antioxidative effect of DMA participates in the cytoprotective effect. Many compounds from natural sources have been reported as antioxidants and are expected to possess protective effects against various disorders of biological systems. For example, it is suggested that a sufficient supply of dietary antioxidants may delay or prevent diabetes complexity including renal or neural impairment by a protective effect against oxidative stress caused by hyperglycemia (Osawa and Kato 2005). If DMA exhibits antioxidative potency in cells, DMA will be expected to protect humans from various disorders induced by oxidative stress.

Salicylic acid (SA), a typical non-steroidal anti-inflammatory drug, induces lipid peroxidation and produces chemiluminescence originating from singlet oxygen and excited carbonyls by its metabolism via CYP (Doi et al. 1998, 2002). tert-Butylhydroperoxide (t-BHP) is used as a model oxidant in isolated hepatocytes (Takayama et al. 2001). In this study, we evaluated the antioxidative effect of DMA against SA- and t-BHP-induced oxidative stress and cytotoxicity of the liver and by using rat liver microsomes and isolated rat hepatocytes.

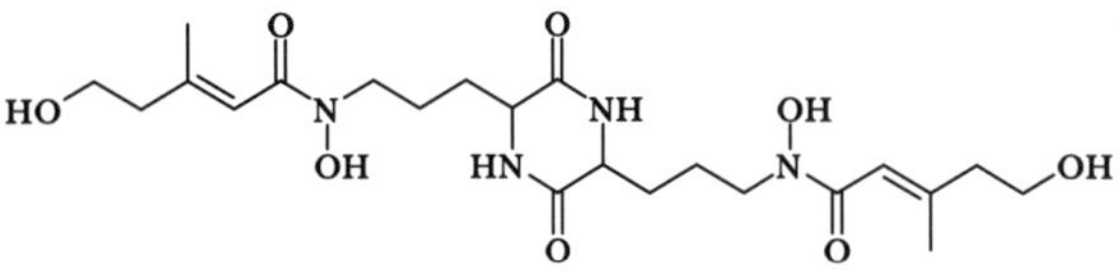

Materials and methods

Chemicals

DMA was extracted from monascus-garlic-fermented extract using *M. pilosus*. SA, 2-thiobarbituric acid (TBA), trichloroacetic acid (TCA), 2,5-dihydroxybenzoic acid (2,5-DHB), 2,4-dihydroxybenzoic acid (2,4-DHB), glutathione (GSH), glutathione oxidized form (GSSG), and lithium pyruvate were purchased from Wako Pure Chemical Industries (Osaka, Japan). Nicotinamide adenine dinucleotide phosphate (reduced form) (NADPH) and β-NADH were obtained from Oriental Yeast (Tokyo, Japan). Collagenase S-1 was from Nitta Gelatin (Osaka, Japan). All other reagents were of analytical grade.

Animals

Male Sprague–Dawley rats aged 6–7 weeks (Japan SLC, Shizuoka, Japan) were used throughout all experiments. The rats were given food and water ad libitum, were housed under a 12-h light/dark cycle, and acclimatized for at least 1 week before experimental use. All procedures described below were approved by the animal care committee of Chiba University.

Preparation of rat liver microsomes

Rats without treatment were sacrificed by decapitation, and the liver was removed. Rat liver microsomes were then prepared according to the method of Omura and Sato (1962). The protein concentration of microsomes was measured according to Lowry et al. (1951) with bovine serum albumin as the standard.

Incubation of rat liver microsomes

Liver microsomes (1 mg protein/ml) were suspended in 154 mM potassium phosphate buffer (pH 7.4) containing 10 mM $MgCl_2$ and 5 mM SA with or without DMA and then preincubated for 5 min at 37°C. The reaction was started by the addition of 0.5 mM NADPH as a

Fig. 1 Chemical structure of dimerumic acid

final concentration. The samples for lipid peroxidation assay were taken from reaction mixtures at 15, 30, and 60 min after the start of the reaction. Desferrioxamine was added in microsomal suspension for the metabolite assay. Samples were taken from reaction mixtures at 15 and 30 min after the start of the reaction and the amount of 2,5-DHB, a metabolite of SA produced in the reaction mixture, was determined by high performance liquid chromatography (HPLC).

Isolation of rat hepatocytes

Isolated rat hepatocytes were prepared by the collagenase perfusion method, as described previously (Horie et al. 1988). The viability of hepatocytes used in this study was more than 85%, as determined by the trypan blue exclusion test. Isolated hepatocytes were suspended in reaction buffer containing 137 mM NaCl, 5.2 mM KCl, 3 mM $NaHPO_4$, 0.9 mM $MgSO_4$, 0.12 mM $CaCl_2$, 5 mM glucose, and 10 mM N-2-hydroxyethylpiperazine-N'-2-ethanesulfonic acid (HEPES) at pH 7.4. This buffer was used for all experiments unless otherwise noted.

Incubation of isolated rat hepatocytes

Hepatocytes (10^6 cells/ml) in the reaction buffer with or without DMA were preincubated for 10 min at 37° C, and then 5 mM SA or 1 mM t-BHP as a final concentration was added to the hepatocyte suspension. Samples from the reaction mixture with added 5 mM SA or 1 mM t-BHP were taken at 2 or 1 h, respectively, after the start of the reaction for the lipid peroxidation assay, chemiluminescence (CL) measurement, glutathione assay, and lactate dehydrogenase (LDH) assay.

Lipid peroxidation assay

The extent of lipid peroxidation was determined by measuring the amount of thiobarbituric acid reactive substances (TBARS) as previously described (Buege and Aust 1978). About 0.5 ml of microsome or hepatocyte samples were added to 0.5 ml of 15% TCA. Then, 2 ml of TBA reagent containing 15% TCA, 0.375% TBA, and 0.25 N HCl were added to the mixture and boiled for 15 min. The absorbance of the supernatant was determined at 535 nm with 1,1,3,3-tetraethoxypropane as the standard.

Metabolite assay

2,5-DHB was determined according to the method of Doi et al. (2002) with some modification. The microsome sample (1 ml) was added to 100 μl of 3 N $HClO_4$ to stop the reaction. The mixture was centrifuged at 15,900×g for 10 min, and then the supernatant (1 ml) was separated. A 50-μl sample of 2.5 mM 2,4-DHB (as an internal standard) and 5 ml of ethyl acetate were added to the supernatant (1 ml) and the mixture was vortexed for 2 min. The mixture was then centrifuged at 1,670×g for 15 min. The organic layer was evaporated to dryness, and the residue was analyzed by HPLC according to the condition of Prasad et al. (1995) with some modifications. TSK-GEL ODS-80$_{TM}$ (4.6 mm inner diameter × 150 mm; TOSOH, Tokyo, Japan) was used for separation. The mobile phase consisted of 30 mM citric acid-sodium acetate buffer (pH 3.6): methanol (17:3, v/v). The flow rate was 0.8 ml/min. A UV spectrophotometer (wavelength, 315 nm) was used for detection.

CL assay

CL was measured using a single photoelectron counting system, CLD-110 and CLC-10 (Tohoku Electronic Industrial, Sendai, Japan). Hepatocyte suspension (1 ml) was placed into a stainless-steel dish (diameter, 20 mm; height, 10 mm) and set inside the detector for 30 s at 37°C. CL intensity was then detected for 1 min.

Glutathione assay

GSH and GSSG were determined by the method of Keller and Menzel (1985) with some modifications (Ji et al. 2002; Ito et al. 2004), in which 1 ml HPO_3/ethylenediaminetetraacetic acid (EDTA) solution (2% HPO_3 and 0.08% EDTA) was added to hepatocytes (10^6 cells) precipitated by centrifugation at 260×g for 1 min. The mixture was then centrifuged at 15,000×g for 15 min. The supernatant was mixed with 3-fluorotyrosine as an internal standard and subsequently filtrated through a 0.45-μm syringe filter (Millex-LH; Millipore, Bedford, MA, USA) for HPLC detection. An Inertsil ODS column (4.6 mm inner diameter × 250 mm; GL Sciences, Tokyo, Japan) was used with a mobile phase (0.1% trifluoroacetic acid/methanol= 20:1) at a flow rate of 1.0 ml/min. The eluate from the column was mixed with solution containing 18.6 mM phthaldialdehyde and 17.1 mM 2-mercaptoethanol in 100 mM carbonate buffer (pH 10.5), delivered at a rate of 0.2 ml/min. The mixture was then passed through a stainless-steel coil at 70°C to facilitate derivatization. A fluorescence detector was used and operated at an excitation wavelength of 355 nm and an emission wavelength of 425 nm. The concentrations of GSH and GSSG were calculated with reference to the area of the standard GSH and GSSG samples.

LDH assay

LDH activity in the supernatant obtained by centrifugation (260×*g* for 1 min) of the hepatocyte suspension was assayed by oxidation of NADH (Wroblewski and Ladue 1955). About 50 mM potassium phosphate buffer containing 0.18 mM β-NADH and 0.62 mM lithium pyruvate (pH 7.5) were preincubated at 37°C for 2 min, and then 20 μl of the supernatant was added to start the reaction. The decrease of absorbance at 340 nm was measured continuously for 2 min. Cytotoxicity was expressed as a percentage of total LDH activity, which was obtained from the cell lysate solubilized by 0.5% Triton X-100.

Statistical analysis

Statistical analysis was performed by analysis of variance (ANOVA) followed by Dunnett's post-hoc test. Differences were considered significant when $P<0.05$.

Results

Effect of DMA on SA-induced lipid peroxidation in rat liver microsomes

The liver microsome suspension (1 mg protein/ml) was incubated at 37°C with 0.5 mM NADPH and 5 mM SA. The production of lipid peroxides was measured as TBARS formation. Microsomal lipid peroxidation was depressed markedly by the addition of 1 μM DMA and completely by 10 μM DMA (Fig. 2), which was almost to the same level as that in the microsome suspension incubated with 10 uM DMA. 2,5-DHB, an SA metabolite, was measured to evaluate whether DMA inhibits CYP activity. SA metabolism in rat liver microsomes was not affected by the presence of 1, 10, and 100 μM DMA (data not shown).

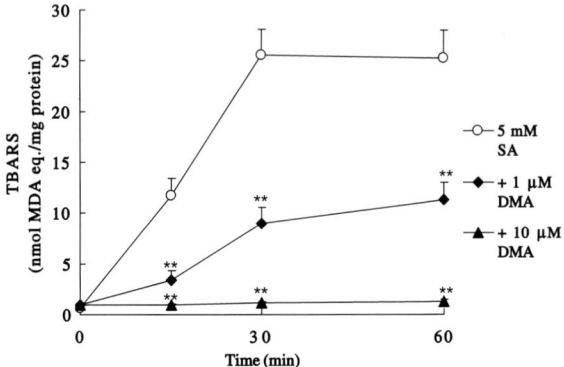

Fig. 2 Effect of DMA on generation of lipid peroxides in rat liver microsomes with SA. Rat liver microsomes with 5 mM SA were incubated for 15, 30, and 60 min with or without DMA. Generation of lipid peroxides was evaluated as TBARS production. Each value represents the mean ± S.D. of three experiments. **P<0.01, significantly different from 5 mM SA

Concentration-dependent effect of DMA on SA-induced oxidative stress in isolated rat hepatocytes

The isolated rat hepatocyte suspension with 5 mM SA was incubated for 2 h with various concentrations of DMA (0.01–10 μM). TBARS produced by SA slightly decreased in the presence of 0.1 μM DMA and was almost completely depressed at more than 1 μM DMA (Fig. 3), which was almost to the same level as that in the hepatocyte suspension incubated with 10 uM DMA. CL generation by SA decreased with 0.1 μM DMA and was significantly depressed with more than 1 μM DMA (Fig. 4). Intracellular GSH/GSSG ratio was used as an indicator of intracellular redox status. The GSH/GSSG ratio in the presence of 1 and 10 μM DMA was significantly higher than that without DMA (Fig. 5).

Effect of DMA on SA-induced cytotoxicity in isolated rat hepatocytes

SA cytotoxicity was evaluated by measuring extracellular LDH. LDH leakage was significantly suppressed by incubating for 3 h with 100 μM DMA and for 2 and 3 h with 1 mM DMA (Fig. 6).

Effect of DMA on t-BHP-induced oxidative stress and cell injury in isolated rat hepatocytes

The isolated rat hepatocyte suspension with 1 mM t-BHP was incubated for 1 h with various concentrations

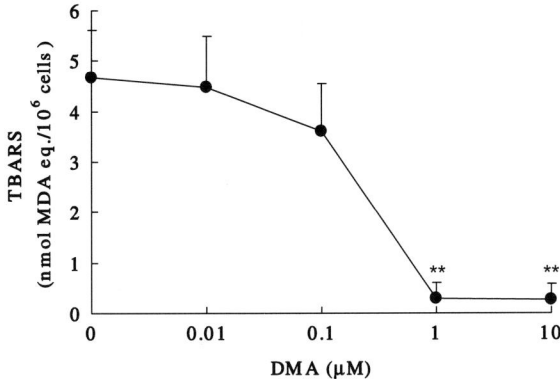

Fig. 3 Effect of DMA on generation of lipid peroxides in isolated rat hepatocytes with SA. The isolated rat hepatocyte suspension with 5 mM SA was incubated for 2 h with or without DMA. Each value represents the mean ± SD of four experiments. **P<0.01, significantly different from 0 μM DMA

of DMA or without DMA. TBARS formation, CL generation, and LDH leakage observed in the isolated rat hepatocyte suspension incubated with 1 mM t-BHP were significantly suppressed by the addition of 100 μM DMA (Fig. 7).

Discussion

DMA is as a siderophore with high affinity for ferric ion (Burt 1982; Frederick et al. 1981). *M. anka* extract was reported to protect against acetaminophen-induced liver toxicity in rats (Aniya et al. 1998) and to prevent H_2O_2-derived lipid peroxidation in rat liver micro-

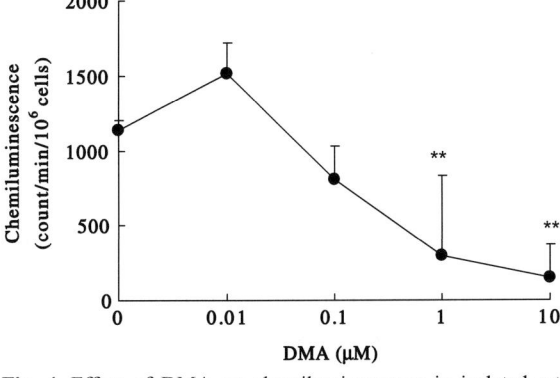

Fig. 4 Effect of DMA on chemiluminescence in isolated rat hepatocytes with SA. The isolated rat hepatocyte suspension with 5 mM SA was incubated for 2 h with or without DMA. Chemiluminescence from hepatocyte suspension was counted for 1 min. Each value represents the mean ± SD of four experiments. **P<0.01, significantly different from 0 μM DMA

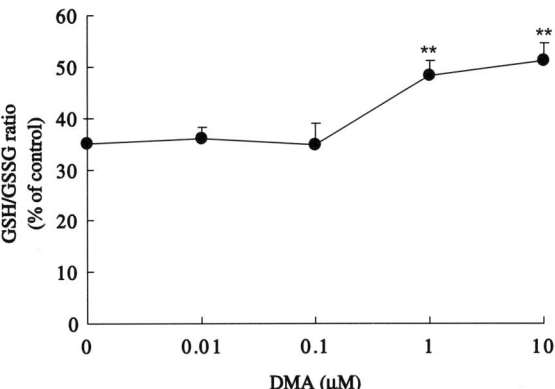

Fig. 5 Effect of DMA on GSH/GSSG ratio in isolated rat hepatocytes with SA. The isolated rat hepatocyte suspension with 5 mM SA was incubated for 2 h with or without DMA. Each value represents the mean ± SD of four experiments. The GSH/GSSG ratio in the hepatocyte suspension without SA and DMA was expressed as 100% (control). **P<0.01, significantly different from 0 μM DMA

somes (Aniya et al. 1999). DMA was identified in *M. anka* extract, and an antioxidative effect was found using electron spin resonance with 1,1-diphenyl-2-picrylhydrazyl (Aniya et al. 2000). Recently, DMA was identified from monascus-garlic-fermented extract, a unique material produced from garlic fermented using *M. pilosus* (Sumioka et al. 2006); however, the antioxidative effect of DMA on intact cells and organs remains to be clarified. Thus, we aimed to confirm its

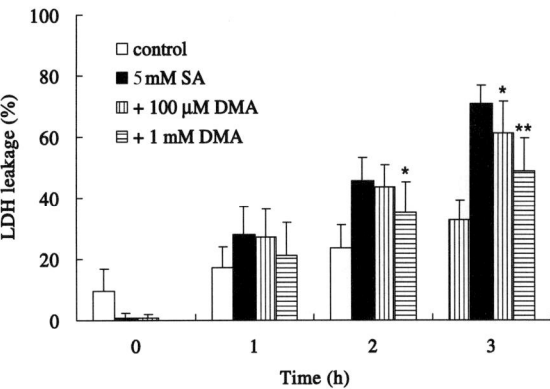

Fig. 6 Effect of DMA on extracellular LDH leakage in isolated rat hepatocytes with SA. The isolated rat hepatocyte suspension with 5 mM SA was incubated for 1, 2, and 3 h with or without DMA. Each value represents the mean ± SD of four experiments. The control means the hepatocyte suspension containing neither SA nor DMA. Cytotoxicity was expressed as a percentage of the extracellular LDH activity of samples to that obtained from cells treated with 0.5% Triton X-100. *P<0.05 and **P<0.01, significantly different from SA-treated hepatocytes without DMA

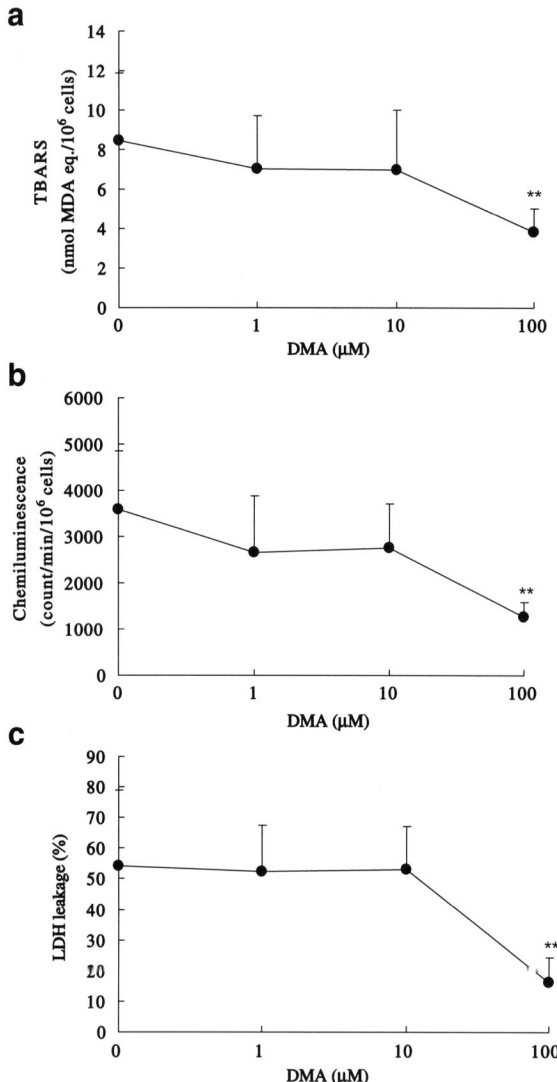

Fig. 7 Effect of DMA on generation of lipid peroxides (**a**), chemiluminescence (**b**) and LDH leakage (**c**) in isolated rat hepatocytes with t-BHP. The isolated rat hepatocyte suspension with 1 mM t-BHP was incubated for 1 h with or without DMA. LDH leakage (%) was expressed as a percentage of extracellular LDH activity of samples to that from hepatocytes treated with 0.5% Triton X-100. Each value represents the mean ± SD of four experiments. $**P<0.01$, significantly different from 0 μM DMA

antioxidative effect on hepatocytes and to investigate whether its antioxidative effect plays a role in the cytoprotective effect.

In the present study, DMA protected against lipid peroxidation and ROS production by oxidants in rat hepatocytes and liver microsomes but did not inhibit the oxidative metabolism of SA. About 1 μM DMA suppressed SA-induced lipid peroxidation in rat liver microsomes (Fig. 2), consistent with a previous report indicating that DMA inhibited NADPH-induced lipid peroxidation at 2 μM in rat liver microsomes, and the concentration of DMA exhibiting an antioxidative effect was about three orders of magnitude lower than that of ascorbic acid (Taira et al. 2002). Thus, DMA has a potent antioxidant effect. Ultraweak CL from living cells is used to measure ROS production in real time because of its non-invasive and direct detection of light emission from singlet molecular oxygen ($^1O_2$) and excited carbonyl compounds (R=O*), as shown in isolated hepatocytes (Cadenas et al. 1981). $^1O_2$ is generated from free radicals and chain reactions of lipid peroxides. R=O* is mainly from chain reactions of lipid peroxides (Cadenas and Sies 1984). Oral administration of SA induced TBARS increase in rat liver (Gunther et al. 1991), and SA-induced oxidative stress occurred in rat liver microsomes (Doi et al. 1998). CYP 3A and 2E isoforms are reported to be involved in the 5-hydroxylation of SA (Dupont et al. 1999). CYP 2E1 is known to be an isoform involved in oxidative stress (Kessova and Cederbaum 2003). SA-induced oxidative stress originated from the CYP metabolic pathway, as it was suppressed by the addition of a CYP inhibitor, SKF-525A (Doi et al. 1998). In the study of isolated rat hepatocytes, 1 μM DMA prevented SA-induced lipid peroxidation and CL generation in isolated rat hepatocytes (Figs. 3 and 4). Furthermore, DMA suppressed the SA-induced decrease of GSH/GSSG ratio (Fig. 5). The DMA concentration exhibiting an antioxidative effect in rat hepatocytes (Figs. 3 and 4) was consistent with that in rat liver microsomes (Fig. 2). Thus, DMA showed an antioxidative effect in intact hepatocytes and in microsomes; however, DMA was considered to be a possible inhibitor of CYP because *M. anka* preparation including DMA was reported to inhibit CYP activity, and an antioxidative effect might be derived from its inhibitor effect (Aniya et al. 1998). The influence of DMA on CYP activity in microsomes was evaluated by measuring the amount of 2,5-DHB, an oxidative metabolite of SA. As it is known that NADPH in microsomes produces free radicals, which inhibit CYP activity, we added desferrioxamine as a radical scavenger in reaction buffer of 2,5-DHB determination experiments to protect CYP from inactivation by NADPH-induced free radicals. As a result, 2,5-DHB production was not changed by the addition of DMA (data not shown), suggesting that DMA does not affect 5-hydroxylation of SA; that is, DMA does not inhibit CYP activity. Thus, the antioxidative effect of DMA was found to come from its own antioxidative property but not from inhibiting CYP, and it is considered that DMA scavenges free radicals generated from oxidative metabolism of SA by CYP before lipid peroxidation. Taira et al. suggested the mechanism of the radical scavenging effect of DMA (Taira et al. 2002). DMA has two hydroxamic acid groups, and these functional groups scavenge free radicals by providing their hydrogen atom through converting the hydroxamic acid group to nitroxide radical. There are many reports about the antioxidative effect of hydroxamic acid derivatives. Desferrioxamine inhibited hydroxyl radical-like peroxynitrite reactivity (Denicola et al. 1995). It was suggested that the protective action of desferrioxamine against tissue damage in vivo was derived from its radical-scavenging ability (Halliwell 1989). DMA acts as siderophore having free iron-binding ability (Burt 1982; Frederick et al. 1981). Free iron stimulates the chain reaction of lipid peroxides and amplifies ROS reactivity by converting hydroperoxide to hydroxyl radical, known as the Fenton reaction. Hydroxyl radical has quite high reactivity to lipids and various proteins followed by its collapse or dysfunction; thus, the iron-binding action of DMA may have some role in its antioxidative effect.

Generation of CL and TBARS in t-BHP-treated hepatocytes was inhibited at 100 µM DMA (Fig. 7a,b). This concentration was two orders of magnitude higher than that of SA-treated hepatocytes. These inconsistent results were derived from the different potency required to induce oxidative stress between SA and t-BHP. As the increase of CL count in t-BHP-treated hepatocytes was higher than that in SA-treated hepatocytes, 1 mM t-BHP was a more potent oxidant than 5 mM SA.

Hepatotoxicity of salicylate including vacuolization and mitochondrial morphological abnormalities was previously reported in cultured rat hepatocytes (Tolman et al. 1978). Salicylate also induces mitochondrial swelling and uncoupling in rat liver mitochondria (Whitehouse 1964; You 1983). In addition, we found that SA induced the depletion of hepatocellular ATP and decrease of mitochondrial oxygen consumption (unpublished data). As shown here, SA-induced LDH leakage was suppressed by DMA addition (Fig. 6), but this concentration was much higher than that exhibiting an antioxidative effect. On the other hand, the concentration of DMA inhibiting t-BHP-induced LDH leakage was consistent with that suppressing lipid peroxidation. These results suggest that cytotoxicity induced by SA may not be caused only by oxidative stress via its oxidative metabolism.

DMA is not a well-studied compound, and its protective effect against disorders derived from oxidative stress is still uncertain; however, there are also many reports suggesting that antioxidants reduce disease risk and many reports indicating a relationship between ROS and various disorders. For example, vitamin E reduces cardiovascular disease risk in humans (Rimm et al. 1993; Stampfer et al. 1993). DMA and *M. anka* preparation protected against CCl_4- and acetaminophen-induced liver injury (Aniya et al. 1998, 2000), respectively. We showed the antioxidant action of DMA in hepatocytes; thus, DMA possibly protects against a variety of diseases caused by oxidative stress.

In conclusion, DMA shows an antioxidative effect on hepatocytes and protects against hepatotoxicity by suppressing oxidative stress without affecting CYP enzymes. This study provides biological evidence supporting the intake of DMA for scavenging free radicals.

References

Aniya Y, Yokomakura T, Yonamine M, Nagamine T, Nakanishi H. Protective effect of the mold Monascus anka against acetaminophen-induced liver toxicity in rats. Jpn J Pharmacol 1998;78(1):79–82.

Aniya Y, Yokomakura T, Yonamine M, Shimada K, Nagamine T, Shimabukuro M, Gibo H. Screening of antioxidant action of various molds and protection of Monascus anka against experimentally induced liver injuries of rats. Gen Pharmacol 1999;32(2):225–31.

Aniya Y, Ohtani II, Higa T, Miyagi C, Gibo H, Shimabukuro M, Nakanishi H, Taira J. Dimerumic acid as an antioxidant of the mold, Monascus anka. Free Radic Biol Med 2000;28(6):999–1004.

Barja G. Free radicals and aging. Trends Neurosci 2004;27(10):595–600.

Buege JA, Aust SD. Microsomal lipid peroxidation. Methods Enzymol 1978;52:302–10.

Burt WR. Identification of coprogen B and its breakdown products from *Histoplasma capsulatum*. Infect Immun 1982;35(3):990–6.

Cadenas E, Sies H. Low-level chemiluminescence as an indicator of singlet molecular oxygen in biological systems. Methods Enzymol 1984;105:221–31.

Cadenas E, Wefers H, Sies H. Low-level chemiluminescence of isolated hepatocytes. Eur J Biochem 1981;119(3):531–6.

Denicola A, Souza JM, Gatti RM, Augusto O, Radi R. Desferrioxamine inhibition of the hydroxyl radical-like reactivity of peroxynitrite: role of the hydroxamic groups. Free Radic Biol Med 1995;19(1):11–9.

Doi H, Masubuchi Y, Narimatsu S, Nishigaki R, Horie T. Salicylic acid-induced lipid peroxidation in rat liver microsomes. Res Commun Mol Pathol Pharmacol 1998;100(3):265–71.

Doi H, Iwasaki H, Masubuchi Y, Nishigaki R, Horie T. Chemiluminescence associated with the oxidative metabolism of salicylic acid in rat liver microsomes. Chem Biol Interact 2002;140(2):109–19.

Dupont I, Berthou F, Bodenez P, Bardou L, Guirriec C, Stephan N, Dreano Y, Lucas D. Involvement of cytochromes P-450 2E1 and 3A4 in the 5-hydroxylation of salicylate in humans. Drug Metab Dispos 1999;27(3):322–6.

Forman HJ, Dickinson DA. Introduction to serial reviews on 4-hydroxy-2-nonenal as a signaling molecule. Free Radic Biol Med 2004;37(5):594–6.

Frederick CB, Bentley MD, Shive W. Structure of triornicin, a new siderophore. Biochemistry 1981;20(9):2436–8.

Gunther T, Grossrau R, Hollriegl V, Vormann J. Effects of Fe, salicylate and Zn on metallothionein and lipid peroxidation in vivo. J Trace Elem Electrolytes Health Dis 1991;5(2):95–100.

Haddad JJ. Redox and oxidant-mediated regulation of apoptosis signaling pathways: immuno-pharmaco-redox conception of oxidative siege versus cell death commitment. Int Immunopharmacol 2004;4(4):475–93.

Halliwell B. Protection against tissue damage in vivo by desferrioxamine: what is its mechanism of action. Free Radic Biol Med 1989;7(6):645–51.

Horie T, Mizuma T, Kasai S, Awazu S. Conformational change in plasma albumin due to interaction with isolated rat hepatocyte. Am J Physiol 1988;254(4 Pt 1):G465–70.

Ito K, Koresawa T, Nakano K, Horie T. Mrp2 is involved in benzylpenicillin-induced choleresis. Am J Physiol Gastrointest Liver Physiol 2004;287(1):G42–9.

Ji B, Ito K, Suzuki H, Sugiyama Y, Horie T. Multidrug resistance-associated protein2 (MRP2) plays an important role in the biliary excretion of glutathione conjugates of 4-hydroxynonenal. Free Radic Biol Med 2002;33(3):370–8.

Kehrer JP. Free radicals as mediators of tissue injury and disease. Crit Rev Toxicol 1993;23(1):21–48.

Keller DA, Menzel DB. Picomole analysis of glutathione, glutathione disulfide, glutathione S-sulfonate, and cysteine S-sulfonate by high-performance liquid chromatography. Anal Biochem 1985;151(2):418–23.

Kessova I, Cederbaum AI. CYP2E1: biochemistry, toxicology, regulation and function in ethanol-induced liver injury. Curr Mol Med 2003;3(6):509–18.

Lowry OH, Rosebrough NJ, Farr AL, Randall RJ. Protein measurement with the Folin phenol reagent. J Biol Chem 1951;193(1):265–75.

Omura T, Sato R. A new cytochrome in liver microsomes. J Biol Chem 1962;237:1375–6.

Osawa T, Kato Y. Protective role of antioxidative food factors in oxidative stress caused by hyperglycemia. Ann N Y Acad Sci 2005;1043:440–51.

Prasad K, Laxdal VA, Yu M, Raney BL. Antioxidant activity of allicin, an active principle in garlic. Mol Cell Biochem 1995;148(2):183–9.

Rimm EB, Stampfer MJ, Ascherio A, Giovannucci E, Colditz GA, Willett WC. Vitamin E consumption and the risk of coronary heart disease in men. N Engl J Med 1993;328(20):1450–6.

Stampfer MJ, Hennekens CH, Manson JE, Colditz GA, Rosner B, Willett WC. Vitamin E consumption and the risk of coronary disease in women. N Engl J Med 1993;328(20):1444–9.

Sumioka I, Hayama M, Shimokawa Y, Shiraishi S, Tokunaga A. Lipid-lowering effect of monascus garlic fermented extract (MGFE) in hyperlipidemic subjects. Hiroshima J Med Sci 2006;55(2):59–64.

Taira J, Miyagi C, Aniya Y. Dimerumic acid as an antioxidant from the mold, Monascus anka: the inhibition mechanisms against lipid peroxidation and hemeprotein-mediated oxidation. Biochem Pharmacol 2002;63(5):1019–26.

Takayama F, Egashira T, Yamanaka Y. Protective effect of Ninjin-yoei-to on damage to isolated hepatocytes following transient exposure to tert-butyl hydroperoxide. Jpn J Pharmacol 2001;85(3):227–33.

Tolman KG, Peterson P, Gray P, Hammar SP. Hepatotoxicity of salicylates in monolayer cell cultures. Gastroenterology 1978;74(2 Pt 1):205–8.

Whitehouse MW. Biochemical properties of anti-inflammatory drugs–Iii. Uncoupling Of oxidative phosphorylation in a connective tissue (Cartilage) and liver mitochondria by salicylate analogues: relationship of structure to activity. Biochem Pharmacol 1964;13:319–36.

Wroblewski F, Ladue JS. Lactic dehydrogenase activity in blood. Proc Soc Exp Biol Med 1955;90(1):210–3.

You K. Salicylate and mitochondrial injury in Reye's syndrome. Science 1983;221(4606):163–5.

JNK and ERK mitogen-activated protein kinases mediate THDA-induced apoptosis in K562 cells

Sheng-Huei Yang · Zchong-Zcho Wu ·
Ching-Ming Chien · Yu-Hsiang Lo ·
Ming-Jung Wu · Long-Sen Chang ·
Shinne-Ren Lin

Originally published in the journal Cell Biology and Toxicology, Volume 24, Nos 4–5, 11–22.
DOI: 10.1007/s10565-007-9038-6 © Springer Science + Business Media B.V. 2007

Abstract 2-(6-(2-thieanisyl)-3(Z)-hexen-1, 5-diynyl) aniline (THDA), an enediyne compound, was identified in our laboratory as a novel antineoplastic agent against human leukemia K562 cells. THDA-induced apoptosis was associated with the upregulation of Bax, downregulation of X-linked inhibitor of apoptosis (XIAP), as well as the activation of caspase-3 and caspase-9. In addition, the mitogen-activated protein family kinases, including c-Jun N-terminal kinase (JNK) and extracellular signal-regulated protein kinase (ERK) kinases, and the transcription factor c-Jun were all activated by phosphorylation after 6 h exposure to THDA. Phosphorylation (activation) of JNK and ERK kinases by THDA was blocked by an ERK inhibitor, PD98059, or a JNK inhibitor, JNK-1, respectively, suggesting that THDA-induced apoptosis in K562 cells is ERK and JNK dependent. Moreover, the blockade of ERK and JNK also attenuated the modulation of Bax and XIAP, as well as the activation of caspase-3 and caspase-9 induced by THDA. These findings suggest that the activation of JNK and ERK is involved in the THDA-induced apoptosis of K562 cells. Therefore, this investigation, for the first time, uncovered the biological properties of this novel antitumor enediyne.

Keywords THDA · JNK · ERK · Apoptosis · K562 cells

Abbreviations

THDA	2-(6-(2-thieanisyl)-3(Z)-hexen-1, 5-diynyl) aniline
MTT	3-(4, 5-dimethylthiazol-2-yl)-2, 5-diphenyl-tetrazolium bromide
MAPK	mitogen-activated protein kinase
ERK	extracellar signal-regulated protein kinase
JNK	c-Jun N-terminal kinase

S.-H. Yang · Z.-Z. Wu · C.-M. Chien · Y.-H. Lo ·
M.-J. Wu · S.-R. Lin
Faculty of Medicinal and Applied Chemistry,
Kaohsiung Medical University,
Kaohsiung 807 Taiwan, Republic of China

L.-S. Chang
Institute of Biomedical Sciences,
National Sun Yat-Sen University,
Kaohsiung 804 Taiwan, Republic of China

L.-S. Chang · S.-R. Lin (✉)
National Sun Yat-Sen University–Kaohsiung Medical
University Joint Research Center,
Kaohsiung, Taiwan, Republic of China
e-mail: shreli@cc.kmu.edu.tw

Introduction

The mitogen-activated protein kinase (MAPK) family consists of extracellular signal-regulated kinase (ERK), c-Jun N-terminal kinase (JNK), and p38 MAPK, which are involved in mediating the processes associated with cell growth, survival, and death (McCawley et al. 1999; Wada and Penninger 2004). JNK and p38 MAPK pathways are activated in response to chemicals and environmental stress (Davis 2000; Minden and Karin 1997; Nagata and Todokoro 1999; Roulston et al. 1998), while the ERK cascade is activated by mitogenic stimuli, such as growth factors, cytokines, and phorbol esters, and is critical for proliferation and survival (Chang and Karin 2001; Johnson and Lapadat 2002). However, ERK signaling has been suggested to be proapoptotic in cells undergoing apoptosis (Bacus et al. 2001; Choi et al. 2003; Wang et al. 2000; Xiao and Singh 2002). In addition, caspase activation is often regulated by various cellular proteins including members of the inhibitor of apoptosis (IAP; Deveraux and Reed 1999) or Bcl-2 families (Adams and Cory 1998; Antonsson and Martinou 2000). Previous reports have demonstrated that some Bcl-2 family members that are located on the mitochondrial membrane can alter the permeability of the mitocondrial membrane and trigger the activation of caspases (Adams and Cory 1998; Antonsson and Martinou 2000; Salvesen and Dixit 1997) leading to apoptotic cell death.

Families of molecules consisting of unique enediyne subdomain cores, which were derived from either natural isolation or synthetic routes, display manifold biological function (Alabugin et al. 2002; Jones et al. 2001; Jones et al. 2000). In our previous study, acyclic enediynes exhibited cytotoxicity toward cancer cells in low range of micromolar concentrations (Lin et al. 2001; Lin 2002; Lo et al. 2004). Recently, the synthesized 2-(6-(2-thieanisyl)-3(Z)-hexen-1,5-diynyl)

aniline (THDA; Fig. 1) was found to show a potent effect against human leukemia cells (Lin et al. 2005). Moreover, THDA induced dose- and time-dependent apoptosis and cell cycle arrest in K562 cells (Wu et al. 2006). Nevertheless, whether the cellular signaling pathway involves the underlying mechanism of this process has not been well elucidated. Considering that MAPKs are usually essential components in the apoptotic mechanism, studies on the role of MAPK pathways in THDA-induced apoptosis in K562 cells are carried out in the present study. Our data suggest that THDA-induced apoptosis is correlated with the activation of JNK- and ERK-signaling pathways. Therefore, this investigation, for the first time, uncovered the biological properties of this novel antitumor enediyne.

Materials and methods

Chemicals

Roswell Park Memorial Institute (RPMI) 1640 medium, fetal calf serum (FCS), trypan blue, penicillin G, and streptomycin were obtained from Gibco BRL (Gaithersburg, MD). 3-(4, 5-Dimethylthiazol-2-yl)-2, 5-diphenyltetrazolium bromide (MTT), dimethylsulfoxide (DMSO), ribonuclease (RNase), and propidium iodide (PI) were purchased from Sigma Chemical (St. Louis, MD). Antibodies against phospho-ERK, ERK, p38, phospho-JNK, JNK, phospho-c-jun, c-jun, and β-actin were obtained from Santa Cruz Biotechnology (Santa Cruz, CA). The antibody of phospho-p38 was obtained from Chemicon (Temecula, CA). PD98059, JNK-1 (JNK inhibitor, a cell-permeable peptide inhibitor), and SB203580 were provided by Calbiochem (San Diego, CA). Anti-poly(adenosine diphosphate–ribose) polymerase (PARP) was purchased from Upstate Biotechnology (Lake Placid, NY), and anti-mouse and anti-rabbit 1 gG peroxidase-conjugated secondary antibody were purchased from Pierce (Rockford, IL). Hybond enhanced chemiluminescence (ECL) transfer membrane and ECL Western blotting detection kit were obtained from Amersham Life Science (Buckinghamshire, UK). The colorigenic synthetic peptide substrate, Ac-DEVD-pNA, Ac-IETD-pNA, and Ac-LEHD-pNA, as well as the Caspase inhibitor Z-VAD-FMK, Z-DEVD-FMK, Z-IETD-FMK, and Z-LEHD-FMK were purchased from Calbiochem-Novabiochem (La Jolla, CA).

Fig. 1 Chemical structure of THDA

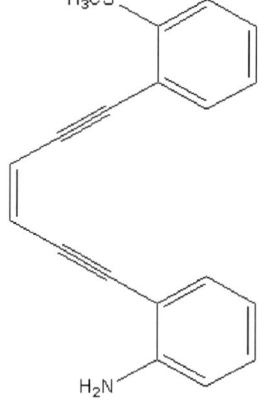

Cell culture

Human leukemia K562 cells were obtained from the American Type Culture Collection (Manassas, VA; Catalogue number, CCL-240). Cells were maintained in RPMI 1640 medium supplemented with 10% FCS, 2 mM glutamine, and antibiotics (100 U/ml penicillin and 100 μg/ml streptomycin) at 37°C in a humidified atmosphere of 5% CO_2.

Preparation of THDA

THDA (Fig. 1) was prepared as previously described, and the structure of this compound has been verified by means of mass spectrometry and spectroscopic techniques (Lin et al. 2005; Lo et al. 2004). THDA (IC_{50}= 53.2±0.5 μM) was dissolved in DMSO (less than 0.01%) and made immediately before experiments.

Cell viability assay

The viability of cells was determined by MTT assay, and the Trypan blue dye exclusion assay was performed to confirm and verify cell viability. Cells were seeded at a density of 1×10^5 cells/3 ml cell culture medium into a 12-well plate. After 24 h of incubation, the cells were treated with vehicle (0.1% DMSO) or 50 μM concentrations of THDA (diluted in DMSO at 0.1% final concentration) in medium for 24 h, respectively. MTT solution was added to each well (1.2 mg/ml) and incubated for 4 h. MTT is reduced by the mitochondrial dehydrogenases of viable cells to a purple formazan product. The MTT–formazan product dissolved in DMSO was estimated by measuring absorbance at 570 nm in an enzyme-linked immunosorbent assay plate reader. As for the Trypan blue dye exclusion assay, cells were seeded at density of 1×10^5 cells/well onto a 12-well plate for 24 h, then THDA was added to the medium at various indicated times and concentrations. After incubation, cells exposed to 0.2% Trypan blue were counted in a hemocytometer.

Annexin V assay for apoptosis

Apoptotic cells were quantified by annexin V and PI double staining by using a staining kit purchased from PharMingen (San Diego, CA). In brief, 10^6 cells were grown in 35-mm-diameter plates and were labeled with Annexin V-flourescein isothiocyanate (10 μg/ml) and PI (20 μg/ml) before harvesting. After labeling, all plates were washed with binding buffer and harvested by scraping. Cells were resuspended in binding buffer as a concentration of 2×10^5 cells/ml before analysis by flow cytometry.

Flow cytometry analysis

Cells (1×10^5 cells/dish) were cultured in cell culture medium in 6-cm dishes. After 24 h incubation, cells were treated with 50 μM of THDA for 0, 12, 24, 36, and 48 h, respectively. Control and treated cells were harvested, washed in cold phosphate-buffered saline (PBS), fixed in 70% ethanol, and stored at 4°C. Deoxyribonucleic acid (DNA) was treated with RNase A solution (500 U/ml) at 37°C for 15 min and stained by PI (50 μg /ml) in 1.12% sodium citrate at room temperature before analysis. Flow cytometric determination of DNA content was analyzed by COULTER EPICS XL Flow Cytometer (Coulter, Miami, FL).

Inhibitor treatment

To investigate the effect of MAPK inhibitors on THDA-induced apoptosis, confluent cell cultures were preincubated for 1 h with one of the following inhibitors before the addition of THDA: 20 μM SB203580 (p38 inhibitor), 20 μM PD98059 (ERK inhibitor), or 20 μM JNK-1 (JNK inhibitor).

Western blotting analysis

Cells (1×10^6/dish) were seeded in 10-cm dishes. After 24 h incubation, cells were treated with 50 μM of THDA for 0, 6, 12, 18, and 24 h, respectively. Control and treated cells were washed in PBS, suspended in lysis buffer containing 50 mM Tris (pH 7.5), 1% NP-40, 2 mM ethylenediamine tetraacetic acid (EDTA), 10 mM NaCl, 20 μg/ml aprotinin, 20 μg/ml leupeptin, and 1 mM phenylmethylsulfonyl fluoride and placed on ice for 30 min. After centrifugation at $20,000 \times g$ for 30 min at 4°C, the supernatant was collected. The protein concentration in the supernatant was determined with a bicinchoninic acid protein assay kit (Pierce, Rockford, IL). Whole lysate (50 μg) were resolved by sodium dodecyl sulfate–polyacrylamide gel electrophoresis (SDS-PAGE), transferred onto polyvinylidene difluoride (PVDF) membranes (Roche) by electroblotting, and probed with anti-PARP, anti-Bax, anti-Bcl-2, anti-X-linked IAP (XIAP), anti-p-JNK, anti-JNK, anti-p-ERK, anti-ERK, anti-p-p38, and anti-c-jun (Santa Cruz Biotechnology). The blot was developed by ECL.

Cellular proteins fractionation for Bax mitochondrial translocation

Mitochondrial and cytosolic fractions were prepared by resuspending cells in ice-cold buffer A (250 mM sucrose, 20 mM hydroxyethyl piperazineethanesulfonic acid, 10 mM KCl, 1.5 mM $MgCl_2$, 1 mM EDTA, 1 mM ethyleneglycoltetraacetic acid [EGTA], 1 mM DTT, 17 µg/ml phenylmethylsulfonylfluoride, 8 µg/ml aprotinin, and 2 µg/ml leupeptin, pH 7.4). Cells were passed through a needle ten times. Unlysed cells and nuclei were pelleted by centrifugation for 10 min at $750 \times g$. The supernatant was then centrifuged at $100,000 \times g$ for 15 min. This pellet was resuspended in buffer A and represents the mitochondrial fraction. The supernatant was again centrifuged at $100,000 \times g$ for 1 h. The supernatant from this final centrifugation step represents the cytosolic fraction. The resulting mitochondrial and cytosolic fractions were used for Western blot analysis with an anti-Bax antibody.

Assays of caspase activity

Cells (1×10^6/dish) were seeded in 10-cm dishes. After 24 h incubation, cells were treated with 50 µM of THDA for 0, 6, 12, 18, and 24 h, respectively. After different treatments, cells were collected and washed three times with PBS and resuspended in 50 mM Tris–HCl (pH 7.4), 1 mM EDTA, and 10 mM EGTA. Cell lysates were clarified by centrifugation at $18,000 \times g$ for 3 min, and clear lysates containing 50 µg of protein were incubated with 100 µM of enzyme-specific colorigenic substrates at 37°C for 1 h. The activity of caspase-3, caspase-8, and caspase-9 was determined as the cleavage of the colorimetric substrate by measuring the absorbance at 405 nm.

Statistical analysis

All data are expressed as the mean±SD. The difference between the treated and the control was analyzed by Student's t test. A probability of $P<0.05$ was considered significant.

Results

Effect of THDA on the expression levels of Bax and XIAP proteins

To explore the possible role of Bcl-2 family members in THDA-induced apoptosis, we examined the effects of THDA on the expression levels of Bcl-2 members by Western blot analysis. Exposure of K562 cells to 50 µM of THDA significantly upregulated the expression of Bax, while the expression level of Bcl-2 protein was unaltered (Fig. 2). Moreover, as shown in Fig. 2b, a time-dependent decrease of Bax in the cytosolic fraction and the increase in Bax in the mitochondrial fraction after THDA treatment were detected, suggesting the translocation of Bax from cytosol to the mitochondria.

In addition to Bcl-2 family proteins, the IAP family proteins regulate apoptotic signaling cascades by blocking caspase activities (Takahashi et al. 1998). The expression levels of XIAP were decreased by treatment with THDA (Fig. 2).

Effects of THDA on caspases activation

The activation of caspases in THDA-treated cells was assessed using colorigenic tetrapeptide substrates, Ac-IETD-pNA, Ac-LEDH-pNA, and Ac-DEVD-pNA, which have been shown to be selective for caspase-8-, caspase-9-, and caspase-3-like enzymatic activities, respectively. Treatment of K562 cells with 50 µM of THDA resulted in the detection of caspase-9 and caspase-3 activation as early as 6 h, whereas caspase-8 was not activated (Fig. 3a). Caspase-3 activation was accompanied by the cleavage of PARP (116 kDa) into an 84-kDa C-terminal fragment that became evident 6 h after THDA treatment (Fig. 2). Moreover, in the presence of caspase-9-specific inhibitor Z-LEDH-FMK and the caspase-3 inhibitor Z-DEVD-FMK, the cell viability was significantly increased from 40 to 80 and 73%, respectively, at 24 h (Fig. 3b). In contrast to inhibition of caspase-3 and caspase-9, pretreatment with the caspase-8-specific inhibitor, Z-IETD-FMK, did not affect THDA-induced cell death (Fig. 3b). To quantify THDA-induced apoptosis of

Fig. 2 a Western blot analyses of expression levels of Bax, Bcl-2, XIAP, and PARP. Cells were treated with 50 μM of THDA in the presence or absence of JNK inhibitor (*JNK-1*) or ERK inhibitor (*PD98059*) for the indicated time points. After treatment, the fractions were resolved by SDS-PAGE, transferred onto PVDF membranes, then probed with specific antibodies and visualized by chemiluminescence ECL kit. The amount of β-actin was measured as an internal control. Intensities of the immunoreactive bands were quantified by densitometric scanning. Data shown are the representative of three independent experiments with similar results. **b** Mitochondrial translocation of Bax induced by THDA. Cells were treated with 50 μM of THDA for the indicated times. The cytosol and mitochondrial fraction proteins were separated on SDS-PAGE, then probed with Bax antibody

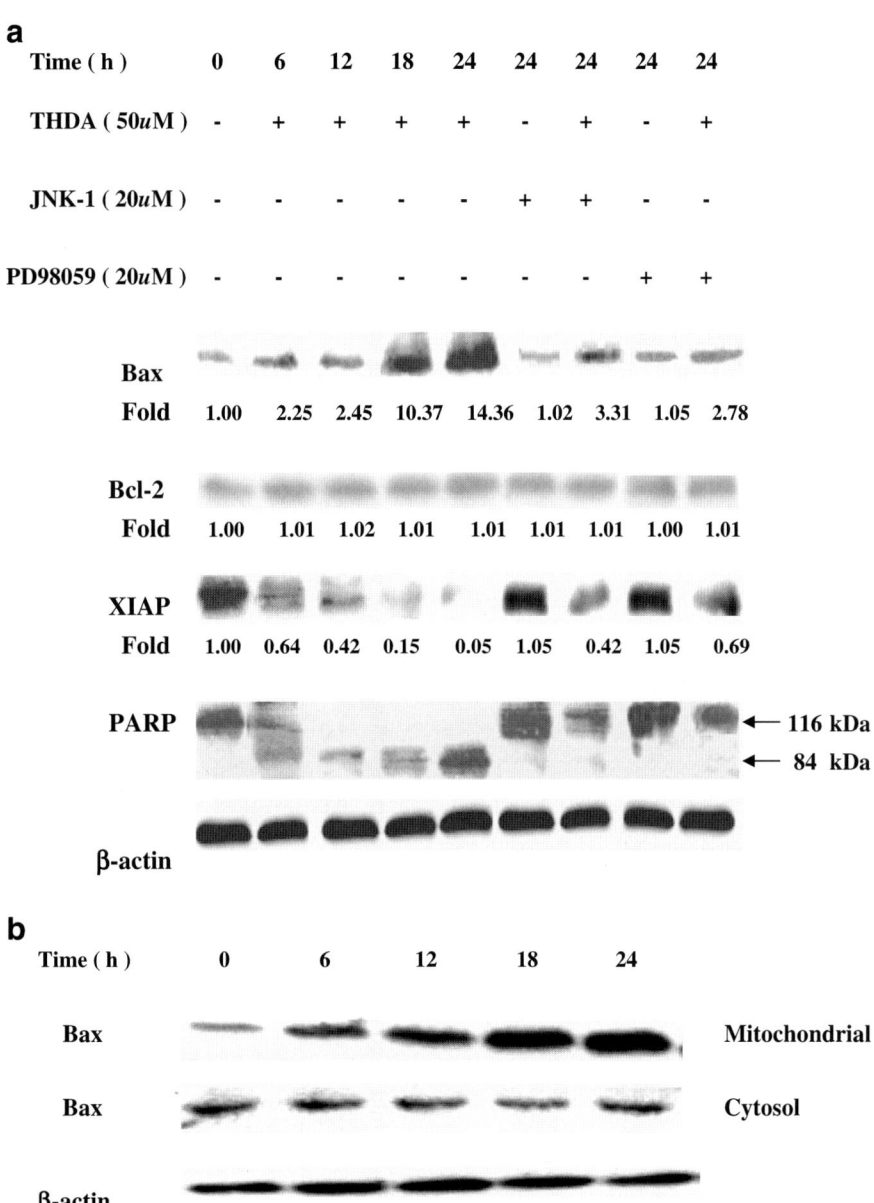

K562 cells, annexin V/PI assay was conducted. Cotreatment of THDA with caspase-9 inhibitor or caspase-3 inhibitor also partially inhibited THDA-induced apoptosis (Fig. 3c), indicating that THDA induces apoptosis through a caspase-9- and caspase-3-mediated pathway.

THDA activated JNK and ERK but not p38 MAPK

To determine the potential involvement of various protein kinase pathways in THDA-induced apoptosis,

MAPK activities were evaluated by measuring phosphorylation of MAPK subfamilies. Phosphorylated JNK was detected earlier after exposure of 50 μM of THDA for 6 h and sustained for 24 h. Pretreatment with JNK-1 (a JNK inhibitor) resulted in an inhibition of THDA-induced JNK activation (Fig. 4b) but not altered by the addition of PD98059 (a specific inhibitor of ERK) and SB203580 (a specific inhibitor of p38; Fig. 4b). Moreover, Western blot analysis on the phosphorylation of the downstream JNK substrate c-Jun by using anti-c-Jun and phospho-c-Jun antibodies showed that expo-

Fig. 3 Effects of THDA on caspase-3, caspase-8, and caspase-9 activations. **a** Activation of caspase-3, caspase-8, and caspase-9 by THDA. Cells were treated with 50 μM of THDA in the presence or absence of JNK inhibitor (*JNK-1*) or ERK inhibitor (*PD98059*) for different time periods. Cell lysates were prepared and enzymatic activities of caspase-3-, caspase-8-, and caspase-9-like protease were determined by incubation of 50 μg of protein with colorigenic substrates, respectively, for 2 h at 37°C. The release of chromophore pNA was monitored spectrophotometrically (405 nm). **b** The cell viability of cells was determined by Trypan blue dye exclusion method. Cells were preincubated with or without the caspase inhibitor, Z-DEVD-FMK, Z-IETD-FMK, Z-LEHD-FMK, for 1 h, and this was followed by treatment with or without 50 μM of THDA for 24 h. *Asterisk*, $P<0.05$, vs the THDA-treated group. **c** Induction of apoptosis was analyzed by annexin V/PI double staining. Cells were preincubated with or without the caspase inhibitor, Z-DEVD-FMK, Z-IETD-FMK, Z-LEHD-FMK, for 1 h, and this was followed by treatment with or without 50 μM of THDA for 24 h. Cells were harvested, washed, stained with annexin V and PI double staining using a kit purchased from PharMingen (San Diego, CA), and analyzed by flow cytometry. The percentage of apoptotic cells corresponds to the number of annexin V-positive cells

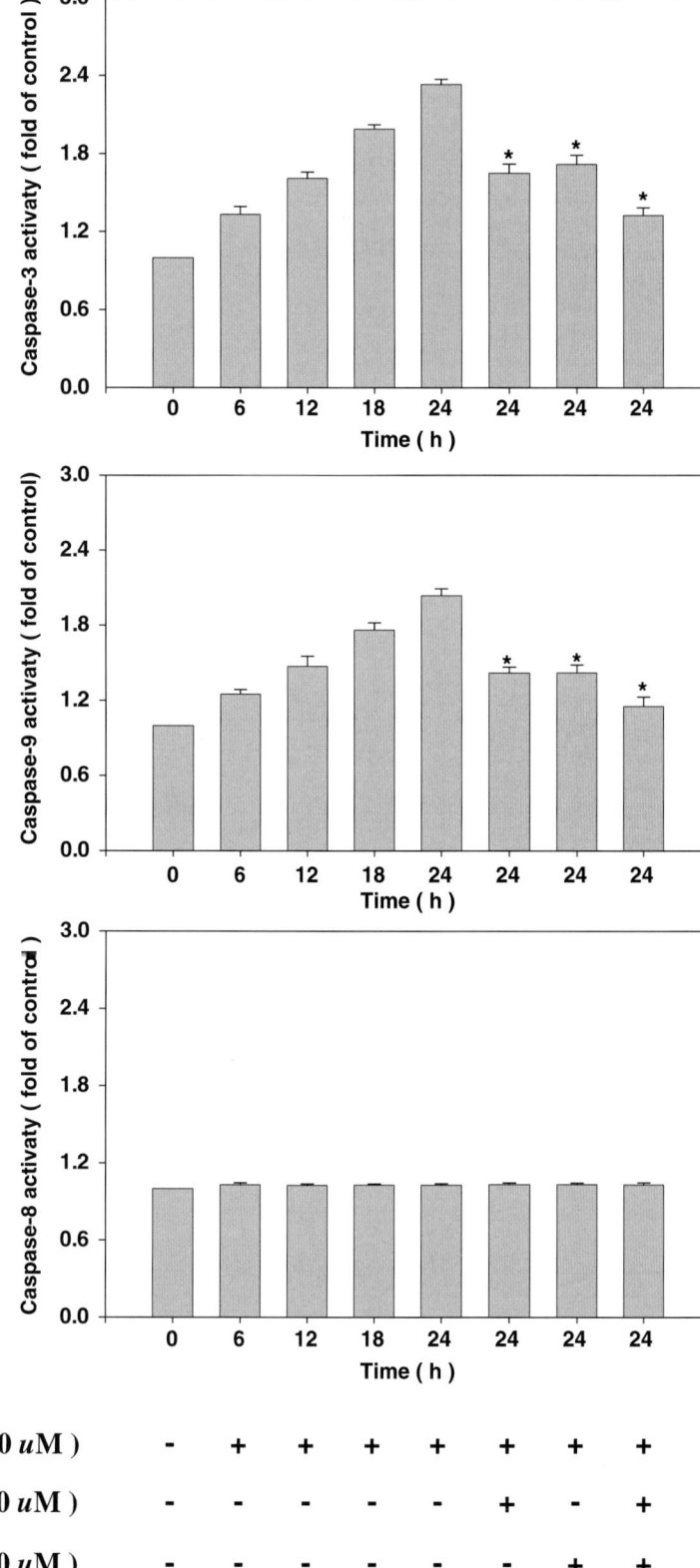

Fig. 3 (continued)

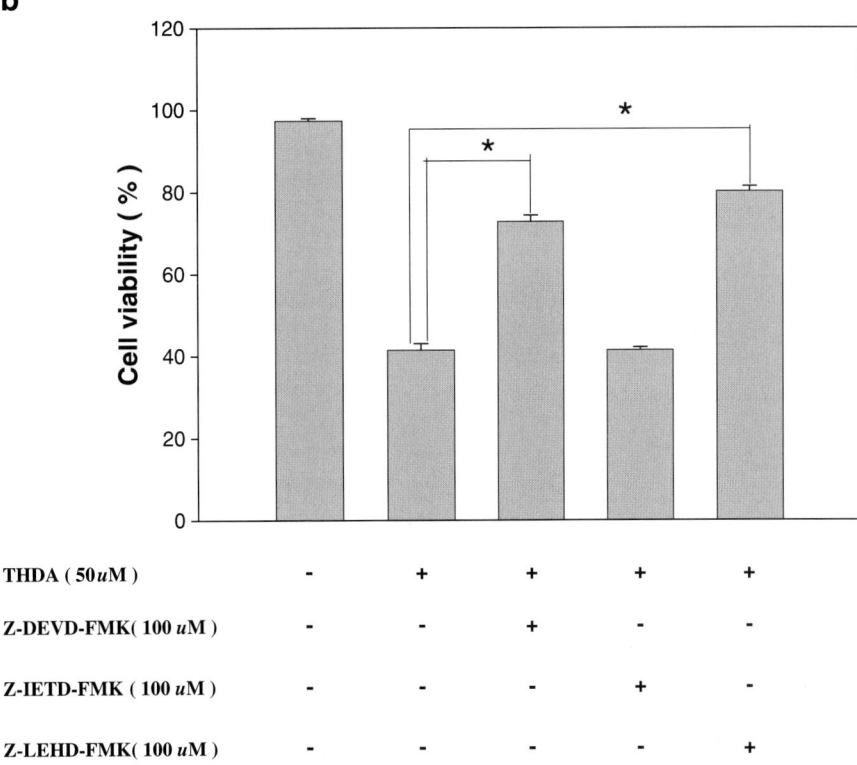

THDA (50 *u*M)	-	+	+	+	+
Z-DEVD-FMK(100 *u*M)	-	-	+	-	-
Z-IETD-FMK (100 *u*M)	-	-	-	+	-
Z-LEHD-FMK(100 *u*M)	-	-	-	-	+

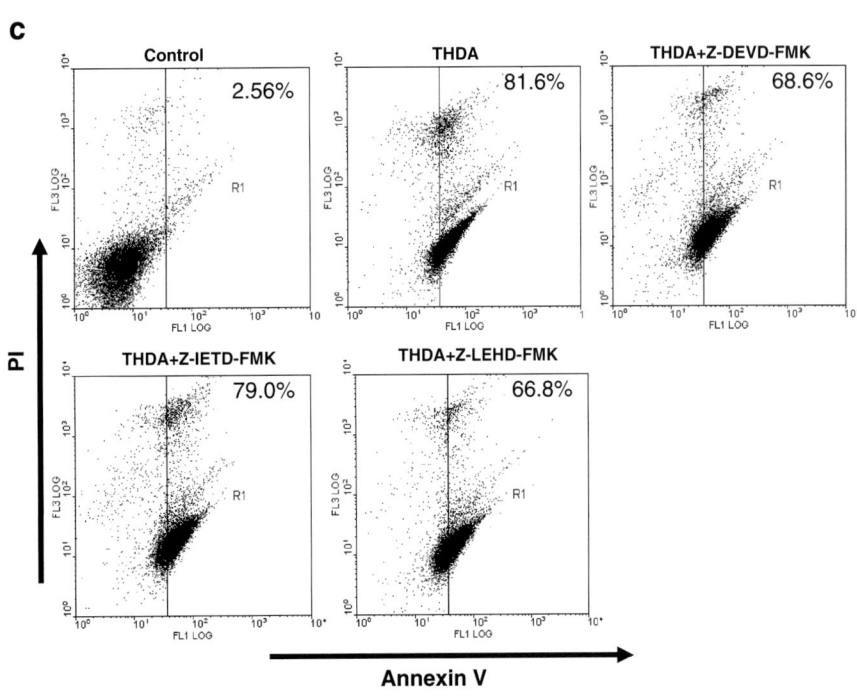

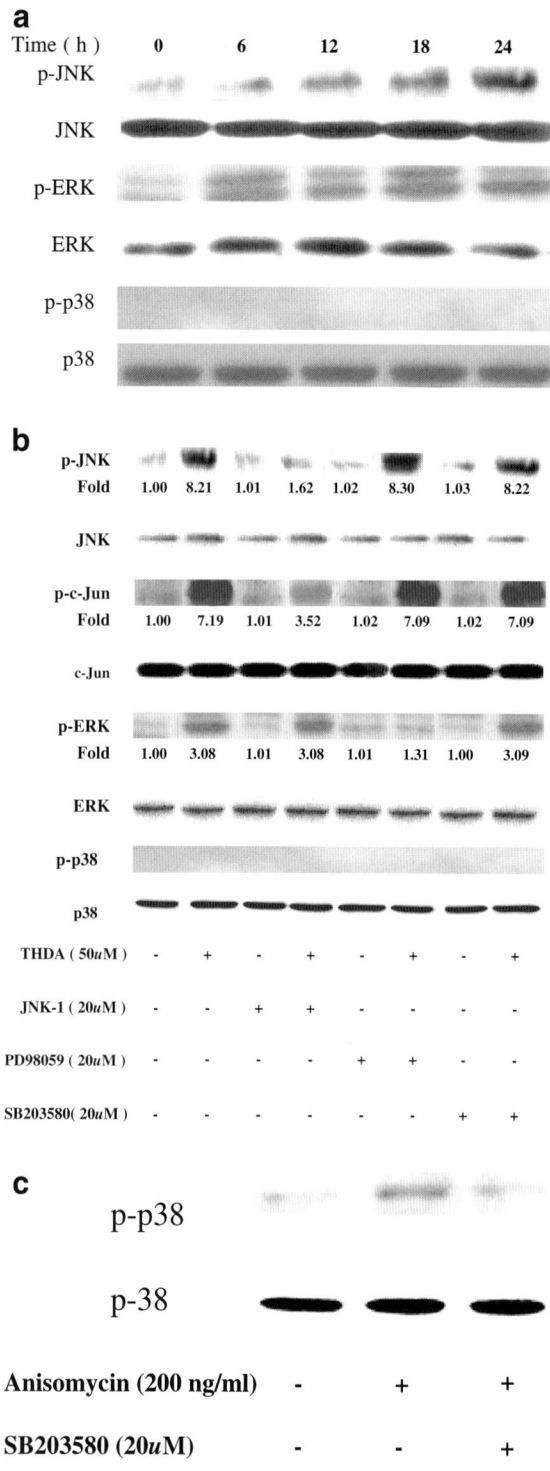

a

Time (h)	0	6	12	18	24

p-JNK

JNK

p-ERK

ERK

p-p38

p38

b

p-JNK

Fold	1.00	8.21	1.01	1.62	1.02	8.30	1.03	8.22

JNK

p-c-Jun

Fold	1.00	7.19	1.01	3.52	1.02	7.09	1.02	7.09

c-Jun

p-ERK

Fold	1.00	3.08	1.01	3.08	1.01	1.31	1.00	3.09

ERK

p-p38

p38

THDA (50uM)	-	+	-	+	-	+	-	+
JNK-1 (20uM)	-	-	+	+	-	-	-	-
PD98059 (20uM)	-	-	-	-	+	+	-	-
SB203580(20uM)	-	-	-	-	-	-	+	+

c

p-p38

p-38

Anisomycin (200 ng/ml)	-	+	+
SB203580 (20uM)	-	-	+

Fig. 4 **a** Effect of THDA on expression of MAP kinases on K562 cells. Cells were cultured overnight, at a density of 1×10^5 ml^{-1} in RPMI 1640 medium without serum and treated the next day with 50 μM of THDA for 0, 6, 12, 18, and 24 h. Equal amounts of whole cell lysate (50 μg) were subjected to electrophoresis and analyzed by Western blot. Activation of MAP kinases, JNK, ERK, and p38 kinase were examined by using respective antibodies against phosphorylated MAP kinases and antibodies against nonphosphorylated proteins as controls. **b** Effect of JNK inhibitor JNK-1 and ERK inhibitor PD98059 on the expression levels of p-c-Jun, p-JNK, and p-ERK. Cells were pretreated with MAPK inhibitors (*PD98059* ERK inhibitor, *JNK-1* JNK inhibitor) for 1 h before exposure to THDA. After 24 h, cells were collected, and equal amounts of whole-cell lysate (50 μg) were subjected to electrophoresis and analyzed by Western blot. Data shown are the representative of three independent experiments with similar results. **c** Anisomycin served as a positive control to verify that the p-p38 antibody was working (Pace et al. 2003). Total protein was isolated from K562 cells treated with the positive control anisomycin (200 ng/ml) for 1 h. Equal amounts of whole-cell lysate (50 μg) were subjected to electrophoresis and analyzed by Western blot

sustained up to 24 h, but THDA did not influence the expression levels of total ERK (Fig. 4a). The PD98059 (an inhibitor of ERK) attenuated the THDA-induced ERK phosphorylation, while the JNK and p38 inhibitors did not suppress the ERK response (Fig. 4b). Collectively, our data showed that ERK and JNK phosphorylations by THDA occurred in a time-dependent manner.

In contrast to ERK and JNK, treatment of K562 cells with THDA did not stimulate the phosphorylation of p38 MAPK (Fig. 4a). These findings indicated that p38 MAPK was not regulated by THDA in K562 cells.

ERK and JNK inhibitors block THDA-induced apoptosis

To clarify which kinase pathway is essential for THDA-induced apoptosis, K562 cells were pretreated with membrane-permeable small-molecular inhibitors for ERK and JNK. The JNK inhibitor JNK-1 or ERK inhibitor PD98059 pretreatment reduced the rate of THDA-mediated cell death (Fig. 5a,b, and c). Furthermore, the use of both inhibitors, JNK-1 and PD98056, together resulted in significant reduction in THDA-induced apoptosis (Fig. 5a,b, and c), suggesting that JNK and ERK inhibitors block THDA-induced apoptosis.

sure to THDA caused c-Jun phosphorylation (Fig. 4b) and the expression of c-Jun was unchanged (Fig. 4b).

Treatment of K562 cells with THDA (50 μM) produced a time-dependent activation of ERK and was

Fig. 5 THDA-induced cell death is abrogated by inhibition of JNK and ERK. **a** Trypan blue dye exclusion assay. Cells were pretreated with MAPK inhibitors (*PD98059* ERK inhibitor, *JNK-1* JNK inhibitor) for 1 h before exposure to THDA. After 24 h, cells were collected, and the cell viability was determined by a hemocytometer. Data are mean±SD of three separate experiments done in triplicate. *Asterisk*, significantly different compared with THDA-treated group (*P*< 0.05). **b** The sub G1 DNA content of cells by flow cytometry. Cells were pretreated with MAPK inhibitors (*PD98059* ERK inhibitor, *JNK-1* JNK inhibitor) for 1 h before exposure to THDA. Cells were collected, and DNA contents were analyzed as described under "Materials and methods." *Asterisk*, *P*<0.05 represents the significant difference between the THDA-treated group and the MAPK inhibitor-treated group. **c** Induction of apoptosis was analyzed by annexin V/PI double staining. Cells were pretreated with MAPK inhibitors (*PD98059* ERK inhibitor, *JNK-1* JNK inhibitor) for 1 h before exposure to THDA, and this was followed by treatment with or without 50 μM of THDA for 24 h. Cells were harvested, washed, and stained with annexin V and PI double staining. The percentage of apoptotic cells corresponds to the number of annexin V-positive cells

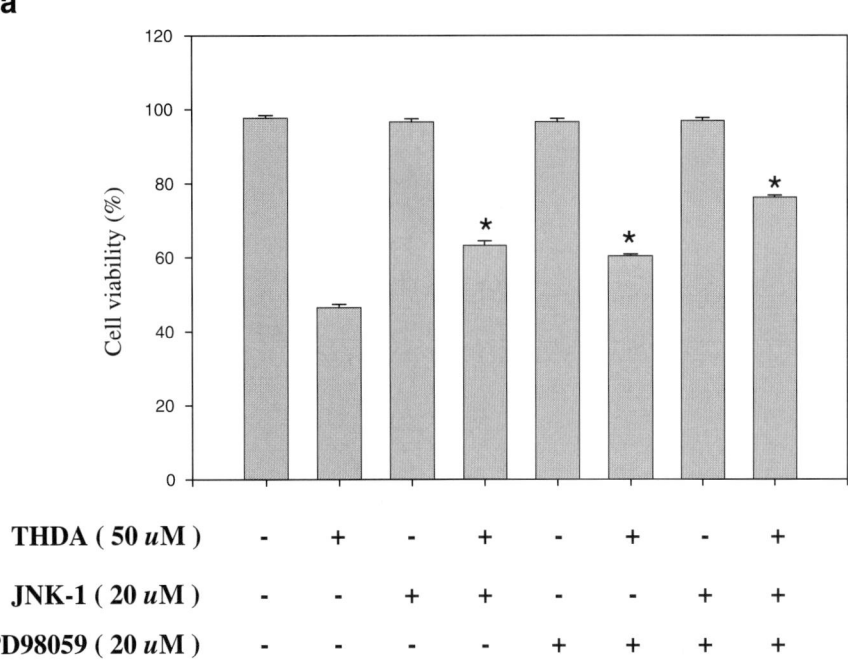

THDA (50 *u*M)	-	+	-	+	-	+	-	+
JNK-1 (20 *u*M)	-	-	+	+	-	-	+	+
PD98059 (20 *u*M)	-	-	-	-	+	+	+	+

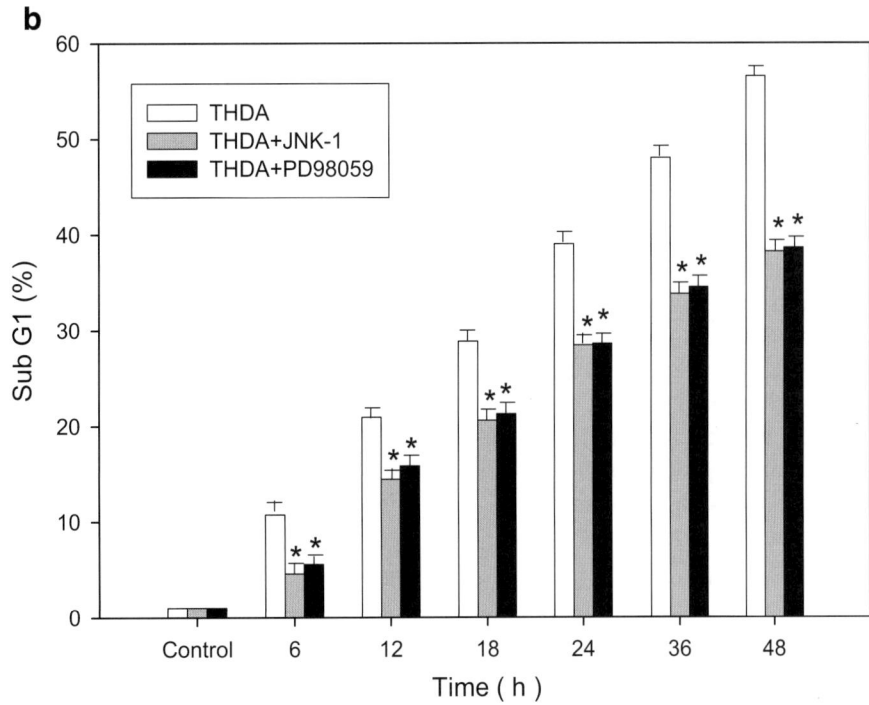

Fig. 5 (continued)

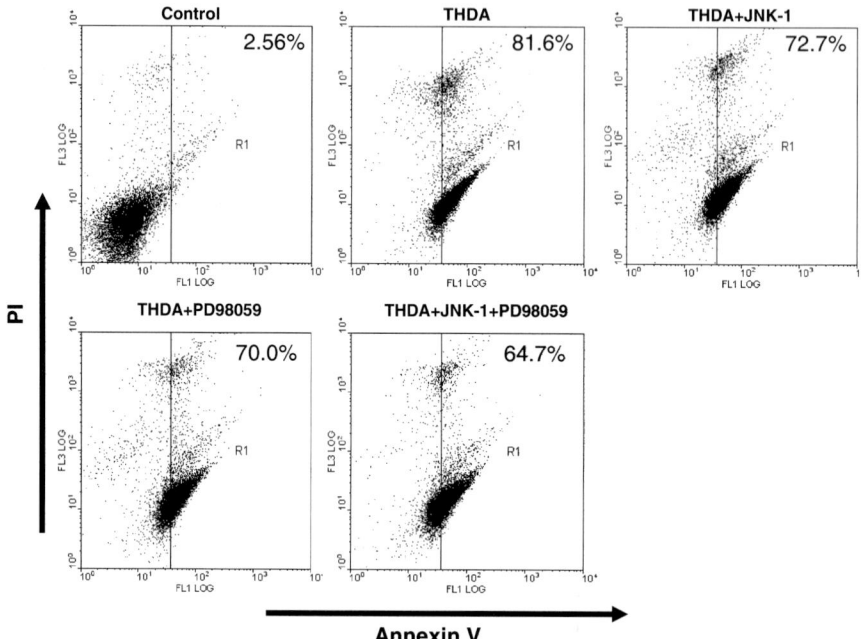

Effect of JNK-1 and PD98059 on THDA-induced changes in the levels of apoptosis-related proteins

To further demonstrate the role of JNK and ERK activation in THDA-induced cell death, we evaluated the effect of JNK and ERK inhibitors on THDA-induced changes in the levels of apoptosis-related proteins. Pretreatment of K562 cells with JNK inhibitor JNK-1 or ERK inhibitor PD98059 effectively prevented the THDA-induced changes in caspase-3 and caspase-9 activation (Fig. 3a) and the level of PARP cleavage (Fig. 2). In addition, THDA-induced XIAP reduction and Bax upregulation were also partially blocked by JNK-1 or PD98059 (Fig. 2). These data support the idea that JNK and ERK activation plays an important role in THDA-induced apoptosis of K562 cells.

Discussion

Members of the Bcl-2 family of proteins are associated with the mitochondrial membrane and regulate membrane integrity (Adams and Cory 1998). Some proteins within this family, including Bcl-2 and Bcl-X_L, inhibit apoptosis, while others, such as Bax and Bid, promote apoptosis (Adams and Cory 1998; Antonsson and Martinou 2000). Bcl-2 and related antiapoptotic pro-

teins seem to dimerize with a proapoptotic molecule, e.g., Bax, and modulate the sensitivity of cells to apoptosis (Pastorino et al. 1998). Hence, an alteration in the levels of anti- and proapoptotic Bcl-2 family proteins influences apoptosis. THDA treatment increases the level of proapoptotic protein Bax but not the Bcl-2 protein, thereby increasing the Bax/Bcl-2 ratio (Fig. 2). This result is consistent with previous observations that apoptosis because of Bax overexpression is caused by a variety of stimuli, including chemotherapeutic agents such as etoposide and paclitaxel (Pastorino et al. 1998).

Several chemotherapeutic and chemopreventive agents have been shown to cause apoptotic cell death through mediation of caspases (Robertson and Orrenius 2000). After K562 cells were cultured with THDA (50 μM), caspase-3 and caspase-9 activation in the cytosol were analyzed. As the duration of culture was extended, the activities of caspase-3 and caspase-9 in the cytosol of THDA-treated cells significantly increased (Fig. 3a). Moreover, incubation with caspase-9-specific inhibitor (Z-LEDH-FMK) or the caspase-3 inhibitor (Z-DEVD-FMK) significantly attenuated THDA-triggered apoptosis in K562 cells (Fig. 3b and c). In contrast to inhibition of caspase-3 and caspase-9, pretreatment with the caspase-8-specific inhibitor, Z-IETD-FMK, did not affect THDA-induced cell death (Fig. 3b), indicating that THDA induces apoptosis through a caspase-9- and caspase-3-mediated pathway. Another factor contributing to caspase activation in THDA-treated K562 cells may be a decreased expression of IAP expression. IAPs have been reported to inhibit apoptosis because of their function as direct inhibitors of activated effector caspases such as caspase-3 and caspase-7. IAPs are also able to inhibit cytochrome *c*-induced activation of caspase-9 (Deveraux and Reed 1999). Our data demonstrated that the expression level of XIAP protein was decreased (Fig. 2), indicating that this protein is linked to inhibit activation of caspases.

Recent evidence indicates that the MAPK family protein kinases are important mediators of apoptosis induced by stressful stimuli (Chang and Karin 2001; Johnson and Lapadat 2002). We therefore attempted to demonstrate whether MAPK-signaling pathways are involved in THDA-induced cytotoxicity of K562 cells. The data presented here showed that THDA caused apoptosis in parallel with the activation of ERK and JNK in K562 cells (Fig. 4a). Although p38 can be activated via phosphorylation induced by diverse cellular stress, THDA did not affect the expression and activation of p38 MAPK (Fig. 4a), indicating that p38 MAPK is not involved in THDA-induced apoptosis.

Several upstream signaling events have been suggested as activators for the mitochondrial translocation of Bax, one of which is JNK activation (Lee et al. 2005). To determine whether activation of JNK is directly associated with the proapoptosis activity of THDA in K562 cells, we sought to block JNK activity using JNK-1 and to determine the effect on the extent of apoptosis induced by THDA. Our results showed that inhibition of the JNK pathway with JNK-1 attenuated the effects of THDA on the activation caspase-3, caspase-9 (Fig. 3a), and the mitochondrial translocation of Bax (Fig. 2b), as well as the XIAP induced by THDA (Fig. 2). Moreover, JNK-1 decreased the THDA-induced apoptosis (Fig. 5). These data demonstrate that JNK is involved in the THDA-induced apoptosis of K562 cells.

Among MAPK subfamilies, ERK is controversial in its role in cell death. While some studies showed that the ERK activation mediates a survival response that counteracts cell death, other studies reported that the ERK activation is associated with apoptotic signaling pathways (Bacus et al. 2001; Choi et al. 2003; Wang et al. 2000; Xiao and Singh 2002). Our data showed that THDA activated ERK, while PD98059 (ERK inhibitor) partially blocked THDA-induced cytotoxicity, caspase-3 and caspase-9 activation, Bax upregulation, and XIAP downregulation (Figs. 2, 3a, and 5), suggesting that ERK activation is involved in the THDA-induced cell death. This notion was further supported by the facts that ERK activation induced apoptosis (Wang et al. 2000; Xiao and Singh 2002).

In conclusion, THDA, a novel enediyne derivative, induced apoptosis of K562 cells. THDA induces JNK and ERK pathways accompanied by increasing the Bax/Bcl-2 ratio and decreasing the protein level of XIAP and leads to activate caspase-9 and caspase-3, followed by PARP cleavage, which are hallmarks of apoptotic cell death. Because a weakly additive effect was observed with JNK and ERK inhibitors, our results suggested that THDA affected JNK and ERK through separate pathways. THDA was a novel compound synthesized in our laboratory. Our previous studies showed that THDA induced dose- ant time-dependent apoptosis and cell cycle arrest in K562 cells (Wu et al. 2006). Present data further showed that THDA-induced cell death engaged certain components of the apoptotic machinery, but detailed signaling pathways still remained to be elucidated in a future study.

Acknowledgments This work was supported by grant NSC 93-2113-M-037–003 from the National Science Council, ROC, and a grant of the National Sun Yat-Sen University–Kaohsiung Medical University Joint Research Center.

References

Adams JM, Cory S. The Bcl-2 protein family: arbiters of cell survival. Science 1998;281:1322–6.

Alabugin IV, Manoharan M, Kovalenko SV. Tuning rate of the bergman cyclization of benzannelated enediynes with ortho substituents. Org Lett 2002;4:1119–22.

Antonsson B, Martinou JC. The Bcl-2 protein family. Exp Cell Res 2000;2561:50–7.

Bacus SS, Gudkov AV, Lowe M, Lyass L, Yung Y, Komarov AP, et al. Taxol-induced apoptosis depends on MAP kinase pathways (ERK and p38) and is independent of p53. Oncogene 2001;202:147–55.

Chang L, Karin M. Mammalian MAP kinase signalling cascades. Nature 2001;410:37–40.

Choi YJ, Lim SY, Woo JH, Kim YH, Kwon YK, Suh SI, et al. Sodium orthovanadate potentiates EGCG-induced apoptosis that is dependent on the ERK pathway. Biochem Biophys Res Commun 2003;305:176–85.

Davis RJ. Signal transduction by the JNK group of MAP kinases. Cell 2000;103:239–52.

Deveraux QL, Reed JC. IAP family proteins—suppressors of apoptosis. Genes Dev 1999;13:239–52.

Johnson GL, Lapadat R. Mitogen-activated protein kinase pathways mediated by ERK, JNK, and p38 protein kinases. Science 2002;298:1911–2.

Jones GB, Hynd G, Wright JM, Purohit A, Plourde GW 2nd, Huber RS, et al. Target-directed enediynes: designed estramycins. J Org Chem 2001;66:3688–95.

Jones GB, Wright JM, Hynd G, Wyatt JK, Yancisin M, Brown MA. Protein-degrading enediynes: library screening of Bergman cycloaromatization products. Org Lett 2000;2: 1863–6.

Lee HJ, Wang CJ, Kuo HC, Chou FP, Jean LF, Tseng TH. Induction apoptosis of luteolin in human hepatoma HepG2 cells involving mitochondria translocation of Bax/Bak and activation of JNK. Toxicol Appl Pharmacol 2005;203: 124–31.

Lin CF, Hsieh PC, Lu WD, Chiu HF, Wu MJ. A series of enediynes as novel inhibitors of topoisomerase I. Bioorg Med Chem 2001;9:1707–11.

Lin CF, Lu WD, Hsieh PC, Kuo YH, Chiu HF, Wang CJ, et al. Cytotoxicities and topoisomerase I inhibitory activities of 2-[2-(2-Alkynylphenyl)ethynyl]benzonitriles, 1-aryldec-3-ene-1,5-diynes, and related bis(enediynyl)arene compounds. Helv Chim Acta 2002;85:2564–75.

Lin CF, Lo YH, Hsieh MC, Chen YH, Wang JJ, Wu MJ. Cytotoxicities, cell cycle and caspase evaluations of 1,6-diaryl-3(Z)-hexen-1,5-diynes, 2-(6-aryl-3(Z)-hexen-1,5-diynyl)anilines and their derivatives. Bioorg Med Chem 2005;13:3565–75.

Lo YH, Lin CF, Hsieh MC, Wu MJ. Remarkable G2/M phase arrest and apoptotic effect performed by 2-(6-aryl-3-hexen-1,5-diynyl) benzonitrile antitumor agents. Bioorg Med Chem 2004;12:1047–53.

McCawley LJ, Li S, Wattenberg EV, Hudson LG. Sustained activation of the mitogen-activated protein kinase pathway. A mechanism underlying receptor tyrosine kinase specificity for matrix metalloproteinase-9 induction and cell migration. J Biol Chem 1999;274:4347–53.

Minden A, Karin M. Regulation and function of the JNK subgroup of MAP kinases. Biochim Biophys Acta 1997; 1333:F85–104.

Nagata Y, Todokoro K. Requirement of activation of JNK and p38 for environmental stress-induced erythroid differentiation and apoptosis and of inhibition of ERK for apoptosis. Blood 1999;94:853–63.

Pace BS, Qian XH, Sangerman J, Ofori-Acquah SF, Baliga BS, Han J, et al. p38 MAP kinase activation mediates γ-globin gene induction in erythroid progenitors. Exp Hematol 2003;31:1089–96.

Pastorino JG, Chen ST, Tafani M, Snyder JW, Farber JL. The overexpression of Bax produces cell death upon induction of the mitochondrial permeability transition. J Biol Chem 1998;273:7770–5.

Robertson JD, Orrenius S. Molecular mechanisms of apoptosis induced by cytotoxic chemicals. Crit Rev Toxicol 2000; 30:609–27.

Roulston A, Reinhard C, Amiri P, Williams LT. Early activation of c-Jun N-terminal kinase and p38 kinase regulate cell survival in response to tumor necrosis factor alpha. J Biol Chem 1998;273:10232–9.

Salvesen GS, Dixit VM. Caspases: intracellular signaling by proteolysis. Cell 1997;91:443–6.

Takahashi R, Deveraux Q, Tamm I, Welsh K, Assa-Munt N, Salvesen GS, et al. A single BIR domain of XIAP sufficient for inhibiting caspases. J Biol Chem 1998;273: 7787–90.

Wada T, Penninger JM. Mitogen-activated protein kinases in apoptosis regulation. Oncogene 2004;23:2838–49.

Wang X, Martindale JL, Holbrook NJ. Requirement for ERK activation in cisplatin-induced apoptosis. J Biol Chem 2000;275:39435–43.

Wu ZZ, Chien CM, Yang SH, Lin YH, Hu XW, Lu YJ, et al. Induction of G2/M phase arrest and apoptosis by a novel enediyne derivative, THDA, in chronic myeloid leukemia (K562) cells. Mol Cell Biochem 2006;292:99–103.

Xiao D, Singh SV. Phenethyl isothiocyanate-induced apoptosis in p53-deficient PC-3 human prostate cancer cell line is mediated by extracellular signal-regulated kinases. Cancer Res 2002;62:3615–9.

Pentoxifylline downregulates α (I) collagen expression by the inhibition of Iκbα degradation in liver stellate cells

E. Hernández · L. Bucio · V. Souza ·
M. C. Escobar · L. E. Gómez-Quiroz · B. Farfán ·
D. Kershenobich · M. C. Gutiérrez-Ruiz

Originally published in the journal Cell Biology and Toxicology, Volume 24, Nos 4–5, 23–34.
DOI: 10.1007/s10565-007-9039-5 © Springer Science + Business Media B.V. 2007

Abstract Overproduction of collagen (I) by activated hepatic stellate cells is a critical step in the development of liver fibrosis. It has been established that these cells express interleukin (IL)-6 and respond to this cytokine with an increase in α(I) collagen. Pentoxifylline, a methylxanthine derivate, has been reported to have antifibrotic properties, but the mechanism responsible for this effect is unknown. The aim of this study was to determine the effect of pentoxifylline on acetaldehyde-induced collagen production in a rat hepatic stellate cell line (CFSC-2G cells). Cells were treated with 100 μM acetaldehyde and 200 μM pentoxifyline for 3 h. IL-6 and α(I) collagen messenger RNA (mRNA) were determined by reverse transcriptase polymerase chain reaction (RT-PCR) assay. NFκB activation was determined by electrophoretic mobility shift assay. To corroborate NFκB participation in pentoxifylline effect, cells were pretreated with 10 μM TPCK, a NFκB inhibitor. IκBα was determined by Western blot. IL-6 expression decreased significantly in acetaldehyde-pentoxifylline-treated cells. Acetaldehyde-treated cells pretreated with an anti-IL-6 monoclonal antibody did not show any increase in α (I) collagen expression. Acetaldehyde-treated cells increased 1.48 times NFκB activation, whereas acetaldehyde-pentoxifylline-treated cells decreased NFκB activation to control values. TPCK pretreated acetaldehyde cells did not present NFκB activation. To corroborate NFκB participation in pentoxifylline effect, IκBα was determined. IκBα protein level decreased 50% in acetaldehyde-treated cells, while acetaldehyde-pentoxifylline-treated cells showed IκBα control cells value. The data suggest that acetaldehyde induced α(I) collagen and IL-6 expression via NFκB activation. Pentoxifylline prevents acetaldehyde-induced α(I) collagen and IL-6 expression by a mechanism dependent on IκBα degradation, which in turn blocks NFκB activation.

Keywords α (I) collagen · HSC · IκB · IL-6 · Liver fibrosis · NFκB · Pentoxifylline

E. Hernández · L. Bucio · V. Souza · M. C. Escobar ·
L. E. Gómez-Quiroz · B. Farfán ·
M. C. Gutiérrez-Ruiz (✉)
Departamento de Ciencias de la Salud,
Universidad Autónoma Metropolitana-Iztapalapa,
Mexico, D.F., Mexico
e-mail: mcgr@xanum.uam.mx

D. Kershenobich
Facultad de Medicina,
Universidad Nacional Autónoma de México,
Mexico, D.F., Mexico

Introduction

Hepatic fibrosis is a scarring response of the liver to chronic liver injury, and it is characterized by an increase in total liver collagen and other matrix proteins content, which alters the architecture of the liver and impairs liver function (Friedman 2000; Pinzani and Rombouts 2004; Albanis et al. 2006). The hepatic stellate cell (HSC) is the primary cell type in the liver responsible for excess collagen synthesis during hepatic fibrosis. After liver injury, the HSC undergoes a complex transformation or activation process where the cell changes from a quiescent, vitamin A storing cell to an activated, myofibroblast-like cell. HSC change their pattern of gene expression, which results in a dramatic increase in the synthesis and deposition of extracellular matrix proteins mainly collagen (I) (Iredale 2004), and the proliferation rate of these cells increase after cellular activation.

Acetaldehyde, first metabolite of alcohol oxidation, enhances α (I) collagen production by HSC (Anania et al. 1996). Several reports indicate that interleukin-6 (IL-6) exerts a profibrogenic action and up-regulates α (I) collagen expression in HSC (Greenwell et al. 1995; Hernández et al. 2002). IL-6 is regulated by nuclear factor κ B (NFκB). This nuclear factor consists principally of homo- and heterodimers of p50 and p65 protein units, which reside normally in the cytoplasm, where they are sequestered by a family of inhibitors of κB (IκB). Upon a stimulus, IκB is phosphorylated and ubiquitinated, which triggers its degradation by proteosoma 26S; NFκB is then released to enter the nucleus and activate the transcription of target genes (Baldwin 2001).

Among the therapeutic strategies against liver fibrosis, some benefit with pentoxifylline (PTX), a nonspecific methylxanthine derived phosphodiesterase inhibitor (Windmeier et al. 1997) has been reported. PTX exerts cytokine/chemokine modulation and presents beneficial action on animal models in liver fibrosis treatment and also exhibits beneficial effect on liver regeneration after portal vein ligation in rats (Kucuktulu et al. 2007). PTX shows an anti-inflammatory action (Sztrym et al. 2004; Desmoliere et al. 1999; Windmier et al. 1997), decreases HSC activation and proliferation (Desmoliere et al. 1999; Lee et al. 1997; Romanelli et al. 1997), and produces antifibrogenic effect (Peterson 1993; Raetsch et al. 2002; Isbrucker and Peterson 1998; Pinzani et al. 1996). Moreover, it has been described that PTX improves survival in human alcoholic liver disease (Akriviadis et al. 2000).

Data from our laboratory shows that PTX is able to decrease acetaldehyde-induced collagen gene expression and secretion in a HSC line (CFSC-2G cells) by reducing IL-6 (Hernández et al. 2002).

NFκB has been involved in a wide range of diseases including fibrosis (Elsharkawy et al. 2005), as its activation up-regulates cytokines, which contributes to liver fibrosis. Recently, it has been reported that phosphodiesterase (PDE) has been implicated in regulating the IκBα/NFκB signaling pathway (Haddad et al. 2002). PTX is considered a non-selective PDEs inhibitor; nevertheless, its mechanism of action in the NFκB signaling pathway has been poorly studied.

Therefore, the aim of this work was to determine the effect of PTX on acetaldehyde-induced collagen production and establish its effects on NFκB in a rat HSC line (CFSC-2G cells).

Materials and methods

Cell culture

All the experiments were performed using the rat HSC line CFSC-2G, which was obtained and kindly donated by Dr Rojkind (Greenwel et al. 1993). Cells were cultured in minimal essential medium (MEM; Gibco) supplemented with 10% bovine fetal serum (Hyclone Laboratories Inc., Logan Utah, USA), 1% non-essential amino acids, penicillin (100 U/ml), and streptomycin (100 mg/ml). The medium prepared in this way will be called complete medium. Cells were grown at 37°C in disposable plastic bottles (Nunc, USA) and in a humidified atmosphere of 5% CO_2/95% air. The medium was replaced twice a week, and cells were harvested and diluted every 3 days at a ratio of 1:3.

Experimental design

CFSC-2G cells were seeded in complete medium. Twenty-four hours later, the medium was changed for one containing acetaldehyde (Ac) 100 μM, or Ac and PTX (Sigma Chemical Co.) 200 μM, and flasks were sealed with film tape to control evaporation. Cells were incubated at 37°C for 3 h and then were washed twice with phosphate buffer saline (PBS), scrapped from the flasks to obtain RNA, and then were stored at −80°C, until experiments were performed.

Control cells were seeded at the same time as treated cells. They were maintained under the same conditions but with no addition of Ac and/or PTX.

RNA isolation

After removing the medium, cells were put on ice and washed twice with ice-cold PBS. Total cellular RNA was isolated by lysing the cells in 1 ml of trizol (Gibco) as described by Chomczynski and Sachi (1987). RNA was treated with chloroform, centrifuged (12,000 rpm, 15 min, 4°C), and finally precipitated with ethanol.

RT-PCR amplification for α (I) collagen and IL-6

CFSC-2G cells were pre-treated with 10 μM of L-1chloro-3-[4-tosylamido]-4-phenyl-2-butanone (TPCK), and sulfasalazine, NFκB inhibitors were added 30 min before Ac/PTX treatment. Total RNA (1.5 μg) was used for the reversal transcription (RT) reaction with 0.5 μg of oligo dT16 (Perkin Elmer), 10 mM of each of the four deoxynucleotides triphosphates, 25 mM $MgCl_2$, 10 U RNAase inhibitor, and 50 U of reverse transcriptase (Perkin Elmer) according to the manufacturer instructions, and were mixed to a final volume of 10 μl. A polymerase chain reaction (PCR) for α (I) collagen was performed with upstream primer 5' GAG TGA GGC CAC GCA TCA GCC GAA GCT AAC-3' and downstream primer 5' AAG AGG AGC AGG AGC CGG AGG TCC ACA AAG-3' in a PCR buffer, 25 mM $MgCl_2$, 5 U DNA polymerase (AmpliTaq polymerase, Perkin Elmer), 3 μl cDNA and 20 pmol of each primer, in a final volume of 65 μl. This reaction mixture was subject to 35 cycles (temperature profile 94°C 1 min, 53 °C 1 min; 72°C 1 min). The PCR for β_2 microglobulin was performed with upstream primer 5' GAT GCT GCT TAC ACG-3' and downstream primer 5' CCA GCA GAG AATGGA AAG TC-3' (temperature profile 94°C 1 min, 53°C 1 min, 72°C 1 min). A PCR for IL-6 was performed with upstream primer 5' TCA ATG AGC AGA CTT GCC TG 3' and downstream primer 5' GAT GAG TTG TCA TGT CCT GC 3' and was subject to 35 cycles (temperature profile 94°C 1 min, 55 °C 1 min, 72 °C 1 min). The PCR products were electrophoresed in 1% agarose gels containing 0.05 μg/ml ethidium bromide. The mRNA expression was quantified using a phosphoimager and the accompanying ImageQuant software, standarized to the β_2 microglobulin housekeeping gene signal to correct any variability in gel loading.

α (I) collagen Northern blot

A Northern blot was developed as described by Nieto et al. (1996). Equal amounts of total RNA (20 μg) from different cell treatments were subject to a Northern blot analysis. RNA blots were prehybridized for 5 h at 65°C in a hybridization solution (0.25M sodium phosphate buffer, pH 7.2 and 7% sodium dodecyl sulfate). Radio-labeled cDNA probes for α (I)collagen and glyceraldehyde 3 phosphate dehydrogenase (GAPDH) were hybridized to blots overnight. The blots were washed three times for 30 min each one at 65°C with a washing buffer solution (49 mM sodium phosphate buffer pH 7.2 and 5% sodium dodecyl sulfate). Membranes were analyzed in a phosphoimager and accompanying Image Quant software. The α (I) collagen signal density was normalized with GAPDH for intra-blot variability in RNA loading.

Preparation of nuclear extracts

Nuclear extracts were prepared as described by Roman et al. (2000). To evaluate if NFκB was involved in IL-6 and α (I) collagen expression, CFSC-2G cells were pre-treated with 10 μM of TPCK, a NFκB inhibitor for 30 min before Ac/PTX treatment. CFSC-2G cells were washed twice with ice-cold PBS and collected with a rubber policeman after treatments. Cells were resuspended in buffer A that contained 10 mM HEPES, pH 7.9, containing 10 mM KCl, 0.1 mM ethylenediaminetetraacetic acid (EDTA), 1 mM dithiothreitol, and 0.5 mM phenol methyl sulfonil fluoride (PMSF) and kept on ice for 15 min. Cells were then lysed with Igepal and the nuclear pellet was recovered after centrifugation at $14,000 \times g$ at 4°C for 30 s. The nuclear pellet was resuspended in ice-cold buffer C of 20 mM HEPES, pH 7.9 containing 0.4 mM NaCl, 1 mM EDTA and was stored at −80°C. Protein concentration was measured by Bradford method using Bio-Rad reagent (Bio-Rad, Hercules, CA, USA).

Electrophoretic mobility shift assays

Activation of NFκB was examined by electrophoretic mobility shift assay (EMSA) using a consensus oligonucleotides probes 5' AGT TGA GGG GAC TTT CCC AGG C 3'. (Promega) The probe was labeled by T4 polynucleotide kinase as described previously (Garcia et al. 1995). Binding reaction included 10 μg of nuclear extracts in incubation buffer (10 mM Tris–HCl, pH 7.5, 40 mM NaCl, 1 mM EDTA and 4% glycerol), 1 μg of poly (dl-deC), and labeled oligonucleotide (30,000 cpm). The mix was electrophoresed. Band specificity was determined by competition experiments using a molar excess of unlabeled NFκB to the nuclear extract 15 min before the addition of labeled probe.

IκB Western blot analysis

IκBα and IκBβ Western blot analysis were performed as described by Roman et al. (2000). HSCs were lysed in 50 mM Tris–HCl, pH 8.0 containing 120 mM NaCl, 0.5% Igepal (Sigma), 10 mM NaF, 200 μM NaVO$_4$, and a complete inhibitor protease cocktail (Roche Diagnostics). Protein concentration was determined by the Bradford method (Bradford 1976), using bovine serum albumin as a standard. Samples were analyzed under reducing conditions on 10% sodium dodecyl sulfate polyacrylamide gel electrophoresis (SDS-PAGE) electrophoresis. The protein bands were transferred (39 V for 12 h) onto polyvinylidene difluoride membranes (Immobilon-P, Amersham Pharmacia Biotech) using a transfer buffer consisting of 25 mM Tris (pH 8.3), 192 mM glycine, 0.05% (w/v) SDS and 20% (v/v) methanol. Membranes were blocked (60 min) with skimmed milk in TBS-Tween (20 mM Tris pH 7.5, 150 mM NaCl, 0.1% (v/v) Tween 20). Primary and secondary antibodies were diluted in the blocking solution to the appropriate dilution as indicated below. For the detection of anti-IκBα antibodies a 1:500 dilution of polyclonal antibody (Sta Cruz, Biotec Inc.) was used and 1:800 of the polyclonal for the IκB-β The membranes were incubated in a 1:2,500 dilution of the secondary antibody mouse antigoat (Santa Cruz, Biotec, Inc). Blots were revealed using supersignal West Pico chemiluminescent substrate (Pierce Chem Co). Protein bands were scanned and intensities quantified using a densitometer and accompanying Molecular Analyst Software.

Data analysis

Data are reported as mean±SD for at least three independent experiments carried out by triplicate. The

SPSS version 10 was used for statistical analysis. Comparisons among groups were done by means of analysis of variance (ANOVA). Tukey's method was used for multiple comparisons. A $p < 0.05$ was considered as statistical significant.

Results

Effect of anti-IL-6 monoclonal antibody on α (I) collagen expression

Previous data (Hernández et al. 2002) indicated that Ac induced α (I) collagen and IL-6 in CFSC-2G cells. To address whether IL-6 was involved in the Ac-induced α (I) collagen increase, cells were exposed to an anti-IL-6 monoclonal antibody 15 min before Ac treatment. α (I) Collagen expression was determined 3 h after by Northern blot and by reverse transcriptase polymerase chain reaction (RT-PCR) analysis as illustrated Fig. (1a, b).

The results obtained were similar with both techniques; anti IL-6 monoclonal antibody-treated cells did not increase α (I) collagen mRNA as a consequence of Ac treatment. The IL-6 monoclonal antibody and IgG alone did not produce any change. This result showed that IL-6 participates in the Ac-induced α (I) collagen expression in CFSC-2G cells. Moreover, these data suggest the presence of another factors besides IL-6, implicated in the Ac-induced α (I) collagen, due to the fact that cells treated with anti-IL-6/Ac did not return to the collagen expression control value.

Effect of pentoxifylline on α (I) collagen expression and IL-6

Once it was determined that IL-6 is involved in α (I) collagen gene expression, the next experiment was focused to determine the effect of PTX in Ac-treated cells. Cells were exposed to Ac (100 μM) and PTX (200 μM) for 3 h (Fig. 2a, b). Cells treated with Ac increased significantly the α (I) collagen expression (1.26±0.05), while cells treated with Ac and PTX diminished 12% mRNA α (I) collagen with respect to Ac-treated cells. Cells treated only with PTX did not change basal expression of α (I) collagen.

IL-6 expression had a significant increase in Ac-treated cells with respect to control cells (1.8-fold± 0.277). PTX by itself did not change the IL-6 basal

Fig. 1 Effect of anti-IL-6 monoclonal antibody on acetaldehyde-induced pro-collagen expression, by Northern blot (**a**) and RT-PCR of α (I) collagen expression (**b**) of CFSC-2G cells. CFSC-2G cells were exposed to anti-IL-6 monoclonal antibody 15 min before 100 μM acetaldehyde (*Ac*) was added to the culture media. α (I) Collagen and collagen expression were measured after 3 h treatment. Values represent the mean±SD of three independent experiments. *Significantly different from control or Ac (*ampersand*) treated cells (*p*<0.05)

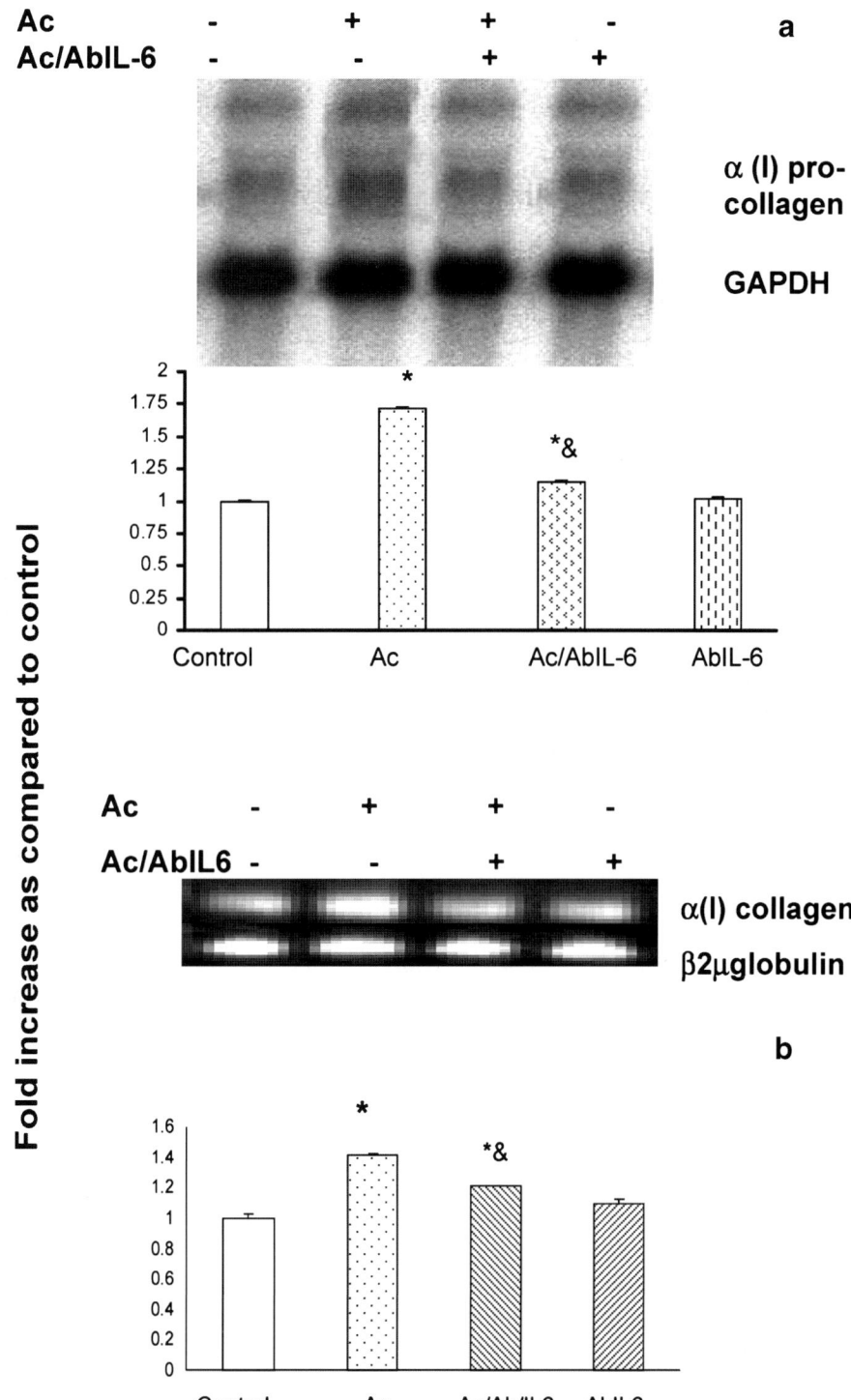

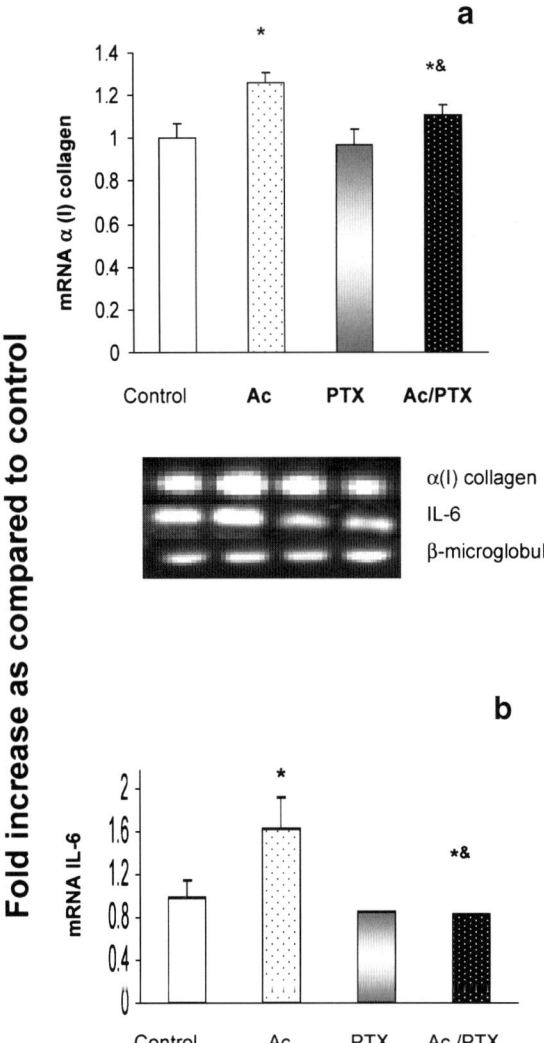

a

b

Fig. 2 α (I) collagen (**a**) and interleukin 6 (IL-6) (**b**) gene expression in CFSC-2G cells. Cells were treated during 3 h with acetaldehyde (*Ac*) 100 μM and/or pentoxifylline (*PTX*) 200 μM. RNA was isolated and RT-PCR was done as described in "Materials and methods". The gene expression of α (I) collagen and IL-6 were quantified using a phosphor imager equipment, standardized to β 2 microgloblin. Values represent the mean±SD of three independent experiments. *Significantly different from control ($p<0.05$)

expression. The value of IL-6 expression was significantly diminished in cells treated with Ac-PTX compared with Ac-treated cells.

Acetaldehyde induces NFκB activation in CFCS-2G cells

To determine the molecular mechanism involved in Ac induced α (I) collagen expression in CFSC-2G cells, NFκB was studied in Ac-treated cells (Fig. 3). An EMSA assay was performed. Cells treated with Ac (100μM) increased 1.5-fold NFκB DNA binding (line 2), while cells exposed to PTX (200 μM) prevented Ac-induced NFκB activation (line 4).

Acetaldehyde induces IκB- α degradation in CFSC-2G cells

IκB-α and IκB-κ degradation after phosphorylation has been described as a predominant pathway for NFκB activation. To evaluate the Ac-induced IκB-α and IκB-β, degradation Western blot was performed. A time course for IκB-α and IκB-β protein levels was determined in Ac-treated CFSC-2G cells. As shown in Fig. 4, Ac induced IκB-α degradation, presenting a 50% decrease 60 min after Ac stimuli compared to untreated cells. Reduced values were maintained until the 240 min. No changes in IκB-β levels were detected (data not shown).

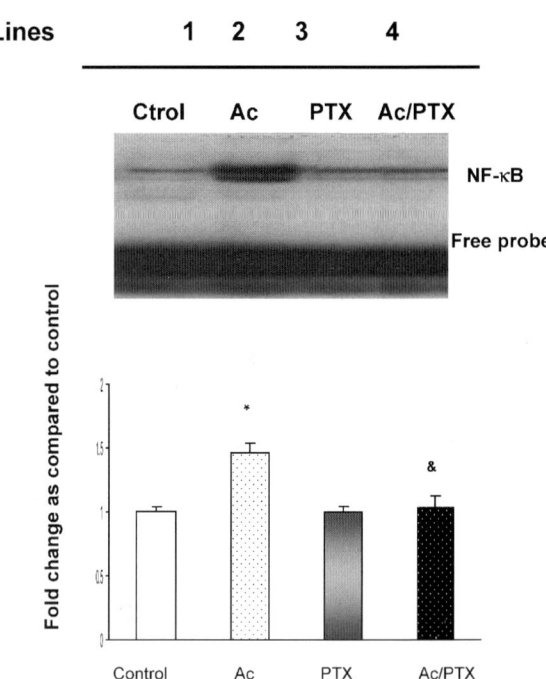

Fig. 3 Effect of pentoxifillyne (*PTX*) on the activation of NFκB in CFSC-2G cells. Nuclear extracts were treated for 1 h with acetaldehyde (*Ac*) 100 μM (*line 2*) or PTX 200 μM (*line 3*) or Ac and PTX (*line 4*) and were analyzed by an electronic mobility shift assays (EMSA). Values represent the mean±SD of three independent experiments. *Significantly different from control or Ac (*ampersand*) treated cells ($p<0.05$)

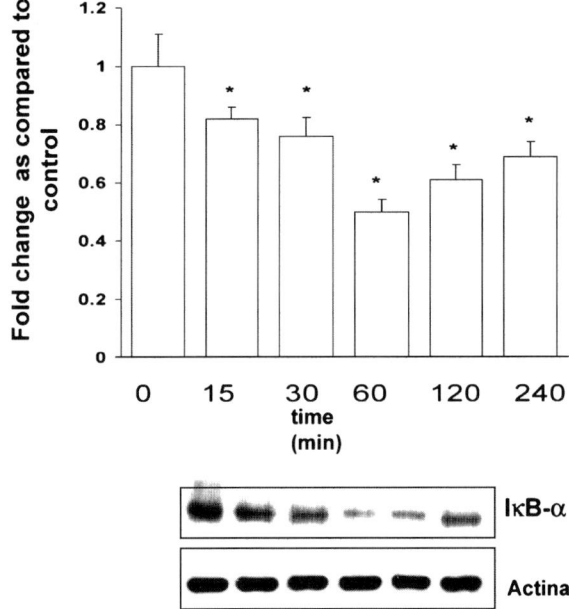

Fig. 4 Time course of IκB-α in CFSC-2G cells treated with acetaldehyde 100 μM as determined by Western blot. CFSC-2G cells were exposed to acetaldehyde during 15, 30, 60, 120, and 240 min. Cellular extracts were prepared for Western blot analyses of IkB-α. Values represent the mean±SD of three independent experiments ($p < 0.05$)

TPCK and PTX blocks NF κB activation

To determine if PTX is involved on preventing NFκB activation, CFSC-2G were pretreated during 30 min with 10 μM TPCK, a NFκB inhibitor (Kim et al 2006; Han et al. 2006). Figure 5 shows that cells treated with Ac, increased 1.48-fold NFκB DNA binding (lane 2) regarding control cells. PTX alone did not have any effect (lane 3). Cells treated with Ac-PTX diminished NFκB activation to value presented in control cells (compared to Ac-treated cells) (line 4). TPCK alone had not any effect in the NFκB basal level (line 5). Cells treated with TPCK and Ac showed a significantly decrease in NFκB compared with Ac cells treatment ($p < 0.05$, line 6).

Effect of PTX and TPCK on IκBα protein levels

Afterward, the next step was to determine how PTX blocks NFκB activation, and IκB-α protein level was quantified. Cellular extracts were subject to Western Blot analysis using a polyclonal antibody against IκB-α after 1 h treatment. Cells treated with Ac-PTX

showed IκBα values similar to control cells. The same results were obtained with Ac and TPCK about the IκB-α protein content. The results obtained suggest that PTX blocked Ac induced α (I) collagen by preventing IκB-α degradation (Fig. 6).

Effect of TPCK and PTX on IL-6 and α (I) collagen expression

To corroborate if NFκB activation is responsible for the Ac-induced in α (I) collagen and IL-6 expression, CFSC-2G cells were pretreated with 10 μM of TPCK, and α (I) collagen and IL-6 expression were determined with or without PTX treatment.

Cells treated with Ac increased α (I) collagen expression (26% compared to control cells), while PTX-treated cells presented values as control cells. Cells pretreated with TPCK did not have any change in α (I) collagen expression, whereas those cells treated with TPCK and Ac showed a 26% decrease in α (I) collagen compared to Ac-treated cells (Fig. 7a).

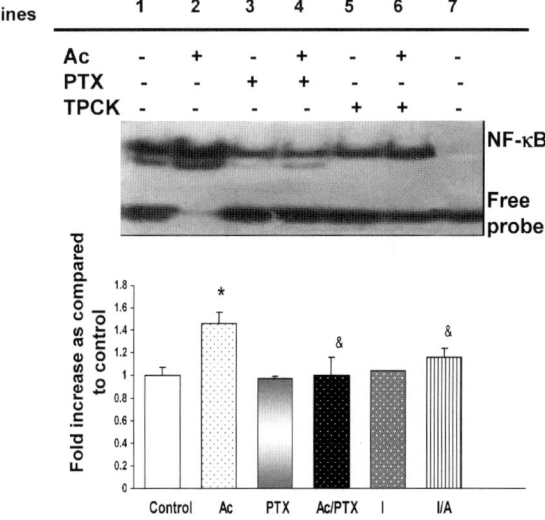

Fig. 5 Activation of NFκB by acetaldehyde (*Ac*) in CFSC-2G cells in presence of L-1chloro 3-[-4-tosylado]-4 phenyl-2-butanone (*TPCK*) a NFκB inhibitor. Nuclear extracts of CFSC-2G cells cultured with Ac and Ac/PTX for 1 h were prepared and analyzed by electronic mobility shift assay. *Line 2* Ac 100 μM treated cells. *Line 3* PTX 200 μM treated cell. *Line 4* Ac/PTX-treated cells. *Line 5* NFκB inhibitor (TPCK 10μM), *line 6* inhibitor and Ac-treated cells. The specificity of NFκB activation by ac was verified using an excess of unlabeled NFκB (*line 7*). Values represent the mean±SD of three independent experiments. *Significantly different from control or Ac (*ampersand*) treated cells ($p < 0.05$)

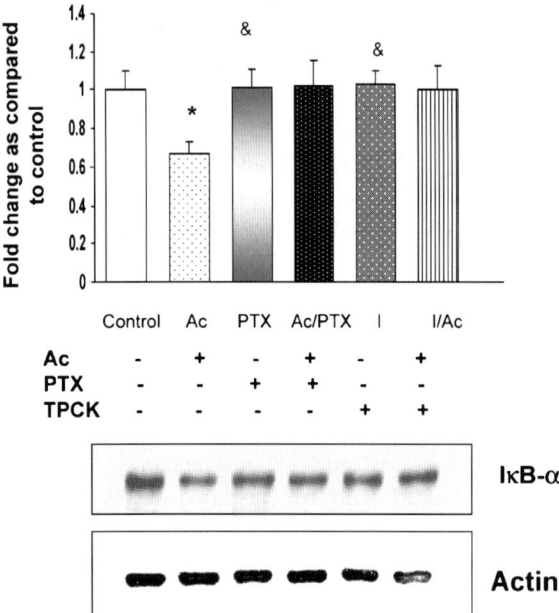

Fig. 6 Effect of pentoxifylline (*PTX*) 200 μM on the IκB-α levels of CFSC-2G cells treated with acetaldehyde (*Ac*) 100 μM, during 1 h. Cellular extract were prepared for Western blot analysis of IκB-α levels. Another cells were treated with TPCK 10 μM an inhibitor of NFκB. Values represent the mean±SD of three independent experiments. *Significantly different from control or Ac (*ampersand*) treated cells ($p<0.05$)

These data were corroborated using another NFκB inhibitor, sulfasalazine (Fig. 7b). Similar results were obtained in both cases.

CFSC-2G cells showed a significant IL-6 increase when cells were treated with Ac (1.64-fold±0.277 compared to control cells). PTX alone did not have any effect on basal IL-6 expression value, while Ac/PTX-treated cells decreased IL-6 expression significantly (0.51 times±0.055). TPCK did not have any effect in the basal IL-6 expression level. However, when cells were pretreated with TPCK and Ac; IL-6 expression was diminished in a significantly way (0.54-fold±0.065 with respect to Ac-treated cells; Fig. 8).

Discussion

Our results demonstrate that, under the experimental conditions of this study, Ac increased α (I) collagen and IL-6 expression in a rat HSC line, (CFSC-2G cells). PTX of 200 μM prevented the increase in α (I)

collagen and IL-6 expression by blocking NFκB activation, protecting the degradation of IκB-α.

Previous work from our laboratory reported that 200 μM PTX did not reduce CFCS-2G cells viability determined by trypan blue (Hernández et al. 2002). Moreover, PTX concentration used in these studies is ten times lower than the one used in other in vitro studies (Preaux et al. 1997).

Acetaldehyde, first metabolite of ethanol, has been proven to be a profibrogenic stimulus in alcohol-induced extracellular matrix increase. α (I) Collagen expression was increased as a result of Ac treatment in CFSC-2G cells. Anania et al. (1996) reported that Ac is highly fibrogenic per se. Recently, it has been reported that IL-6 is implicated in extracellular matrix proteins regulation and in liver fibrosis. Our findings indicate that IL-6 acts as a profibrogenic cytokine because treatment with the monoclonal IL-6 antibody assays prevents α (I) collagen production in Ac-treated CFSC-2G cells. Greenwell et al. (1995) reported that IL-6 plays an important role in liver fibrogenesis by inducing the expression of α(I) collagen. Experiments developed in rats showed that IL-6 has been associated with liver stellate cells activation in acute and chronic injuries, indicating that IL-6 is a factor involved in liver fibrosis (Zhang et al. 2004). IL-6 has also been reported to play a role in hepatic collagenesis in the presence of other toxics, such as arsenic (Das et al. 2005).

It is well known that PTX spread out anti-inflammatory properties, including downregulation of IL-6 and TNF-α synthesis (Coimbra et al. 2005a, b). Our data showed that PTX diminished Ac-induced IL-6 expression. Hoebe et al. (2001) reported that PTX showed differentially effects in the endotoxin-induced inflammatory response in primary porcine liver cell cultures by suppressing TNF-α and IL-6 synthesis while enhancing nitric oxide production. Ji et al. (2004) reported that PTX decreased IL-6 expression in rat intestine cells stimulated with lipopolysaccharide and downregulates IL-6 and TNF-α secretion in alveolar epithelial cells (Haddad et al. 2002).

Cellular signaling pathways that mediate the immunoregulatory potential of PTX have not been well characterized. Many effector genes, including those encoding IL-6 and α (I) collagen, are in turn regulated by NFκB (Ghosh 2002) because the regulatory regions of those genes are NFκB-responsive.

Fig. 7 α (I) Collagen gene expression in CFSC-2G treated with NFkB inhibitors. **a** Cells were pretreated with 10 μM L-1chloro 3-[-4-tosylado]-4 phenyl-2-butanone (*TPCK*), 200 μM pentoxifillyne (*PTX*), and 100 μM acetaldehyde (*Ac*). **b** Cells were pretreated with 0.05 μM of sulfasalazine and 100 μM Ac. RNA was isolated and reverse transcription polymerase chain reaction (*RT-PCR*) was done as described in "Material and methods". The α (I) collagen gene expression was quantified using a phosphor imager equipment, significantly different from control (*asterisk*) or Ac (*ampersand*) treated cells ($p<0.05$)

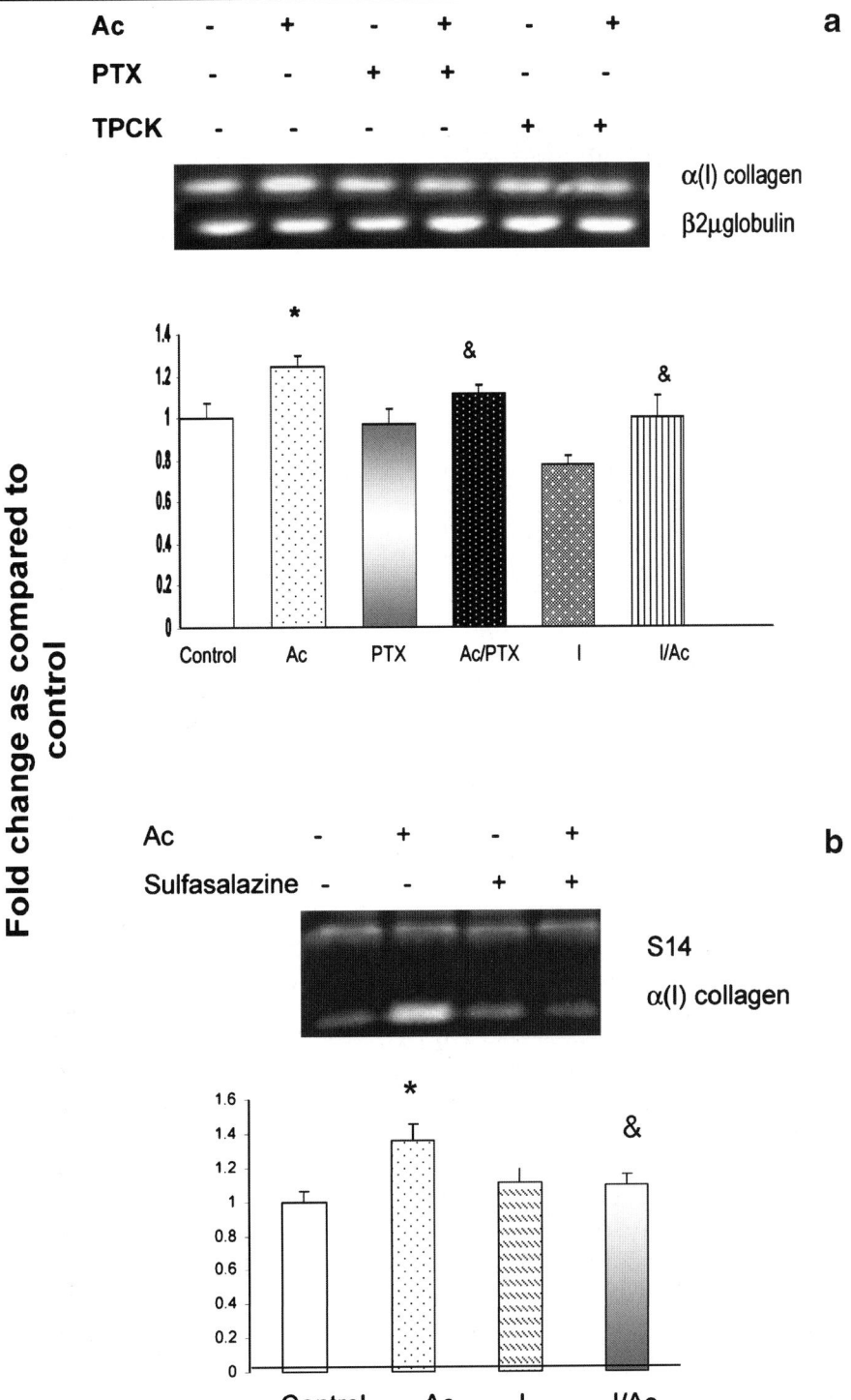

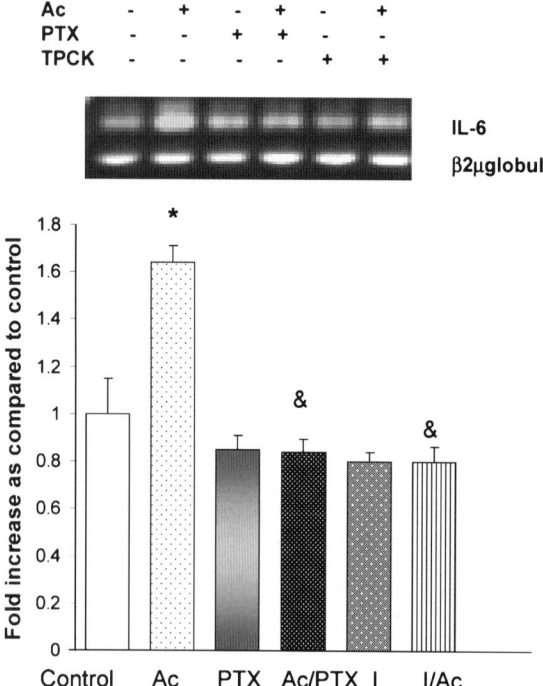

Fig. 8 IL-6 gene expression in CFSC-2G. Cells pretreated with 10 μM L-1chloro 3-[-4-tosylado]-4 phenyl-2-butanone (*TPCK*) a NFκB inhibitor, 200 μM pentoxifilyne (*PTX*), and 100 μM acetaldehyde (*Ac*). RNA was isolated and reverse transcription polymerase chain (*RT-PCR*) was done as described in "Material and methods". The IL-6 gene expression was quantified using a phosphor imager equipment, standardized to β 2 μglobulin. *Significantly different from control or Ac (*ampersand*) treated cells ($p < 0.05$)

IL-6 gene promoter is dynamically regulated at the NFκB site by equilibrium of a co-activator complex (including CBP/p300) interacting with NFκB (Vanden et al. 2002).

NFκB is typically a heterodimeric protein of p50 and p65 subunits, which in unstimulated cells resides in the cytoplasm through association with one of the IκB inhibitory proteins, such as IκBα or IκBβ. Following a specific cellular stimuli, IκB is phosphorylated by a specific kinase complex (IKK), which leads its ubiquination and subsequent proteolysis by proteosome 26S (Delhalle et al. 2004; Shoonbroodt et al. 2000). Degradation of IκB releases active NF-κB, which translocates to the nucleus and regulates gene expression by interacting with other transcription factors (Schreiber et al. 1998; Dixit and Mak 2002).

Our data showed that Ac activates NFκB in CFSC-2G cells. It has been reported that Ac increased nuclear NFκB (p65) protein in stellate cells. Several reports have been showed that ethanol and its metabolite, Ac, activate NF-κB in HepG2 cells. (Roman et al. 1999; Gómez Quiroz 2005).

Thus, data obtained in this work showed that Ac activated NFκB by IκBα degradation, while IκB-β was not affected. Although IκBα and IκBβ share 52% sequence identity in their primary structure (Zandi et al. 1997), only IκBα is necessary for phosphorylation of IκB's (Delhase et al. 1999). Novitskyi et al. (2004) reported that Ac increased IκB kinase activity and phosphorylated IκB-α indicating that Ac enhances the translocation of NFκB to the nucleus by increasing the degradation of IκB α in HSCs and in Hep-2G cells (Gómez-Quiroz et al. 2005; Román et al. 2000).

Our data suggests that PTX blocks NFκB activation, by a mechanism mediated by IκB α degradation protection. Coimbra et al. (2005a, b) reported that PTX decrease IKB-β phosphorylation and NFκB nuclear translocation in lipopolysaccharide-stimulated human peripheral blood mononuclear cells. Similar results were obtained using thalidomide in cirrhotic HSCs treated with CCl_4 (Peng et al. 2007).

It has been reported that other products inhibit NFκB activation preventing the degradation of IκB's protein such as the natural product gliotoxin (Pahl et al. 1996; Umezawa et al. 2000) and IL-10 (Lentsch and Ward 1999), or some synthetic products like aspirin and cyclosporine A (Marienfel et al. 1997). Habbans et al. (2005) reported the recovery of liver fibrosis by the inhibition of NFκB activation by sulfasalazin, which inhibits the autophosphorylation of IKKα and IKKβ.

Theophylline, an analogue of PTX, suppresses the production of proinflammatory cytokines via inhibition of NFκB activation through preservation of the IκBα protein in human pulmonary epithelial cells (Ichiyama et al. 2001) and in monocytes, macrophages, and T cells (Umeda et al. 2001).

We conclude that Ac induces α (I) collagen gene expression upregulating IL-6 via NFκB activation in CFSC-2G cells. PTX decreases Ac-induced collagen and IL-6 gene expression inhibiting NFκB activation through preservation of the IκBα. Drugs that selectively target inhibition of IκB's phosphorylation could be considered as a possible antifibrotic drugs. PTX could have therapeutic potential in alcohol-mediated liver damage.

References

Akriviadis E, Botla E, Briggs W, Han S, Reynolds T, Shakil O. Pentoxifylline improves shorter survival in severe acute alcoholic hepatitis: a double-blind placebo controlled trial. Gastroenterology 2000;119(6):1637–48.

Albanis E, Friedman SL. Antifibrotic agents for liver disease. Am J Transplant 2006;6(1):12–9.

Anania F, Potter J, Rennie-Tankersley L, Mezey E. Activation by acetaldehyde of the promoter of the mouse alpha 2 (I) collagen gene when transfected into rat activated stellate cells. Arch Biochem Biophys 1996;331:187–93.

Baldwin AS. Series Introduction: The transcription factor NF-κB and human disease. J Clin Invest 2001;105(1):3–6.

Bradford AM. A rapid and sensitive method for the quantification of microgram quantities of protein utilizing the principle of protein-dye binding. Anal Biochem 1976;72:248–54.

Chomczynski P, Sacchi N. Reagent for the single step simultaneous isolation of RNA. Anal Biochem 1987;162: 536–7.

Coimbra R, Melbostad H, Loomis W, Tobar M, Hoyt DB. Phosphodiesterases inhibition decreases factor-k B activation and shifts the cytokine response toward anti-inflammatory activity in acute endotoxemia. J Trauma 2005;59(3):575–82.

Coimbra R, Porcides RD, Melbostad H, Loomis W, Tobar M, Hoyt DB, et al. Nonspecfic phosphodiesterases inhibition attenuates liver injury in acute endotoxemia. Surg Infect 2005;1:73–85.

Das S, Santra A, Lahiri S, Guha-Mazuder DN. Implications of stress and hepatic cytokine (TNF-alpha and IL-6) response in the pathogenesis of hepatic collagenesis in chronic arsenic toxicity. Toxicol Appl Pharmacol 2005;1:18–26.

Delhalle S, Blasius R, Dicato M, Diederich M. A beginner's guide to NFκB signaling pathways. Ann NY Acad Sci 2004;1030:1–13.

Delhase M, Hayakawa M, Chen Y, Karin M. Positive and negative regulation of IκB kinase activity through IKKb subunit phosphorylation. Science 1999;284(5412):309–13.

Desmoliere A, Xu G, Costa A, Yousef I, Gabbiani G, Tucweber B. Effect of pentoxyfilline on early proliferation and phenotypic modulation on fibrogenic cells in two rat models of liver fibrosis and cultured hepatic stellate cells. J Hepatol 1999;30:621–31.

Dixit V, Mak T. NFkappaB signaling. Many roads lead to Madrid. Cell 2002;111:615–9.

Elsharkawy AM, Oakley F, Mann DF. The role and regulation of hepatic stellate cell apoptosis reversal of liver fibrosis. Apoptosis 2005;10:927–39.

Friedman SL. Molecular regulation of hepatic fibrosis, an integrated cellular response to tissue injury. J Biol Chem 2000;274:2247–50.

García R, Colell A, Morales A, Kaplowitz N, Fernández-Checa JC. Role of oxidative stress generated from the mitochondrial electron transport chain and mitochondrial glutathione status in loss of mitochondrial function and activation of transcription factor nuclear factor-kappa B: studies with isolated mitochondria and rat hepatocytes. Mol Pharmacol 1995;48(5):825–34.

Ghosh A. Factors involved in the regulation of type I collagen gene expression: implication in fibrosis. Exp Biol Med 2002;227(5):301–14.

Gómez-Quiroz L, Paris R, Lluis JM, Bucio L, Souza V, Hernández E, et al. Differential modulation of interleukin 8 by interleukin 4 and interleukin 10 in HepG2 cells treated with acetaldehyde. Liver Int 2005;25:122–30.

Greenwel P, Rubin J, Scwartz M, Hertzberg E, Rojkind M. Liver fat storing cells clones obtained from a CCl_4 cirrhotic rat are heterogeneous with regard to proliferation, expression of extracellular matrix components, interleukin-6 and connexin 43. Lab Invest 1993;69:210–6.

Greenwel P, Iraburo MJ, Reyes-Romo M, Meraz-Cruz N, Casado E, Soliz-Herruzo JA, Rojkind M. Induction of an acute phase response in rats stimulates the expression of alpha 1(I) procollagen Messenger ribonucleic acid in the livers. Possible role of interleukin-6. Lab Invest 1995;72:83–91.

Habans F, Srinvasan N, Oakley FD, Mann DA, Ganesan A, Packham G. Novel sulfasalazine analogues with enhanced NFκB inhibitory and apoptosis promoting activity. Apoptosis 2005;10(3):481–90.

Haddad JJ, Land S, Tarnow-Mordi W, Zembala M, Kowalczyk D, Lauterbach R. Immunopharmacological potential of selective phosphodiestererase inhibition. Differential regulation of lipopolyshaccharide-mediated proinflammatory cytokine (Interleukin-6 and tumor necrosis factor α) biosynthesis in alveolar epithelial cells. J Pharmacol Exp Ther 2002;300:559–66.

Han Y, Know Jh, Yu D, Moon E. Inhibitory effect of peroxiredoxin II (PrxII) on Ras-Erk-NFkappaB pathway in mouse embryonic fibroblast (MEF) senescence. Free Radic Res 2006;40(11):1182–9.

Hernández E, Correa A, Bucio L, Souza V, Kershenobich D, Gutierrez-Ruiz MC. Pentoxifylline diminished acetaldehyde-induced collagen production in hepatic stellate cells by decreasing interleukin-6 expression. Pharmacol Res 2002;46:435–43.

Hoebe KH, Ganzález-Ramón N, Nijmeijer SM, Wikamp RF, van Leengoed LA, van Miert AS, Monshouwer M. Differential effects of pentoxifylline on the hepatic inflammatory response in porcine liver cell cultures. Increase in inducible nitric oxide synthase expression. Biochem Pharmacol 2001;9:1137–44.

Ichiyama T, Hasegawa S, Matsubara T, Hayashi T, Furukawa S. Theophyllline inhibits NFκB activation and IκBα degradation in human pulmonary epithelial cells. Naunyn-Shmiedeberg's Arch Pharmacol 2001;364:558–61.

Iredale JP. A cut above the rest? MMP-8 and liver fibrosis gene therapy. Gastroenterology 2004;126(4):1199–201.

Isbrucker RA, Peterson TC. Plateled-derived growth factor and pentoxifylline modulation of collagen synthesis in myofibroblasts. Toxicol Appl Pharmacol 1998;25:120–26.

Ji Q, Zhang L, Jia H, Yang J, Xu J. Pentoxifylline inhibits endotoxin-induced NFκB activation and associated production of proinflammatory cytokines. Ann Clin Lab Sci 2004;34:427–36.

Kim S, Hwang C, Juhnn Y, Park W, Song Y. GDD153 mediates celecoxib-induced apoptosis in cervical cancer cells. Carcinogenesis 2006;10:1961–9.

Kucuktulu U, Alhan E, Tekelioglu Y, Ozekin A. The effects of pentoxifylline on liver regeneration after portal vein ligation in rats. Liv Int 2007;27(2):274–9.

Lee K, Cottam H, Houglum K, Wasson B, Carson D, Chockier M. Pentoxifylline blocks hepatic stellate cell activation independently of phosphodiesterase inhibitory activity. Am J Physiol 1997;273:G1094–G100.

Lentsch AB, Ward PA. Activation and regulation of NFκB during acute inflammation. Clin Chem Lab Med 1999;37 (3):205–8.

Lv P, Luo HS, Zhou XP, Xiao YJ, Paul SC, Si XM, et al. Reversal effect of thalidomide on established hepatic cirrhosis in rats via inhibition of nuclear factorkB/inhibitor of nuclear factor kB pathway. Arch Med Res 2007;38: 15–27.

Marienfel R, Neumann M, Chuvpilo S, Escher C, Kneitz B, Avots A, et al. Cyclosporin A interferes with the inducible degradation of NFκB inhibitors, but not with the processing of p105/NF-kappa B1 in T cells. Eur J Immunol 1997;27:1601–09.

Nieto N, Friedman S, Greenwel P, Cederbaum A. CYP2E1 mediated oxidative stress induces collagen type I expression in rat hepatic stellate cells. Hepatology 1996;30: 987–96.

Novitsky G, Potter J, Rennie-Tankersley L, Mezey E. Identification of a novel NFκB binding site with regulation of the murine α (I) collagen promoter. J Biol Chem 2004;279: 15639–44.

Pahl HL, Krauss B, Schulze-Ozthoff K, Decker T, Traenckner EB, Vogt M, et al. Muhlbacher A. The immunosuppressive fungal metabolite gliotoxin specifically inhibits transcription factor Nfkappab. J Exp Med 1996;183(4):1829–40.

Peterson T. Pentoxifylline prevents fibrosis in an animal model and inhibits plateled –derived growth factor driven proliferation of fibroblast. Hepatology 1993;17(3):486–93.

Pinzani M, Rombouts K. Liver fibrosis: from the bench to clinical targets. Dig Liver Dis 2004;36(4):231–42.

Pinzani M, Marra F, Caligiuri A, DeFranco R, Gentilini A, Faili P, et al. Inhibition by pentoxifylline of extracellular signal-regulated kinase activation by plateled-derived growth factor in hepatic stellate cells. Br J Pharmacol 1996;119: 1117 24.

Preaux A, Mallat A, Rosenbaum J, Zafrani E, Mavier P. Pentoxifylline inhibits growth and collagen synthesis of cultured human hepatic myofibroblast cells. Hepatology 1997;26(2):315–22.

Raetsch C, Jia J, Boigk G, Bauer M, Hahn EG, Riecken E, et al. Pentoxifylline downregulates profibrogenic cytokines and procollagen I expression in rat secondary biliary fibrosis. Gut 2002;50:241–7.

Román J, Colee A, Blasco C, Caballeria J, Parés A, Rodés J, et al. Differential Role of ethanol and acetaldehyde in the induction of oxidative stress in HepG2 cells: effect on transcription factors AP-1 and NFκB. Hepatology 1999; 30:1473–80.

Román J, Giménez A, Lluis J, Gassó M, Rubio M, Caballeria J, et al. Enhanced DNA binding and activation of transcription factors NFκB and AP-1 by acetaldehyde in HepG2 cells. J Biol Chem 2000;275:14684–90.

Romanelli R, Caliguri A, Carloni V, De Franco R, Montalto P, Ceni E, et al. Effect of pentoxiffylline on the degradation of procollagen type I produced by human hepatic stellate cells in response to transforming growth factor-beta1. Br J Pharmacol 1997;122(6):1047–54.

Schreiber S, Nikolaus S, Hampe J. Activation of nuclear factor kappa B inflammatory bowel disease. Gut 1998;42(4): 477–84.

Shoonbroodt S, Piette J. Oxidative stress interference with the nuclear factor κB activation pathways. Biochem Pharmacol 2000;60:1075–83.

Sztrym FB, Rabiller A, Nunes H, Savale L, Lebrec D, Le Pape A, et al. Prevention of hepatopulmonary syndrome and hyperdinamic state by pentoxifylline in cirrhotic rats. Eur Respir 2004;23:752–8.

Umeda M, Ichiyama T, Hasehawa S, Kaneko M, Matsubara T, Furukawa S. Theophylline inhibits NFκB activation in human peripheral blood mononuclear cells. Int Arch Allergy Immunol 2001;128:130–5.

Umezawa K, Ariga A, Matsumoto N. Naturally occurring and synthetic inhibitors of NF-κB functions. Anticancer Drug Des 2000;15:239–144.

Vanden W, Vermeulen L, De Wilde G, De Bosscher K, Boone E, Haegeman G. Signal transduction of the inflammatory cytokine interleukin-6. Biochem Pharmacol 2002;60(8): 1185–95.

Windmeier C, Gressner A. Pharmacological aspects of pentoxifylline with emphasis on its inhibitory actions on hepatic fibrogenesis. Gen Pharmacol 1997;29(2):181–96.

Zandi E, Rothwart DM, Delhase M, Hayakawa M, Karin M. The IκB kinase complex (IKK) contains two kinase subunits, IKKα, and IKKβ necessary for IκB phosphorylation and NFκB activation. Cell 1997;17/91(2):243–52.

Zhang LJ, Yu JP, Huang YH, Chen Z, Wang X. Effects of cytokines on carbon tetrachloride-induced hepatic fibrogenesis in rats. World J Gastroenterol 2004;10:77–81.

Correlation of visual in vitro cytotoxicity ratings of biomaterials with quantitative in vitro cell viability measurements

Sujata K. Bhatia · Ann B. Yetter

Originally published in the journal Cell Biology and Toxicology, Volume 24, Nos 4–5, 35–39.
DOI: 10.1007/s10565-007-9040-z © Springer Science + Business Media B.V. 2007

Abstract Medical devices and implanted biomaterials are often assessed for biological reactivity using visual scores of cell–material interactions. In such testing, biomaterials are assigned cytotoxicity ratings based on visual evidence of morphological cellular changes, including cell lysis, rounding, spreading, and proliferation. For example, ISO 10993 cytotoxicity testing of medical devices allows the use of a visual grading scale. The present study compared visual in vitro cytotoxicity ratings to quantitative in vitro cytotoxicity measurements for biomaterials to determine the level of correlation between visual scoring and a quantitative cell viability assay. Biomaterials representing a spectrum of biological reactivity levels were evaluated, including organo-tin polyvinylchloride (PVC; a known cytotoxic material), ultra-high molecular weight polyethylene (a known non-cytotoxic material), and implantable tissue adhesives. Each material was incubated in direct contact with mouse 3T3 fibroblast cell cultures for 24 h. Visual scores were assigned to the materials using a 5-point rating scale; the scorer was blinded to the material identities.

Quantitative measurements of cell viability were performed using a 3-(4,5-dimethylthiozol-2-yl)-2,5-diphenyltetrazolium bromide (MTT) colorimetric assay; again, the assay operator was blinded to material identities. The investigation revealed a high degree of correlation between visual cytotoxicity ratings and quantitative cell viability measurements; a Pearson's correlation gave a correlation coefficient of 0.90 between the visual cytotoxicity score and the percent viable cells. An equation relating the visual cytotoxicity score and the percent viable cells was derived. The results of this study are significant for the design and interpretation of in vitro cytotoxicity studies of novel biomaterials.

Keywords 3T3 cell line · Adhesives · Biomaterials · Cytotoxicity · Fibroblasts

Abbreviations
MTT   3-(4,5-dimethylthiozol-2-yl)-2,5-diphenyltetrazolium bromide

S. K. Bhatia · A. B. Yetter
Biochemical Sciences and Engineering, Central Research and Development, DuPont Experimental Station, Wilmington, DE 19880, USA

S. K. Bhatia (✉)
DuPont Experimental Station,
E328/140B, P.O. Box 80328, Wilmington, DE 19880, USA
e-mail: sujata.k.bhatia@usa.dupont.com

Introduction

To possess clinical value, medical devices and implanted biomaterials must be non-toxic, eliciting no adverse response from the application site or surrounding tissues. There is great necessity for reliable in vitro cytotoxicity assays, so that medical biomaterials can be correctly evaluated before preclinical or clinical studies. An accurate and precise in vitro cytotoxicity assay can reduce the number of animal studies needed to develop a new medical device. At the same time, it is desirable that in vitro cytotoxicity evaluations be sufficiently rapid to allow the screening of large numbers of potential biomaterial candidates. For this reason, visual scoring systems are often used to report cytotoxic effects of medical biomaterials. In such systems, biomaterials are assigned cytotoxicity ratings based on visual evidence of morphological cellular changes, including cell lysis, rounding, spreading, and proliferation. A visual grading method requires only microscopic inspection of cell–material interactions, in contrast to quantitative methods for cytotoxicity measurement, which require time-consuming colorimetric assays and spectrophotometer equipment. While visual cytotoxicity scoring provides advantages in terms of speed and convenience, it is critical to ensure that accuracy is not compromised.

Important disparities exist in regulatory recommendations for cytotoxicity testing of new medical devices. The International Organization for Standardization has set forth ISO-10993-5 guidelines for "Biological Evaluation of Medical Devices" that allow for the use of visual grading systems in cytotoxicity determinations (ISO 10993-5 1999). The US Food and Drug Administration guidelines for medical device evaluation are largely in concordance with ISO-10993 requirements (FDA G95-1 1995) so that medical device cytotoxicity may be evaluated according to ISO-10993-5 recommendations, with a visual scoring method. In contrast, the Japanese Ministry for Health and Welfare applies a more stringent standard for medical device approval and specifies that medical device cytotoxicity be evaluated using a quantitative assessment of surviving cells (MHW notification no. 99 1995). Thus, there is disagreement between regulatory bodies regarding the appropriateness of visual scoring methods for cytotoxicity assessment of new medical devices.

The objective of the present study is to compare visual in vitro cytotoxicity ratings to quantitative in vitro cytotoxicity measurements for biomaterials to determine the level of correlation between visual scoring and a quantitative cell viability assay. Biomaterials representing a spectrum of biological

reactivity levels were evaluated, including organo-tin polyvinylchloride (PVC; a known cytotoxic material), ultra-high molecular weight polyethylene (a known non-cytotoxic material), and implantable tissue adhesives. Polyethylene and organo-tin PVC were chosen for the dynamic cytotoxicity assay because these two materials typically represent the extremes of non-toxicity and toxicity, respectively, in ISO 10993-5 standardized static cytotoxicity tests of medical devices (AAMI 2003). Tissue adhesives were chosen for the study as representative biomaterials intended for use in the abdominal space. A total of 33 material assessments were performed. The mouse fibroblast cell line NIH 3T3 was chosen for the cytotoxicity study, as fibroblasts are the main cellular component of dense connective tissues and are the typical cell line used for cytotoxicity studies of biomaterials. Biomaterial samples were placed in direct contact with 3T3 fibroblasts to more closely mimic the physiological situation (Ratner et al. 1996). Each material was incubated in direct contact with mouse 3T3 fibroblast cell cultures for 24 h. Visual scores were assigned to the materials using a 5-point rating scale; the scorer was blinded to the material identities. Quantitative measurements of cell viability were performed using a 3-(4,5-dimethylthiozol-2-yl)-2,5-diphenyltetrazolium bromide (MTT) colorimetric assay; again, the assay operator was blinded to material identities. The results of this study are significant for the selection and interpretation of in vitro cytotoxicity studies for medical biomaterials.

Materials and methods

Biomaterial samples

Organo-tin PVC strips were obtained from Smiths Medical (Kent, UK). Polyethylene samples were obtained from the US Pharmacopeia (Rockville, MD). Polysaccharide-based tissue adhesives composed of dextran aldehyde and multi-arm polyethylene glycol (PEG) amine were obtained from Dr. George Kodokian at DuPont; the synthesis of these adhesives has been previously described (Kodokian and Arthur 2006). The commercial cyanoacrylate-based tissue adhesive Dermabond™ was obtained from Johnson & Johnson/Ethicon (Somerville, NJ).

Cell culture and reagents

The mouse fibroblast NIH 3T3 cell line was obtained from American Type Culture Collection (ATCC). Cells were grown at 37°C in a 5% (*v/v*) CO_2 incubator in Dulbecco's modified Eagle's medium (DMEM) supplemented with 10% (*v/v*) fetal bovine serum (Invitrogen; Carlsbad, CA).

Cytotoxicity assay with visual scoring

Biomaterial samples were randomized, and the assay operator was blinded to material identities. A 30-mg sample of biomaterial was placed into an empty well of a six-well culture plate. Mouse 3T3 fibroblast cells were then seeded into the well at a density of 50,000 cells per well. The plate was incubated at 37°C for

Table 1 Visual cytotoxicity ratings and quantitative cell viability data for 33 medical biomaterial samples

Visual cytotoxicity rating	% Cell viability
1	3
1	3
1	3
1	27
1	30
1	43
2	25
2	26
2	25
2	45
2	49
2	54
2	50
2	53
2	50
3	32
3	32
3	31
4	76
4	77
4	76
4	79
4	85
4	79
4	83
4	82
4	83
5	100
5	95
5	84
5	100
5	94
5	84

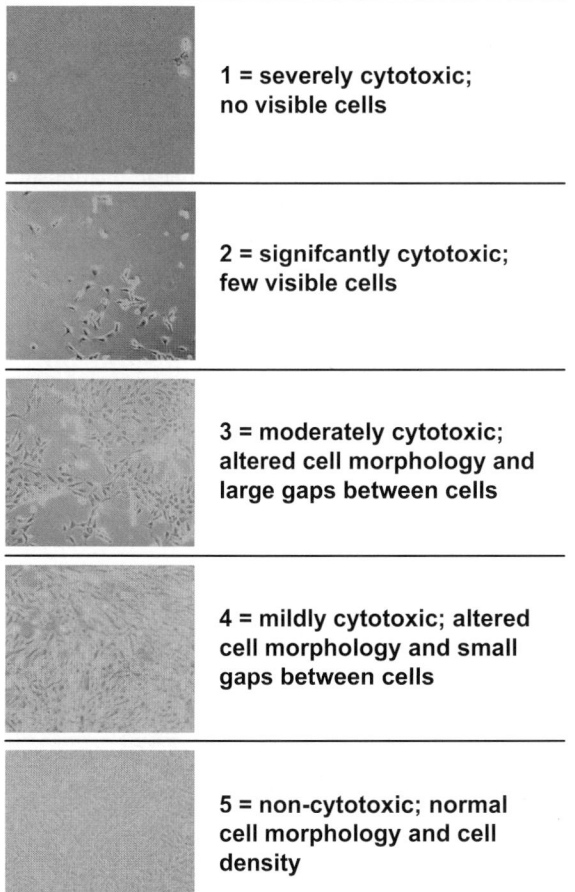

1 = severely cytotoxic; no visible cells

2 = signifcantly cytotoxic; few visible cells

3 = moderately cytotoxic; altered cell morphology and large gaps between cells

4 = mildly cytotoxic; altered cell morphology and small gaps between cells

5 = non-cytotoxic; normal cell morphology and cell density

Fig. 1 Scheme for assigning visual cytotoxicity scores to biomaterials

24 h. After the incubation, fibroblast cell growth and morphology were visualized directly, using a Nikon microscope with a 10× objective, equipped with a Nikon 35-mm camera. A visual cytotoxicity score was assigned according to a 5-point rating scale, ranging from 1=cytotoxic to 5=non-cytotoxic, based on observable characteristics of cell spreading and cell lysis (Fig. 1). A score of 5 is assigned for a confluent monolayer of well-defined cells exhibiting cell-to-cell contact; cell morphology and cell density are not altered by the presence of a biomaterial, and discrete intracytoplasmic granules are observed. No cell lysis is observed, indicating a non-cytotoxic reaction. A

score of 4 is assigned when occasional lysed cells are present; not more than 20% of the cells appear to be round, loosely attached, and without cytoplasmic granules. A score of 3 is assigned when cell lysis becomes more prevalent, but no more than 50% of the cells are round and devoid of intracytoplasmic granules. A score of 2 is assigned when the majority of cells are affected, but not more than 70% of the cells are rounded or lysed. A score of 1 is assigned when destruction and lysis of cells is nearly complete; considerable open areas between cells indicate that extensive cell lysis has occurred, indicating a cyto-toxic reaction.

Cytotoxicity assay with quantitative cell viability measurement

Biomaterial samples were randomized, and the assay operator was blinded to material identities. A 30-mg sample of biomaterial was placed into an empty well of a six-well culture plate. Mouse 3T3 fibroblast cells were then seeded into the well at a density of 50,000 cells per well. The plate was incubated at 37°C for 24 h. After the incubation, the cell viability was determined using a MTT colori-metric assay kit from ATCC; the protocol for the MTT assay has been extensively described (Sgouras and Duncan 1990).

Results

Thirty-three biomaterial samples were assessed for cytotoxicity using both a visual rating scale and a quantitative MTT colorimetric assay. The results are summarized in Table 1. The results indicate a high degree of correlation between the visual cytotoxicity rating and the quantitative cell viability measurement (Fig. 2). When the data are plotted to show the relationship between the visual cytotoxicity score and the MTT colorimetric technique for quantifying cell viability, a linear relationship is suggested. The visual rating and quantitative cell viability are related by the following equation:

% cell viability = 18.8(visual score)

A Pearson's correlation gives a correlation coeffi-cient of 0.90 between the visual cytotoxicity score and the percent viable cells.

Discussion

The above results indicate that a linear relationship exists between visual in vitro cytotoxicity ratings and quantitative in vitro cell viability measurements for medical biomaterials. When mouse 3T3 fibroblasts

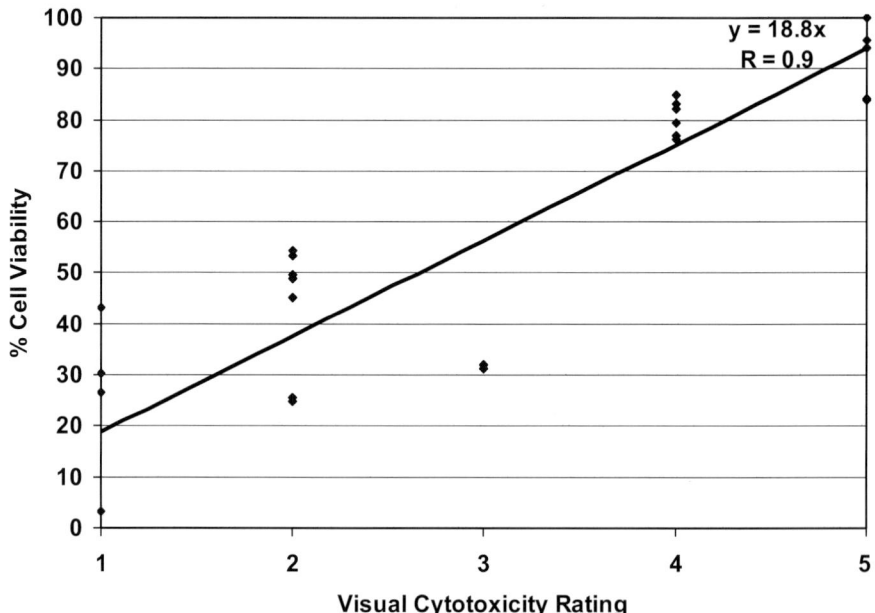

Fig. 2 Relationship between quantitative cell viability and visual cytotoxicity ratings for medical biomaterials. Fibroblast cells were incubated in direct contact with material samples for 24 h at 37°C. Visual cytotoxicity scores were assigned according to a 5-point rating scale. Quantitative cell viability measurements were performed using an MTT colorimetric assay. Linear correlation was performed with Pearson's linear correlation, with the equation of the line and *r* value shown

are incubated in direct contact with biomaterial samples, visual cytotoxicity scores are predictive of the percentage of viable cells. This finding is significant because it suggests that visual scoring is a valid method for rapidly estimating the cytotoxicity of new materials to clinically relevant cell lines. Visual inspection can be performed more quickly than a colorimetric assay and avoids the necessity for additional equipment, so the visual rating method may be particularly advantageous for screening a large number of biomaterial samples. It is important to note, however, that the medical biomaterial samples given a visual rating of 3 (in the middle of the rating scale) all demonstrated quantitative cell viabilities well below 50%, suggesting that special caution should be used in interpreting visual ratings in the middle of the rating scale. The visual rating system used in the present study suggests that biomaterials should raise serious concern for cytotoxicity when the visual rating is 3 or lower.

It is critical that in vitro assays for cytotoxicity accurately assess the potential of biomaterials to damage cells; a lack of stringency during in vitro testing can lead to unnecessary and harmful animal studies and disastrous results during in vivo preclinical testing and clinical use. Indeed, cyanoacrylate-based adhesives have been widely used in medical and surgical procedures, yet concerns have recently been raised regarding the hazards of cyanoacrylate use to both patients and healthcare workers (Leggat et al. 2007). Cyanoacrylate adhesives have been shown to cause inflammation and tissue necrosis in vivo (Toriumi et al. 1991; Kim et al. 1995). In another instance, a commercial albumin/glutaraldehyde tissue adhesive was shown to cause significant damage to lung and liver tissue, and investigators have recommended that its use be restricted to emergency procedures (Furst and Banerjee 2005). Direct contact testing of novel biomaterials with in vitro cell cultures may provide an early indicator of potential problems in vivo. We therefore recommend that any subjective in vitro cytotoxicity assessment that utilizes visual rating scales be validated against a quantitative in vitro cell viability assay before routine use of the visual inspection scheme. The visual rating system

must be validated for the specific cell lines and biomaterials being examined. Such an assessment increases the likelihood of regulatory approval for novel biomaterials, and more importantly, it represents responsible product stewardship.

Acknowledgements This study was performed as part of a DuPont Six Sigma project. We are grateful to Deana DiCosimo, Harvey Gold, and Lourdes Puig from the DuPont Six Sigma organization for their guidance and suggestions.

References

AAMI (Association for the Advancement of Medical Instrumentation). Biological evaluation of medical devices–Part 5: Tests for *in vitro* cytotoxicity. Arlington, VA; 2003.

Food and Drug Administration, US Department of Health and Human Services. Use of International Standard ISO 10993, biological evaluation of medical devices–Part 1: Evaluation and testing; G95-1. Rockville, MD; 1995.

Furst W, Banerjee A. Release of glutaraldehyde from an albumin-glutaraldehyde tissue adhesive causes significant in vitro and in vivo toxicity. Ann Thorac Surg. 2005; 79:1522–8.

International Organization for Standardization. Biological evaluation of medical devices – ISO 10993, Part 5: Tests for *in vitro* cytotoxicity. Geneva, Switzerland; 1999.

Kim JC, Bassage SD, Kempski MH, del Cerro M, Park SB, Aquavella JV. Evaluation of tissue adhesives in closure of scleral tunnel incisions. J Cataract Refract Surg. 1995;21:320–5.

Kodokian GK, Arthur SD. Polysaccharide-based polymer tissue adhesive for medical use. U.S. Patent Application 11/244,756;2006.

Leggat PA, Smith DR, Kedjarune U. Surgical applications of cyanoacrylate adhesives: a review of toxicity. ANZ J Surg. 2007;77:209–13.

Ministry of Health and Welfare, Pharmaceutical Affairs Bureau. Japanese guidelines for basic biological tests for medical devices and materials, notification no. 99. Tokyo, Japan; 1995.

Ratner BD, Hoffman AS, Schoen FJ, Lemons JE (eds) Biomaterials science, 2nd ed. New York: Academic; 1996.

Sgouras D, Duncan R. Methods for the evaluation of biocompatibility of soluble synthetic polymers which have potential for biomedical use: 1 – Use of the tetrazolium-based colorimetric assay (MTT) as a preliminary screen for evaluation of in vitro cytotoxicity. J Mater Sci Mater Med. 1990;1:61–8.

Toriumi DM, Raslan WF, Friedman M, Tardy ME. Variable histotoxicity of histoacryl when used in a subcutaneous site: an experimental study. Laryngoscope. 1991;101:339–43.

Effect of dietary selenium deficiency on the in vitro fertilizing ability of mice spermatozoa

M. Sánchez-Gutiérrez · E. A. García-Montalvo · J. A. Izquierdo-Vega · L. M. Del Razo

Originally published in the journal Cell Biology and Toxicology, Volume 24, Nos 4–5, 41–49.
DOI: 10.1007/s10565-007-9044-8 © Springer Science + Business Media B.V. 2007

Abstract Selenium is an essential micronutrient for mammals, being integral part of antioxidant system. The aim of the study was to evaluate the effect of selenium deficiency on in vitro fertilization (IVF) capacity of spermatozoa and on oxidative stress in these cells. Male C57BL/6N mice were maintained on selenium-deficient or selenium-sufficient diets (0.02 or 0.2 ppm of selenium as selenomethionine, respectively) for 4 months. Liver glutathione peroxidase activity measurements were used to confirm selenium deficiency. Sperm quality and IVF capability among both groups were evaluated. To assess oxidative damage, lipid peroxidation as malondialdehyde production was determined in spermatozoa as well as the testes. Ultrastructural analyses of spermatozoa nuclei using transmission electron microscopy were also performed. The percentage of eggs fertilized with sperm from selenium-deficient mice was significantly decreased by approximately 67%. This reduced fertilization capacity was accompanied by increased levels of lipid peroxidation in both the testes and sperm, indicating that selenium deficiency induced oxidative stress. Consistent with this finding, spermatozoa from selenium-deficient animals exhibited altered chromatin condensation. Deficiency in dietary selenium decreases the reproductive potential of male mice and is associated with oxidative damage in spermatozoa.

Keywords Selenium deficiency · In vitro fertilization · Oxidative damage · Mice spermatozoa · Reproduction

M. Sánchez-Gutiérrez
Área Académica de Medicina,
Instituto de Ciencias de la Salud,
Universidad Autónoma del Estado de Hidalgo,
Pachuca, Hidalgo 42000, México

E. A. García-Montalvo · J. A. Izquierdo-Vega ·
L. M. Del Razo (✉)
Sección Externa de Toxicología,
Centro de Investigación y de Estudios Avanzados del
Instituto Politécnico Nacional (CINVESTAV-IPN),
Av. IPN 2508, Col. Zacatenco,
México, DF 07360, México
e-mail: ldelrazo@cinvestav.mx

J. A. Izquierdo-Vega
FES-Cuautitlán. UNAM,
Cuautitlán Izcalli, Estado de México, México

Introduction

Selenium is an essential trace element for mammals and is an integral part of antioxidant systems. Selenium, which commonly replaces sulfur in proteins, is normally incorporated into the body through selenoamino acids (L-selenomethionine, L-selenocysteine, selenium–methylselenocysteine), taken up mainly from cereals, plants, and meat. It has been reported that SeMet can substitute for Met during translation, since tRNA^{Met} is incapable of discriminating between these two amino acids in the growing peptide chain (Schrauzer 2000). This process has been described in detail in prokaryotes (Böck 2000), whereas in mammals it is increasingly becoming better understood (Hatfield and Gladyshev 2002).

An important aspect of selenium is its nutritional significance as lower levels of selenium in the body decreases the expression of the seleno-proteins and thereby impairs selenium's biological functions resulting in nutritional deficiency of the element. Estimated intakes of selenium by US residents exceed the recommended dietary allowance value of 55 µg/day for healthy adults (NAS 2000); however, the selenium intake of some Europeans is as low as 35 µg/day (Broadley et al. 2006) or dramatically as low as 17 µg/day or ≤10 µg/day, respectively, in other geographic areas such as Africa and China (Benemariya et al. 1993; Moreno-Reyes et al. 1998).

Selenium has potential relevance to the reproductive system, as evidenced by reports of selenium deficiency causing impaired reproductive abilities in both sexes (Harrison et al. 1984). In females, disturbances caused by selenium deficiency remain unclear, whereas in males, impaired spermatogenesis has been reported in several species including pigs (Edwards et al. 1977), rats (Wu et al. 1979), and mice (Wallace et al. 1983). Selenium deficiency has been associated with impaired sperm motility, flagellar defects, and structural alterations in the sperm midpiece, which normally contains mitochondria embedded in a keratinous matrix called the mitochondrial capsule (Ursini et al. 1999; Olson et al. 2004).

Selenium plays an important role in cellular antioxidant defenses, since it forms the catalytic site of antioxidant enzymes (mainly as selenocysteine) such as glutathione peroxidase (GPx) and thioredoxin reductase. Thus, selenium deficiency may compromise the functional activity of the GPx and/or thioredoxin systems in sperm, resulting in oxidative damage, alterations of the cauda epididymidis, and impaired spermiogenesis (Olson et al. 2004).

Oxidative stress results when cellular antioxidant defenses become overwhelmed by reactive oxygen species (ROS). In comparison to somatic cells, germ cells are more susceptible to oxidative stress. Spermatozoa, in particular, are highly susceptible to oxidative damage due to high concentrations of polyunsaturated fatty acids and low concentrations of cytoplasmic antioxidants (Jones 1979). ROS positively regulate capacitation and the acrosome reaction, both of which are required for spermatozoa to acquire fertilizing ability (Aitken et al. 1998; O'Flaherty et al. 2005). However, when present in excess, particularly as a result of the H_2O_2-generating oxidase system in spermatazoa, ROS attack polyunsaturated fatty acids in the sperm plasma membrane, initiating lipid peroxidation cascades (Aitken 1994; Aitken and Krausz 2001; Kaur and Bansal 2004) that might be responsible for reducing fertility.

Although there are several studies that show the importance of selenium levels in male reproduction, the direct influence of selenium deficiency on in vitro fertilization (IVF) has not yet been quantified. In the current study, we investigated the effect of selenium deficiency on the reproductive capability of male mice and its relationship with oxidative damage.

Materials and methods

Chemicals

Bovine serum albumin fraction V (BSA), butylated hydroxytoluene (BHT), desferrioxamine (DFA), hyaluronidase, human chorionic gonadotropin (hCG), lactic acid, sodium pyruvate, and thiobarbituric acid (TBA) were from Sigma Chemical Co. (St. Louis, MO, USA). Pregnant mare serum gonadotropin (PMSG; Folligon) was from Intervet, International B.V. (Boxmeer, Holland). Trichloroacetic acid (TCA) and formaldehyde were from J.T. Baker (Phillipsburg, NJ, USA). Spurr's resine was from Electron Microscopic Sciences (Fort Washington, PA, USA). All other chemicals used were of analytical grade or better.

Animals

Four-week-old male C57BL/6N mice and five-week-old female C57BL/6N mice were obtained from Cinvestav-IPN, México animal house. All animal procedures were approved by Cinvestav Animal Care and Use Committee in compliance with international guidelines for use and care of laboratory animals. The animal room was kept on a 12/12-h light/dark cycle at $22\pm1°C$ with a humidity of $50\pm5\%$ filtered air (filter efficiency, 95%). Noise levels did not exceed 85 db. The animals were housed in polycarbonate cages ($43\times27\times$

15 cm, Nalgene, Rochester, NY) in groups of six animals per cage. The C57BL/6N strain was selected since it is commonly used in fertilization and dietary studies (Kamjoo et al. 2002; Fenton and Hord 2006).

Diets

The mice were fed for 4 months with one of two diets, prepared in pellets by Bio-Serv Co. (Frenchtown, NJ, USA) and were given free access to distilled water. The base diet was composed of 14.60% protein, 4.90% fat, 2.20% fiber, 5.08% ash, 5.90% humidity, and 67.21% carbohydrates. The base diet was supplemented with L-(+)-SeMet (Sigma Number S3875), to achieve final concentrations of 0.2 mg Se/kg (selenium sufficient group or Se–Suf) or 0.02 mg Se/kg (selenium deficient group or Se–Def). Sufficient dietary selenium levels were selected based on NAS (2000) recommendations. Selenium concentration for each diet was evaluated by the supplier Bio-Serv Co. using hydride atomic absorption spectroscopy. The certificate of analysis showed concentrations of 0.021 ± 0.009 and 0.19 ± 0.013 mg Se/kg for Se–Def and Se–Suf diet, respectively.

Gamete retrieval

Sperm isolation and assessment of sperm parameters

The sperm parameters assessed included sperm concentration, viability, and progressive motility. These parameters were evaluated according to World Health Organization guidelines (2001). Briefly, the mice were killed by cervical dislocation. The testis–epididimus–vas deferens complex were dissected, spermatozoa were obtained by flushing the lumen of the vas deferens and cauda epididymis with 1 ml of M-16 medium supplemented with 3 mg/ml of BSA at 37°C. Media M-16 was comprised of 100-mM NaCl, 25-mM NaHCO$_3$, 5.5-mM glucose, 2.6-mM KCl, 1.56-mM Na$_2$HPO$_4$, 0.5-mM sodium piruvate, 1.8-mM CaCl$_2$, 0.5-mM MgCl$_2$, and 20-mM sodium lactate, pH 7.4 (Whittingham 1971). All media were prepared with deionized water (Milli-Q Plus water system, Millipore).

Spermatozoa motility was assessed in ten random fields as percentage of motile cells using optical microscope. The spermatozoa viability was determined using tripan blue exclusion. Sperm concentration was measured in a hemocytometer and expressed as million/ml of suspension. From each sample, three aliquots (100–200 cells each) were separately counted.

Sperm capacitation

Spermatozoa concentration was adjusted to 10×10^6 cells/ml, and 200 µl of sperm suspension was processed for transmission electron microscopy (see below). For capacitation, remaining suspension was incubated for 2 h in cell culture medium M-16 supplemented with BSA at 37°C in a high-humidity incubator under a 5% CO$_2$–95% air atmosphere.

Egg recovery

Eggs were obtained from immature female mice C57BL/6. Superovulation was induced by i.p. injection of 10 IU PMSG and 48 h later, 10 IU hCG. Approximately 14–16 h after hCG injection, the animals were killed by cervical dislocation. The uterine ovary–salpinge–horn complex was dissected and suspended in M-16 medium. In each oviduct, the ampulla was punctured, and the cumulus–egg complex was extruded and placed in 0.1% (*w/v*) hyaluronidase in M-16 medium for 7 min at 37°C to remove cumulus cells. Then, cumulus free eggs were pooled and washed with M-16 medium, to remove hyaluronidase; approximate 50 eggs by female were obtained. Only mature eggs showing polar body and with zone intact were used to fertilization assay.

Insemination of zone-intact eggs

In vitro fertilization was carried out in 40 random eggs resuspended in 200 µl M-16 medium and seeded in a standard slide with two polished spherical depressions of approximately 0.5–0.8 mm depth (VWR International). The eggs were then inseminated with 10 µl suspension of Se–Suf or Se–Def spermatozoa (1×10^5 cells), which had been previously capacitated. Gametes were coincubated for 20 h at 37°C in a high-humidity incubator under a 5% CO$_2$–95% air atmosphere. The eggs were examined for the presence of the two-cell-stage embryos as an indication of successful fertilization. The cells were fixed in 3% formaldehyde–PBS (*v/v*) and observed by phase contrast microscopy. Three independent experiments with different batches of cells, each one in duplicate were performed.

Glutathione peroxidase (GPx) activity assay

In a previous report, we found that 24 h cumulative urinary selenium excretion in mice fed for 2 months with the same diets used herein clearly showed that levels of dietary selenium supplementation were directly proportional to levels of selenium urinary excretion (0.006 ± 0.0048 and 0.035 ± 0.010 μg/day for Se–Def diet and Se–Suf diet, respectively; Vega et al. 2007).

The activity of GPx was measured by the Paglia and Valentine (1967) method, using a Ransel kit (RANDOX, CA, USA). Briefly, the liver was removed and a representative piece was rinsed in saline solution and homogenized in phosphate buffer (pH 7.4). The homogenates was centrifuged at $10,000 \times g$ for 30 min at 4°C. The supernatant fraction of each sample was removed, 20 μl of supernatant were added to a mixture containing phosphate buffer (0.05 M, pH 7.2), ethylenediamine tetraacetic acid (4.3 mM), GSH (4 mM), glutathione reductase ($\geq$0.5 U/l), NADPH (0.28 mM), and cumene hydroperoxide (0.18 mM). GPx catalyzes the oxidation of GSH, using cumene hydroperoxide as a substrate. In the presence of glutathione reductase and NADPH, the oxidized glutathione is immediately converted to the reduced form with the concomitant oxidation of NADPH to NADP. Decreases in NADPH were monitored by measuring absorbance at 340 nm with a spectrophotometer (Vitalabe Eclipse, The Netherlands). Three independent experiments were carried out, each one in duplicate.

Lipid peroxidation assay

The amount of thiobarbituric acid reactive substances (TBARS) was used as an index of lipid peroxidation (Buege and Aust 1987). Briefly, testes homogenates or sperm suspensions (2×10^6 spermatozoa/ml) were added to a mixture containing 1 ml of 0.5% TBA, 5 μl of 3.75% BHT in methanol, and 5 μl of 1.5 mM DFA. The samples were heated in a boiling water bath for 20 min and then cooled. Absorbance at 532 nm was then measured. Three independent experiments, each one by duplicate, were performed.

Transmission electron microscopy

Sperm samples were fixed with 3% (v/v) glutaraldehyde in PBS buffer for 1 h at room temperature.

Samples were then postfixed in 1% osmium tetroxide in PBS buffer for 1 h. The cells were rinsed in PBS, dehydrated through a graded ethanol series, and embedded in Spurr's resin. Resin blocks were thin-sectioned and double-stained with uranyl acetate and lead nitrate. The samples were examined using a JEM-1200 EXII transmission electron microscope at 60 keV (Jeol LTD; Tokyo, Japan). From each sample, three thin sections were separately analyzed (~40 cells each).

Data analysis

Comparisons of group means were performed using paired or unpaired two-tailed t tests as appropriate. Values of $p < 0.05$ were considered significant. All data are expressed as mean ± standard deviation (SD). All analyses were performed using the statistical software Stata 8.0 (Stata Corp., College Station, TX, USA).

Results

Selenium deficiency effects on mice body weight

Mice with Se–Def levels in diet exhibited lesser food consumption (~19%) versus those with Se–Suf diet (data not shown). In consequence, the body weight of mice fed with Se–Def was lower than animals with Se–Suf dietary (Fig. 1). However, no significant differences were observed in the relative weight of organs as testes (data not shown). No obvious indications of poor health such as, hair loss, low fur quality, or bloated abdomen were observed in mice with selenium deficiency.

Selenium deficiency negatively affects spermatozoa quality

As shown in Table 1, spermatozoa quality was significantly reduced in mice maintained on a Se–Def diet as compared to their control counterparts. There was a slight, but significant, decrease in sperm concentration in Se–Def animals ($p=0.025$ vs Se–Suf), and sperm motility was reduced in these animals by approximately 40% ($p=0.017$ vs Se–Suf). A trend towards decreased sperm viability was also observed in the Se–Def group ($p=0.057$ vs Se–Suf). These results confirm that selenium is an essential dietary

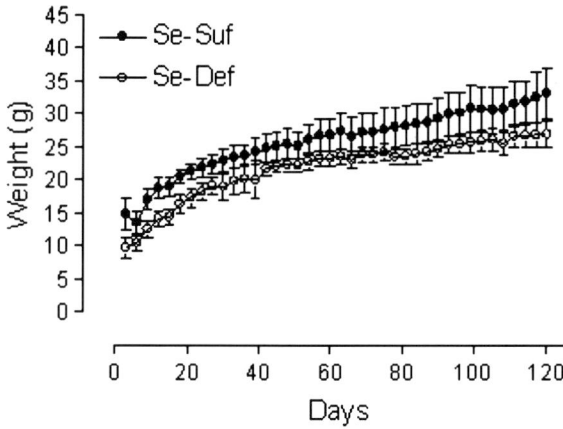

Fig. 1 Effect of selenium deficiency on body weight. Body weight of mice fed with Se–Def and Se–Suf during 120 days; $n=6$. A significant difference was observed during the time of study ($p<0.01$)

micronutrient required for maintenance of spermatozoa quality.

Selenium deficiency increases oxidative damage in the testes and spermatozoa

The bioavailability of selenium from selenium-rich SeMet was assessed in selenium-deficient mice by measuring GPx activity in the liver (Beckett et al. 1990; Burk et al. 1981).The liver was selected since it harbors the largest pool of selenium and is one of the main sites of selenium action (Levander 1985). Liver GPx activity was reduced by fourfold in animals maintained on a Se–Def diet ($p<0.0001$ vs Se–Suf; Table 2), confirming selenium deficiency in these animals.

Table 1 Assessment of sperm parameters in mice fed Se-deficient and Se-sufficient diets

Sperm parameters	Selenium diet	
	Deficient ($n=6$)	Sufficient ($n=6$)
Concentration (10^6/ml)	14.7±0.47*	17.0±0.8
Motility (%)	59±17.5*	97±5.7
Viability (%)	79±3.9	95±0.57

Values are mean ± SD

*$p<0.05$ vs Se-sufficient diet

Table 2 Selenium deficiency effect on liver glutathione peroxidase (GPx) activity

Selenium diet	GPx activity (U/g protein)
Deficient ($n=6$)	155.47±42.52*
Sufficient ($n=6$)	633.60±121.12

Values are mean ± SD

*$p<0.05$ vs Se-sufficient diet

Lipid peroxidation was also evaluated, as an oxidative damage marker, in the testes and sperm (Table 3). Lipid peroxidation levels in Se–Def spermatozoa and testes were increased by 62-fold ($p=0.008$ vs Se–Suf) and 2-fold ($p=0.036$ vs Se–Suf), respectively.

Selenium deficiency altered in vitro fertilization capability of spermatozoa

A well-known marker assessment of fertility is the IVF test, which measures the ability of sperm cells to fertilize eggs. Assessment of the fertilization capacity of Se–Def and Se–Suf sperm using the IVF test revealed that the former less efficiently fertilized zone-intact eggs (Figs. 2 and 3). Approximately 80% of eggs were fertilized by Se–Suf spermatozoa, whereas only 25% were fertilized by Se–Def spermatozoa (Fig. 2). Figure 3a shows an inseminated egg with Se–Suf spermatozoa, which is in division process, whereas Fig. 3b shows an inseminated egg with Se–Def spermatozoa, which was not fertilized. This result clearly shows that selenium deficiency adversely affects sperm fertilization capability in mice.

Selenium deficiency alters chromatin condensation in spermatozoa

Ultrastructural evaluations of Se–Suf and Se–Suf spermatozoa nuclei were performed via transmission electron microscopy, and representative images are shown in Fig. 4. Nuclei of all Se–Suf spermatozoa exhibited a normal morphology characterized by homogenous electron-dense chromatin bound by an intact nuclear envelope (Fig. 4a). This normal appearance was visibly altered in nuclei of Se–Def spermatozoa. Nuclei showed heterogeneous electron-dense chromatin, which was frequently associated with a disrupted nuclear envelope (Fig. 4b).

Table 3 Effects of selenium deficiency on lipid peroxidation in the spermatozoa and testes

Selenium diet	TBARS concentration	
	Spermatozoa (nmol/2×10^6 sperm)	Testes (nmol/g tissue)
Deficient ($n=6$)	93.13±5.2*	0.0107±0.0017*
Sufficient ($n=6$)	1.52±1.0	0.0067±0.0014

Values are mean ± SD

*$p<0.05$ vs Se-sufficient diet

Discussion

Recent advances in the understanding of male infertility have implicated oxidative stress as a major causative factor (Aitken et al. 1998). The present study was carried out to evaluate the effect of selenium deficiency on the oxidative damage of the testes and sperm and its consequences on of the IVF of male mice. Here, we demonstrate that spermatozoa quality is significantly reduced as a result of selenium deficiency. Consistent with this result, others have reported that selenium deficiency is associated with flagellar defects in spermatids and epididymal spermatozoa as well as with a reduction in the number of post-meiotic germ cells, spermatids, and spermatozoa (Shalini and Bansal 2006). These effects were attributable to the decreased expression, of both levels mRNA and protein of cJun and cFos in the testicular germ cells. These proteins comprise the transcription factor AP1, which regulates cellular growth and differentiation and also exerts a regulatory role in steroidogenesis and spermatogenesis (Shalini and Bansal 2006). It has recently been shown that selenium deficiency also induces the expression of

NFκB, which is known to positively regulate iNOS expression (Shalini and Bansal 2007).

Alterations in cellular redox status toward oxidative conditions may occur as a result of over production of ROS or a deficiency in antioxidant systems. Lipid peroxidation is considered the main indicator of oxidative stress-induced loss of cellular function (Storey 1996). One of the most recognized products of lipid peroxidation are TBARS, which were increased in testes as a result of selenium deficiency (Kaushal and Bansal 2007). Results of present study show a notable increase of lipid peroxidation in mice sperm (Table 3).

Selenium forms the catalytic center of antioxidant enzymes such as cytosolic GPx or membrane bound GPx (PHGPx). GPx plays an important role in the defense against oxidative damage by catalyzing the reduction in a variety of hydroperoxides, using glutathione as the reducing substrate (Brigelius-Flohé et al. 2002). PHGPx undergoes physical modification and acquires alternate biological functions during sperm maturation. PHGPx exists as a soluble peroxidase in spermatids but persists in mature spermatozoa as an enzymatically inactive, oxidatively cross-linked, insoluble protein (Ursini et al. 1999). In rats, this selenoenzyme is present in the mature sperm head and in tail midpiece mitochondria and it is capable of oxidizing reduced sperm protamines (Godeas et al. 1997). PHGPx is highly expressed in the nuclei of late spermatids, where the reorganization and condensation of DNA take place.

In the present study, we found that selenium deficiency caused a 67% decrease in sperm fertilization capability. This decrease in fertility might result from oxidative damage to the plasma membrane, which would lead to a total loss of the membrane fluidity and integrity. This, in turn, would be expected to reduce the number of spermatozoa available to compete in the membrane fusion events associated with fertilization

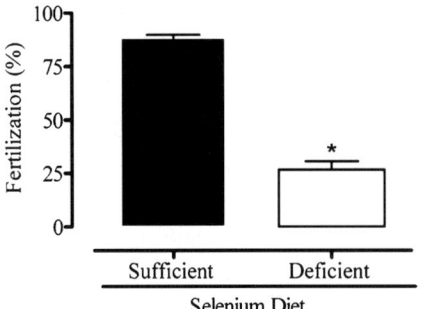

Fig. 2 Effect of selenium deficiency on fertilization. Spermatozoa isolated from mice maintained on Se–Suf or Se–Def diets were tested for their ability to fertilize zone-intact eggs. A total of 102 eggs were examined, in each experimental group, over the course of three independent experiments; *asterisk*, $p<0.001$

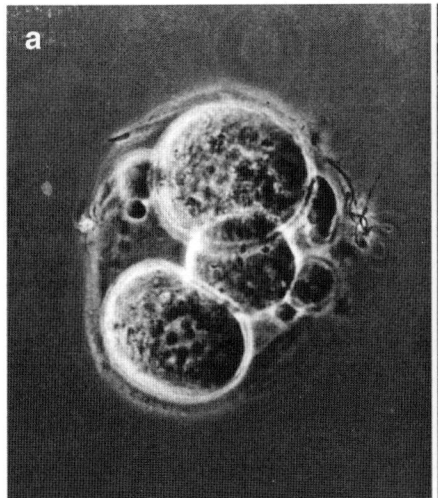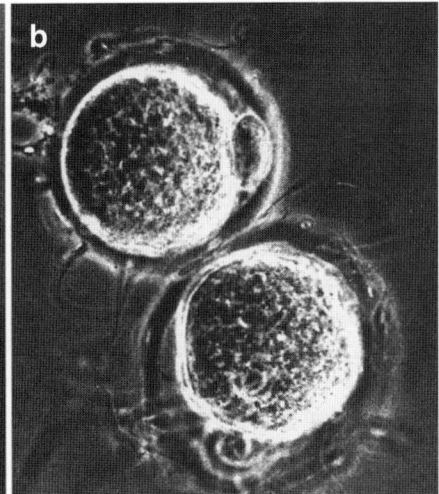

Fig. 3 Phase contrast microscopy of in vitro fertilization by selenium deficient spermatozoa. Zone-intact eggs were incubated with spermatozoa from mice maintained on Se–Suf or Se–Def or diets. Representative images are shown (×400). **a** Se–Suf spermatozoa were clearly able to inseminate eggs, as shown by fertilized egg in process of division. **b** Two eggs incubated with Se–Def spermatozoa showed no evidence of fertilization. A total of 102 eggs were examined, in each experimental group, over the course of three independent experiments

(Aitken 1994; Levander 1985). In agreement with this, human spermatozoa that have been exposed to very high levels of oxidative stress exhibit a sudden decline in both the quality of sperm movement and sperm–egg fusion (Aitken and Fisher 1994).

In addition to inflicting oxidative damage to the sperm plasma membrane, ROS are also know to attack DNA, inducing strand breaks and oxidative base damage in rodent and human spermatozoa (Huges et al. 1996; Kumar et al. 2002). Accordingly,

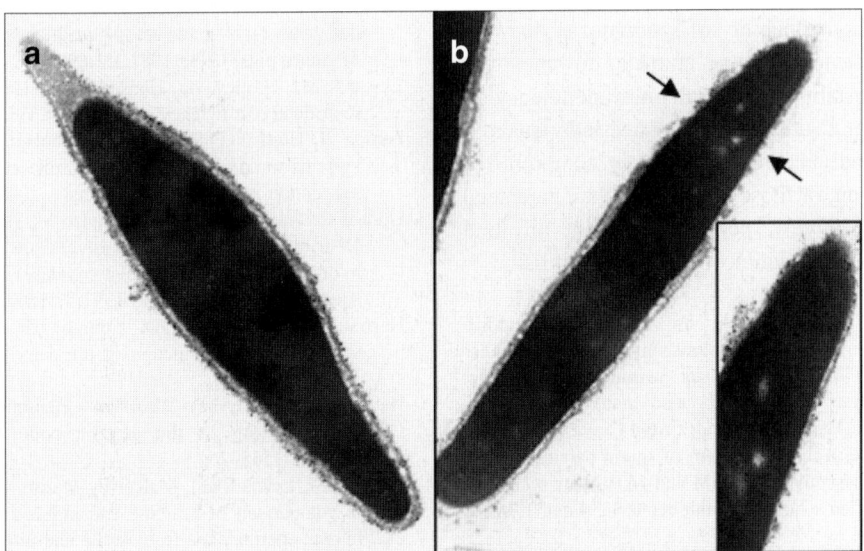

Fig. 4 Effect of selenium deficiency on the ultrastructure of spermatozoa nuclei. Spermatozoa from mice maintained on **a** Se–Suf or **b** Se–Def diets were examined by transmission electron microscopy (×15,000). Nuclei of spermatozoa from selenium-sufficient animals were uniformly electron-dense, and the nuclear envelope was intact. On the other hand, nuclei of spermatozoa from selenium-deficient animals exhibited heterogeneous electron dense density, and the nuclear envelope was frequently disrupted (*arrows*). *Inset* in **b** shows a portion of the nucleus under higher magnification (×20,000)

it has been demonstrated that a lipid peroxidation occurs concurrently with oxidative damage to testicular DNA (Kumar et al. 2002).

DNA strand breaks and denaturation are inversely correlated with the fertilizing potential of spermatozoa (Aravindan et al. 1997). Here, impaired fertility was associated with alteration on chromatin condensation, as seen by electron microscopy. The process of chromatin condensation seems to be crucial not only for maturation of sperm cells, but also for fertility and genesis of offspring. It has been suggested that nuclear PHGPX plays a role in chromatin condensation and in the protection of sperm DNA against oxidative damage (Pfeifer et al. 2001). In vitro experiments with murine sperm showed that a condensed sperm nucleus with a stable matrix is needed to ensure normal embryonic development (Ward et al. 1999). Our results suggest that selenium deficiency may elicit alteration on chromatin condensation via oxidative damage. The assessment of sperm chromatin is relevant because it is completely reorganized during the late stages of spermatogenesis when histones, small proteins rich in cysteine residues, are replaced by protamines. Thus, additional studies examining some markers of DNA integrity will be required to evaluate the effects of selenium deficiency on embryo development.

In the present work, we showed an important effect on the fertilization capability of spermatozoa due to a severe Se deficiency in these animals, however it is important to establish that selenium deficiency is relatively rare in healthy well-nourished individuals. It can occur in individuals with severely compromised intestinal function, or those undergoing total parenteral nutrition. Alternatively, people dependent on food grown from selenium-deficient soil are also at risk.

Acknowledgement The authors are thankful to Rodolfo Paredes-Díaz from Electronic Microscopic Unit of Cellular Physiology of UNAM, México for helping with electron microscopic analysis. The authors also thank Belem Piña-Guzmán and Angel Barrera-Hernández from Cinvestav, México for their assistance in the assessment of sperm parameters and care of animals, respectively. EAGM and JAIV were recipients of a Conacyt-México scholarship number 163334 and 170210, respectively.

References

Aitken RJ. A free radical theory of male infertility. Reprod Fertil Dev 1994;6:19–24.

Aitken RJ, Fisher H. Reactive oxygen species generation and human spermatozoa: the balance of benefit and risk. Bioessays 1994;6:259–67.

Aitken RJ, Krausz C. Oxidative stress DNA damage and the Y chromosome. Reproduction 2001;122:497–506.

Aitken RJ, Gordon E, Harkiss D, Twigg JP, Milne P, Jennings Z. Relative impact of oxidative stress on the functional competence and genomic integrity of human spermatozoa. Biol Reprod 1998;59:1037–46.

Aravindan GR, Bjordahl J, Jost LK, Evenson DP. Susceptibility of human sperm to in situ DNA denaturation is strongly correlated with DNA strand breaks identified by single cell electrophoresis. Exp Cell Res 1997;236:231–7.

Beckett GJ, Nicol F, Proudfoot D, Dyson K, Loucaides G, Arthur JR. The changes in the hepatic enzyme expression caused by selenium deficiency and hypothyroidism in rats are produced by independent mechanism. Biochem J 1990;266:743–7.

Benemariya H, Robberecht H, Deelstra H. Daily dietary intake of copper, zinc and selenium by different population groups in Burundi, Africa. Science Total Environ 1993;136:49–76.

Böck A. Biosynthesis of selenoproteins – an overview. Biofactors 2000;11:77–8.

Brigelius-Flohé R, Wingler K, Muller C. Estimation of individual types of glutathione peroxidases. Methods Enzymol 2002;347:101–12.

Broadley MR, White PJ, Bryson RJ, Meacham MC, Bowen HC, Johnson SE, Hawkesford MJ, McGrath SP, Zhao FJ, Breward N, Harriman M, Tucker M. Biofortification of UK food crops with selenium. Proc Nutr Soc 2006;65:169–81.

Buege JA, Aust SD. Microsomal lipid peroxidation. Methods Enzymol 1987;52:302–10.

Burk RF, Lane JM, Lawrence RA, Gregory PE. Effect of selenium deficiency on liver and blood glutathione peroxidase activity in guinea pigs. J Nutr 1981;111:690–93.

Edwards MJ, Hartley WJ, Hansen EA. Selenium and lowered reproductive efficiency in pigs. Aust Vet J 1997;53:553–4.

Fenton JI, Hord NG. Stage matters: choosing relevant model systems to address hypotheses in diet and cancer chemoprevention research. Carcinogenesis 2006;27:893–902.

Godeas C, Tramer F, Micali F, Soranzo M, Sandri G, Panfili E. Distribution and possible novel role of phospholipid hydroperoxide glutathione peroxidase in rat epididymal spermatozoa. Biol Reprod 1997;57:1502–8.

Harrison JH, Hancock DD, Conrad HR. Vitamin E and selenium for reproduction of the dairy cow. J Dairy Sci 1984;67:123–32.

Hatfield DL, Gladyshev VN. How selenium has altered our understanding of the genetic code. Mol Cell Biol 2002;22:3565–76.

Huges CM, Lewis SEM, McKelvey-Martin VJ, Thompson W. A comparison of baseline and induced DNA damage in human spermatozoa from fertile and infertile men using a modified comet assay. Mol Hum Reprod 1996;2:613–20.

Jones WR. The investigation of immunological infertility. Med J Aust 1979;2:188–92.

Kamjoo M, Brison DR, Kimber SJ. Apoptosis in the preimplantation mouse embryo: effect of strain difference and in vitro culture. Mol Reprod Dev 2002;61:67–77.

Kaur P, Bansal MP. Effect of selenium induced-oxidative stress on the oxidation reduction system and reproductive ability of male mice. Biol Trace Elem Res 2004;97:83–93.

Kaushal N, Bansal MP. Inhibition of CDC2/Cyclin B1 in response to selenium-induced oxidative stress during spermatogenesis: potential role of Cdc25c and p21. Mol Cell Biochem 2007;298:139–50.

Kumar R, Doreswamy K, Shrilatha B, Muralidhara. Oxidative stress associated DNA damage in testis of mice: Induction of abnormal sperms and effects of fertility. Mutat Res 2002;513:103–11.

Levander OA. Considerations on the assessment of selenium status. Fed Proc 1985;44:2579–83.

Moreno-Reyes R, Suetens C, Mathieu F, Begaux F, Zhu D, Rivera MT, Boelaert M, Nève J, Perlmutter N, Vanderpas J. Kashin-Beck osteoarthropathy in rural Tibet in relation to selenium and iodine status. N Engl J Med 1998;339:1112–20.

National Academy of Sciences (NAS). Dietary reference intakes for vitamin C, vitamin E, selenium and carotenoids. New York: Academic; 2000.

O'Flaherty C, Breininger E, Beorlegui N, Beconi MT. Acrosome reaction in bovine spermatozoa: role of reactive oxygen species and lactate dehydrogenase C4. Biochim Biophys Acta 2005;1726:96–101.

Olson GE, Winfrey VP, Hill KE, Burk RF. Sequential development of flagellar defects in spermatids and epididymal spermatozoa of selenium-deficient rats. Reproduction 2004;127:335–42.

Paglia DE, Valentine WN. Studies on the quantitative and qualitative characterization of erythrocyte glutathione peroxidase. J Lab Clin Med 1967;70:158–69.

Pfeifer H, Conrad M, Roethlein D, Kyriakopoulos A, Brielmeier M, Bornkamm, GW, Behne D. Identification of a specific sperm nuclei selenoenzyme necessary for protamine thiol cross-linking during sperm maturation. FASEB J 2001;15:1236–8.

Schrauzer GN. Selenomethionine: A review of its nutritional significance, metabolism and toxicity. J Nutr 2000;130:1653–6.

Shalini S, Bansal MP. Role of selenium in spermatogenesis: differential expression of cjun and cfos in tubular cells of mice testis. Mol Cell Biochem 2006;292:27–38.

Shalini S, Bansal MP. Alterations in selenium status influences reproductive potential of male mice by modulation of transcription factor NFkappaβ. Biometals 2007;20:49–59.

Storey KB. Oxidative stress: animal adaptations in nature. Braz J Med Biol Res 1996;29:1715–33.

Ursini F, Heim S, Kiess M, Maiorino M, Roveri A, Wissing J, Flohe L. Dual function of the selenoprotein PHGPx during sperm maturation. Science 1999;285:1393–6.

Vega L, Rodríguez-Sosa M, García-Montalvo EA, Del Razo LM, Elizondo G. Non-optimal levels of dietary selenomethionine alter splenocyte response and modify oxidative stress markers in female mice. Food Chem Toxicol 2007;45:1147–53.

Wallace E, Calvin HI, Cooper GW. Progressive defects observed in mouse sperm during the course of three generations of selenium deficiency. Gamete Res 1983;4:377–87.

Ward WS, Kimura Y, Yanagimachi R. An intact sperm nuclear matrix may be necessary for the mouse paternal genome to participate in embryonic development. Biol Reprod 1999;60:702–6.

Whittingham DG. Culture of mouse ova. J Reprod Fertil 1971;14:7–21.

World Health Organization (WHO). Laboratory manual for the examination of human semen and semen-cervical mucus interaction, 4th edn. University Press, Cambridge, New York; 2001.

Wu AS, Oldfield JE, Shull LR, Cheeke PR. Specific effect of selenium deficiency on rat sperm. Biol Reprod 1979;20:793–8.

Comparative studies of the antioxidant effects of a naturally occurring resveratrol analogue – *trans*-3,3′,5,5′-tetrahydroxy-4′-methoxystilbene and resveratrol – against oxidation and nitration of biomolecules in blood platelets

Beata Olas · Barbara Wachowicz · Pawel Nowak ·
Anna Stochmal · Wieslaw Oleszek ·
Rafal Glowacki · Edward Bald

Originally published in the journal Cell Biology and Toxicology, Volume 24, Nos 4–5, 51–60.
DOI: 10.1007/s10565-007-9045-7 © Springer Science + Business Media B.V. 2007

Abstract The action of two phenolic compounds isolated from the bark of *Yucca schidigera*: *trans*-3,3′,5,5′-tetrahydroxy-4′-methoxystilbene and its analogue - resveratrol (*trans*-3,4′,5-trihydroxystilbene, present also in grapes and wine) on oxidative/nitrative stress induced by peroxynitrite ($ONOO^-$, which is strong physiological oxidant and inflammatory mediator) in human blood platelets was compared. The *trans*-3,3′,5,5′-tetrahydroxy-4′-methoxystilbene, like resveratrol, significantly inhibited protein carbonylation and nitration (measured by enzyme-linked immunosor-bent assay method) in the blood platelets treated with peroxynitrite (0.1 mM) and markedly reduced an oxidation of thiol groups of proteins (estimated with 5,5′-dithio-bis(2-nitro-benzoic acid)] or glutathione (measured by high performance liquid chromatography method) in these cells. The *trans*-3,3′,5,5′-tetrahydroxy-4′-methoxystilbene, like resveratrol, also caused a distinct reduction of platelet lipid peroxidation induced by peroxynitrite. The obtained results indicate that in vitro *trans*-3,3′,5,5′-tetrahydroxy-4′-methoxystilbene and resveratrol have very similar protective effects against peroxynitrite-induced oxidative/nitrative damage to the human platelet proteins and lipids. Moreover, *trans*-3,3′,5,5′-tetrahydroxy-4′-methoxystilbene proved to be even more potent than resveratrol in antioxidative tests. We conclude that the novel tested phenolic compound – trans-3,3′,5,5′-tetrahydroxy-4′-methoxystilbene isolated from *Y. schidigera* bark possessing Generally Recognized As Safe label given by the Food and Drug Administration and allows their human dietary use – seems to be a promising candidate for future evaluations of its antioxidative activity and may be a good candidate for scavenging peroxynitrite.

B. Olas (✉) · B. Wachowicz · P. Nowak
Department of General Biochemistry,
Institute of Biochemistry, University of Lodz,
Banacha 12/16,
90-237 Lodz, Poland
e-mail: olasb@biol.uni.lodz.pl

B. Wachowicz
e-mail: wachbar@biol.uni.lodz.pl

A. Stochmal · W. Oleszek
Institute of Soil Science and Plant Cultivation,
State Research Institute,
Czartoryskich 8,
24-100 Pulawy, Poland

R. Glowacki · E. Bald
Department of Environmental Chemistry,
University of Lodz,
Pomorska 163,
90-236 Lodz, Poland

Keywords *trans*-3 · 3′ · 5 ·
5′-tetrahydroxy-4′-methoxystilbene · Resveratrol ·
Peroxynitrite · Oxidative stress · Blood platelets ·
Yucca schidigera

Introduction

Apples, onions, chocolate, red wines, green tea, and other plant extracts are good sources of phenolics. Resveratrol (3,4′,5-trihydroxystilbene) is a naturally occurring stilbene derivatives, found mainly in skin of grapes and red wine (Calderon et al. 1993; Jeandet et al. 1995), mulberries and peanuts (Langcake and Pryce 1976), and in some medicinal plants (Hata et al. 1979; Jayatilake et al. 1993; Kimura et al. 1995; Orsini et al. 1997; Ogungbamila et al. 1997; Chen et al. 1999). The oxyresveratrol (piceatannol, 2,3′,4,5′-tetrahydroxystilbene) was found as a naturally occurring compound in *Morus alba* (Shin et al. 1998) and in *Scirpus maritimus* (Powell et al. 1987). Resveratrol oligomers were identified in *Gnetum* species (Lins et al. 1982) and resveratrol trimers were reported in *Sophora leachiana* (Ohyama et al. 1994). Recently, the high concentration of resveratrol and its derivative, *trans*-3,3′,5,5′-tetrahydroxy-4′-methoxystilbene, was also reported in the bark of *Yucca schidigera* (Oleszek et al. 2001), the plant growing widely in Mexico and well known because of its very high content of steroidal saponins and phenolic compounds (Oleszek et al. 2001; Piacente et al. 2005). Because *Y. schidigera* products have been generally recognized as a safe label and were approved by the US Food and Drug Administration to be used as food additives, this plant can be a good source of active stilbenic compounds. The *trans*-3,3′,5,5′-tetrahydroxy-4′-methoxystilbene was identified for the first time in the stem of *Phoenix dactylifera* (Fernandez et al. 1983), and its presence was later confirmed in the roots of *Cassia pudibunda* (Messana et al. 1991). A chemical synthesis of this compound was also performed (Fernandez et al. 1983).

Resveratrol has been shown to have various biological activities in different test systems (Rotondo et al. 1996; Daniel et al. 1999; Fremont et al. 1999; Savouret and Quesne 2002; Dong 2003; Hakimudin et al. 2004; Signorelli and Ghidoni 2005). Our previous studies showed that antioxidative activity of this compound might reduce oxidative stress and damage to cellular biomolecules (lipids, proteins, and DNA) induced by platinum compounds used as anticancer drugs (strong synthetic oxidants; Olas and Wachowicz 2004; Olas et al. 2004a, 2005a) or by a strong biological oxidant, peroxynitrite (ONOO$^-$; Olas et al. 2004b, c, 2006a, b). Moreover, our preliminary results

showed that trans-3,3′,5,5′-tetrahydroxy-4′-methoxystilbene is even a stronger antioxidant [in human blood cells treated with platinum compounds: cisplatin (*cis*-diamminedichloroplatinum II, *cis*-Pt) used in chemotherapy and selenium-cisplatin conjugate ([NH$_3$]$_2$Pt (SeO$_3$))], than resveratrol (Olas et al. 2006c). The aim of our present study was to investigate in vitro the changes in human blood platelets induced by peroxynitrite, which is compound of particular importance for vascular thrombosis and inflammatory process (Mondoro et al. 1997; Sabetkar et al. 2002; Lufrano and Balazy 2003; Nowak et al. 2003), in the presence of trans-3,3′,5,5′-tetrahydroxy-4′-methoxystilbene. The changes were determined by various biomarkers such as levels of thiol groups, carbonyl groups, and nitrotyrosine residues in proteins; a level of glutathione (GSH) and the level of thiobarbituric acid reactive substances (TBARS). In this study, we compared the properties of trans-3,3′,5,5′-tetrahydroxy-4′-methoxystilbene in blood platelets with well-known antioxidant, resveratrol. Blood platelets are not only involved in hemostasis but they also have many of the features of classic inflammatory cells.

The concentration of stilbenes used in this study lies within the physiological range of resveratrol in plasma. The concentration of peroxynitrite (0.1 mM) used in our experiments was relatively high. The lifetime of peroxynitrite at physiological pH is very short; its half-time being of the order of 1 s. Exposure to a bolus of 250 μM peroxynitrite is equivalent of 7-min exposure to a steady-state ONOO$^-$ concentration of 1 μM. This concentration could be readily formed at sites of inflammation, where production of rates of NO$^·$ and superoxide radicals considerably increases (Bartosz 1996).

Materials and methods

Materials

Resveratrol (*trans*-3,4′,5-trihydroxystilbene), 5,5′-dithio-bis(2-nitro-benzoic acid) (DTNB), rabbit anti-DNP antibody and 2,4-dinitrophenylhydrazine (DNPH) were purchased from Sigma. The *trans*-3,3′,5,5′-tetrahydroxy-4′-methoxystilbene from bark of *Y. schidigera* was isolated and identified according to previously described procedure (Oleszek et al.

2001). Peroxynitrite was synthesized according to the method of Pryor and Squadrito (1995). Freeze fractionation ($-70°C$) of the peroxynitrite solution formed a yellow top layer, which was retained for further studies. The top layer typically contained 80–100 mM peroxynitrite as determined spectrophotometrically at 302 nm in 0.1 M NaOH ($\varepsilon_{302\ nm}=$ 1,679 $M^{-1}\ cm^{-1}$). Some experiments were also performed with decomposed $ONOO^{-}$, which was prepared by allowing the $ONOO^{-}$ to decompose at neutral pH (7.4) in 100 mM potassium phosphate buffer (15 min, room temperature). All other reagents were of analytical grade. Stock solution of resveratrol and *trans*-3,3′,5,5′-tetrahydroxy-4′-methoxystilbene were made in 50% dimethylsulfoxide at the concentration of 5 mg/ml and kept frozen.

Blood platelets isolation

Peripheral blood [collected into ACD solution (citric acid/citrate/dextrose; 5:1; *v/v*; blood/ACD)] was obtained from young (23–35 years), non-smoking men. Platelet-rich plasma was prepared by centrifugation of fresh human blood at $250\times g$ for 10 min at room temperature. Platelets were then sedimented by centrifugation at $500\times g$ for 10 min at room temperature, and the platelet pellet was washed twice with Tyrode's buffer containing 10 mM *N*-2-hydroxyethylpiperazine-*N*′-2-ethanesulfonic acid, 140 mM NaCl, 3 mM KCl, 0.5 mM $MgCl_2$, 5 mM $NaHCO_3$, and 10 mM glucose, pH 7.4. Concentration of platelets in cell suspensions was estimated spectrophotometrically and equaled to $2.5–3.8\times10^{8}$/ml (Walkowiak et al. 1989). Washed human platelet suspensions were incubated (30 min, 37°C) with resveratrol and its derivative *trans*-3,3′,5,5′-tetrahydroxy-4′-methoxystilbene at dose of 0.1 mM and then with $ONOO^{-}$ (0.1 mM, 2 min, 37°C).

Detection of thiol groups in blood platelet proteins

Washed human platelet suspensions in Tyrode's buffer were incubated with *trans*-3,3′,5,5′-tetrahydroxy-4′-methoxystilbene or resveratrol with our without peroxynitrite at 37°C for 30 min. To frozen control or tested compounds-treated platelets (1 ml of platelet suspension), 1 ml of protein-precipitating solution was added (30% NaCl, 0.85% H_3PO_4, 0.2% ethylenediaminetetraacetic acid). Acid-soluble (GSH) and acid-insoluble (proteins) platelet fractions were separated according to Ando and Steiner (1973a, b), and then the amount of free thiol groups in the acid-insoluble (proteins) fraction was estimated with DTNB (Ando and Steiner 1973a, b). To the pellet (the acid-precipitable fraction), 5 ml of H_2O and 3 ml of 10% sodium dodecyl sulfate were added. After solubilization, 0.5 ml of samples were taken, and free thiol groups were determined (Ando and Steiner 1973a, b). A standard -SH curve was prepared for GSH.

Detection of carbonyl groups in blood platelet proteins by ELISA method

Detection of carbonyl groups by an enzyme-linked immunosorbent assay (ELISA) method in blood platelets (control or incubated with *trans*-3,3′,5,5′-tetrahydroxy-4′-methoxystilbene or resveratrol and/or peroxynitrite at 37°C for 30 min) was carried out according to the procedure of Buss et al. (1997), with modifications as described previously (Olas et al. 2006a).

Determination of nitrotyrosine in the proteins of blood platelets by a competition ELISA method

Detection of nitrotyrosine-containing proteins by a competition ELISA (C-ELISA) method in blood platelets (control or antioxidants and $ONOO^{-}$ treated platelets) was performed according to the procedure of Khan et al. (1998) as described previously (Olas et al. 2006a). The nitro-fibrinogen (at concentration of 0.5 μg/ml and 3–6 mol nitrotyrosine/mol protein) was prepared for use in the standard curve. The linearity of the method was confirmed by the construction of a standard curve ranging from 10 to 500 nM nitrotyrosine-fibrinogen equivalent. The concentrations of nitrated proteins that inhibit anti-nitrotyrosine antibody binding were estimated from the standard curve and are expressed as nitro-Fg equivalents. The amount of nitrotyrosine present in fibrinogen after treatment with peroxynitrite (at final concentration of 1 mM) was determined spectrophotometrically (at pH 11.5, $\varepsilon_{430\ nm}=4400\ M^{-1}\ cm^{-1}$).

Production of TBARS in blood platelets

Incubation of blood platelets suspensions (control and incubated with *trans*-3,3′,5,5′-tetrahydroxy-4′-methoxystilbene or resveratrol and/or peroxynitrite)

was stopped by cooling the samples in an ice-bath. Samples of platelets were transferred to an equal volume of 20% (*v/v*) cold trichloroacetic acid in 0.6 M HCl and centrifuged at 1,200×*g* for 15 min. About 1 volume of clear supernatant was mixed with 0.2 volume of 0.12 M thiobarbituric acid in 0.26 M Tris at pH 7.0 and immersed in a boiling water bath for 15 min. Absorbance at 532 nm was measured, and results were expressed as nanomoles of TBARS (Wachowicz 1984).

Determination of GSH in blood platelets by HPLC method

The classical technique high performance liquid chromatography (HPLC) has been used to separation and analysis of GSH from human blood platelets treated with tested compounds. HPLC analysis was performed with a Hewlett-Packard 1100 Series system according to Glowacki et al. (2001) and Bald et al. (2004). The analytes (acid soluble platelet fraction) were derivatized with thiol-specific ultraviolet labeling reagent, 2-chloro-1-methylquinolinium tetrafluoroborate (CMQT), and separated from each other and reagent excess and platelet constituents by reversed-phase HPLC with detection at 355 nm.

Data analysis

The statistical analysis was done by several tests. To eliminate uncertain data, the Q-Dixon test was performed. All the values in this study were expressed as mean±SD. The statistically significant differences were also assessed by applying the paired Student's *t* test.

Results

Formation of carbonyl groups in the platelet proteins in the absence and presence of tested phenolics (*trans*-3,3′,5,5′-tetrahydroxy-4′-methoxystilbene or resveratrol) and/or peroxynitrite was assayed by ELISA method, which is based on the covalent reaction of the carbonyl groups with DNPH. The results are presented in Table 1. The trans-3,3′,5,5′-tetrahydroxy-4′-methoxystilbene and resveratrol at the concentration of 0.1 mM had no effect on the carbonyl level in control platelet proteins (*p*>0.05). The phenolics significantly (*p*<0.05) inhibited peroxynitrite-induced carbonylation of platelet proteins. A better protective effect (63% of inhibition) was shown in the presence of *trans*-3,3′,5,5′-tetrahydroxy-4′-methoxystilbene than resveratrol (45% of inhibition) at the same concentration in blood platelets treated with peroxynitrite (Table 1).

Table 1 The effect of *trans*-3,3′,5,5′-tetrahydroxy-4′-metoxystilbene or resveratrol (0.1 mM, 30 min, 37°C) on the level of free thiol groups, carbonyl groups, and 3-nitrotyrosine of platelet proteins treated with peroxynitrite (0.1 mM, 2 min, 37°C)

Blood platelets treated with	The level of thiol groups in proteins (nmol/2.5×10^8 platelets)	The level of 3-nitrotyrosine in proteins (μM)	The level of carbonyl groups in proteins (nmol/2.5×10^8 platelets)
Control	80.1±5.5	0.05±0.06	8.8±0.7
trans-3,3′,5,5′-tetrahydroxy-4′-metoxystilbene (*p*>0.05, with respect to control platelets)	78.3±4.4	0.05±0.03	8.4±0.5
Resveratrol (*p*>0.05, with respect to resveratrol – untreated control platelets)	81.4±5.1	0.06±0.02	8.2±0.6
Peroxynitrite (*p*<0.01, with respect to peroxynitrite – untreated control platelets)	40.9±6.3	5.1±1.2	21.4±5.6
trans-3,3′,5,5′-tetrahydroxy-4′-metoxystilbene+ peroxynitrite (*p*<0.05, with respect to peroxynitrite-treated platelets; *p*<0.05, with respect to peroxynitrite plus resveratrol-treated platelets)	76.4±7.8	1.7±0.9	8.0±2.0
resveratrol+peroxynitrite (*p*<0.05, with respect to peroxynitrite-treated platelets)	55.2±9.1	3.3±0.7	9.6±3.2

Results are means±SD of three experiments

Our studies demonstrated that exposure of blood platelets to peroxynitrite resulted in an increase of nitrotyrosine amount in platelet proteins, as determined by a competition C-ELISA method (Table 1). We have shown that both tested phenolics diminished tyrosine nitration in platelet proteins (Table 1). In the presence of resveratrol, inhibition of tyrosine nitration was about 36% (Table 1), but *trans*-3,3′,5,5′-tetrahydroxy-4′-methoxystilbene had stronger protective effect (about 67% inhibition; Table 1).

Exposure of blood platelets to peroxynitrite at the concentration of 0.1 mM resulted in a distinct depletion of free thiol groups in platelet proteins ($p<0.01$; Table 1). After 2 min incubation of blood platelets with ONOO⁻ (0.1 mM), the amount of thiol groups in proteins decreased by about 50% ($p<0.01$; Table 1). The presence of tested phenolic antioxidants – *trans*-3,3′,5,5′-tetrahydroxy-4′-methoxystilbene and resveratrol – protected platelet protein thiols from oxidation induced by ONOO⁻ (Table 1). In the presented experiments, the interaction of *trans*-3,3′,5,5′-tetrahydroxy-4′-methoxystilbene, like resveratrol with thiol groups in platelet proteins, was not observed (Table 1).

We observed that incubation of blood platelets with peroxynitrite at the concentration of 0.1 mM results in the changes of low molecular weight thiol, GSH ($p<0.01$; Fig. 1). Our studies demonstrated that the presence of antioxidants protects -SH groups of low molecular platelet thiol, GSH, from oxidation induced by peroxynitrite (Fig. 1). In platelets treated with ONOO⁻, the level of GSH is about 0.8 nmol GSH/2.5×10^8 platelets, but in the presence of *trans*-3,3′,5,5′-tetrahydroxy-4′-methoxystilbene, GSH level increased to about 3.5 nmol/2.5×10^8 platelets (Fig. 1). Resveratrol has less protective effects against ONOO⁻ action on GSH in platelets than *trans*-3,3′,5,5′-tetrahydroxy-4′-methoxystilbene (Fig. 1). Peroxynitrite also changed in blood platelets the GSH/GSSG ratio (Table 2). We showed that after ONOO⁻ treatment, GSH/GSSG ratio in platelets was distinctly decreased from 0.231 (control platelet) to 2.147 (Table 2).

We have observed that tested phenolics compounds did not change the level of GSH (data are not presented).

Moreover, we observed that *trans*-3,3′,5,5′-tetrahydroxy-4′-methoxystilbene, like resveratrol, suppresses peroxynitrite toxicity measured by the thiobarbituric acid technique (expressed as TBARS; Fig. 2).

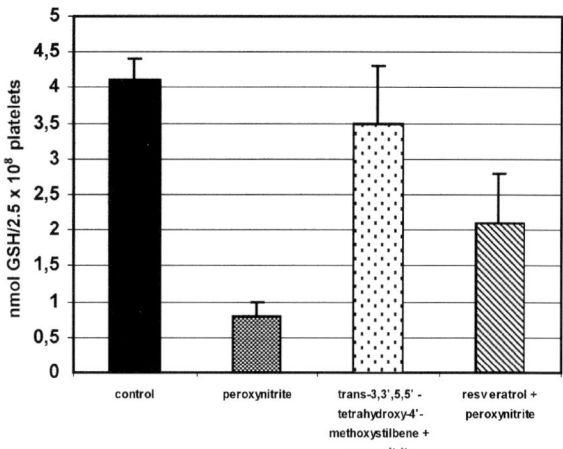

Fig. 1 The effects of trans-3,3′,5,5′-tetrahydroxy-4′-methoxystilbene and resveratrol (0.1 mM, 30 min, 37°C) on the level of GSH in human blood platelets treated with peroxynitrite (0.1 mM, 2 min, 37°C). The results are representative of three independent experiments and are expressed as means±SD. The presented results are three distinct paired comparisons. The effects were statistically significant according to the paired Student's t test [peroxynitrite-treated blood platelets vs control ($p<0.01$); phenolic compound (trans-3,3′,5,5′-tetrahydroxy-4′-methoxystilbene or resveratrol) + peroxynitrite-treated blood platelets vs peroxynitrite-treated blood platelets ($p<0.05$); trans-3,3′,5,5′-tetrahydroxy-4′-methoxystilbene+peroxynitrite-treated blood platelets vs resveratrol+peroxynitrite-treated blood platelets ($p<0.05$)]

In control experiments, we have observed that the decomposed ONOO⁻ did not change the level of TBARS and GSH. It also did not cause the tyrosine nitration in platelet proteins nor did protein oxidation (measured by carbonyl groups and thiol groups; data are not presented).

Table 2 Change of the GSSG/GSH ratio in blood platelets treated with peroxynitrite (0.1 mM, 2 min, 37°C) in the absence and the presence of *trans*-3,3′,5,5′-tetrahydroxy-4′-metoxystilbene or resveratrol (0.1 mM, 30 min, 37°C)

Blood platelets treated with	GSSG/GSH
Untreated platelets	0.231
ONOO⁻	2.147**
trans-3,3′,5,5′-tetrahydroxy-4′-metoxystilbene+peroxynitrite	0.322*
Resveratrol+peroxynitrite	0.534*

$n=3$

*$p<0.05$ ONOO⁻-treated platelets with antioxidant vs ONOO⁻-treated platelets

**$p<0.01$ ONOO⁻-treated platelets versus untreated platelets

Discussion

The blood platelets, like the other circulating blood cells can produce a reactive oxygen species (ROS) and reactive nitrogen species (RNS). In the blood platelets, the peroxynitrite may also be formed (Lufrano and Balazy 2003) during a rapid reaction between superoxide anion (O_2^-) and nitric oxide ($^{\cdot}$NO). Peroxynitrite not only decreases $^{\cdot}$NO bioavailability but also induces oxidation and/or nitration of different platelet components, including the lipids and proteins as well as a low-molecular weight biomolecules (Nowak et al. 2003; Olas et al. 2004b, 2006b). Peroxynitrite and its active derivatives are responsible for changes in a structure and functions of various platelet proteins. Peroxynitrite causes also an oxidation of amino acids (especially cysteine), tyrosine residues nitration, and carbonyl formation in blood platelets (Kato et al. 1997; Nowak et al. 2003; Olas et al. 2004b, 2006b). The reactions triggered by peroxynitrite, firstly oxidation and secondly nitration, are competitive processes. A nitrated tyrosine residues in proteins are thought to be an indicator of the peroxynitrite activity in vivo. Nitration of biomolecules may play an important role in pathology. The level of a nitrated proteins, although normally low, severely increases in patients with an inflammation based diseases (like atherosclerosis, rheumatoid arthritis, chronic renal failure, septic shock, diabetes, or lung injuries), when an extraordinary generation of peroxynitrite is apparent (Ischiropoulos and Al-Mehdi 1995; Mondoro et al. 1997; Ducrocq et al. 1999).

The defense mechanisms against the reactive nitrogen species, especially peroxynitrite, are crucial for a normal cellular function. There are three basic strategies against the dangerous action of ONOO$^-$: (1) the prevention of reactive species formation, (2) the interception with its damaging targets, and (3) the repair of a damage done (Sies 1993; Arteel et al. 1999; Klotz and Sies 2003).

Due to the increasing importance of oxidative/ nitrative stress in a pathology and the efficacy displayed by phenolics components in canceling the effects of peroxynitrite, we decided to conduct a comparative study of two different phenolics: resveratrol and its analogue, trans-3,3′,5,5′-tetrahydroxy-4′-methoxystilbene. The role of polyphenolic antioxidants in cellular biomolecules protection against oxidative/nitrative stress induced by peroxynitrite is still unclear. (−)-

Epicatechin, a polyphenolic antioxidant, present in a high amounts in a dietary sources, particularly in the green tea, a certain chocolate, and the red wine is active against a peroxynitrite action (Fiala et al. 1996; Pannala et al. 1997; Wippel et al. 2004), but only against nitration and not oxidation of thiols (Fiala et al. 1996; Pannala et al. 1997; Wippel et al. 2004; Schroeder et al. 2001). Wippel et al. (2004) suggest that epicatechin preferentially inhibits the $^{\cdot}$NO-related nitration and oxidation reactions without affecting the $^{\cdot}$NO synthesis and a cyclic GMP signaling. Epicatechin in vitro protects also against peroxynitrite-induced oxidation of dihydrorhodamine 123 and the nitration of tyrosine with efficiencies similar to those of ebselen, which is a well-known scavenger of peroxynitrite. It suggests that the interaction of epicatechin with peroxynitrite alone does not exist, but the reaction intermediate, the tyrosyl radical with epicatechin, may occur. This hypothesis is based on an efficiency of epicatechin in preventing the peroxynitrite-induced dimerization of tyrosine equal to that of preventing its nitration (Schroeder et al. 2001). Some flavonoids can act as scavengers of $^{\cdot}$NO (van Acker et al. 1995) and O_2^- (Robak and Gryglewski 1988), but the underlying mechanisms are still unclear. It has been proposed that flavonoids, like epicatechin, act as a potent scavenger of $NO_2^{\cdot}$ (Kostyuk et al. 2003). Bouaziz et al. (2007) showed that another phenolic compound with antioxidant activity, cinnamtannin B-1, had the inhibitory effect of the production of H_2O_2 in blood platelets, platelet functions, and the development of apoptotic events.

Results of our earlier study in vitro indicate that plant antioxidant present in human diet, resveratrol (used at doses corresponding to physiological level in plasma), protects against toxicity of ONOO$^-$ on platelets (Olas et al. 2004b, c) and on plasma (Olas et al. 2006a). We also observed that resveratrol suppresses the peroxynitrite toxicity measured as a protein nitration in platelet or plasma (Olas et al. 2006a) and the level of carbonyl groups in proteins (Olas et al. 2006a, b).

Blood platelets play a central role in hemostasis, and their hyperactivity is observed in cardiovascular diseases. The reaction in platelets involving thiol groups play an important role in the platelet functions, but little is known about the role of intracellular GSH in these processes. The blood platelets contain a relative low GSH level of about 11–15 nmol of GSH/ 10^9 platelets, with more than 90–95% of intraplatelet

GSH being maintained in the reduced form (Giustarini et al. 2000). Our results on GSH level in platelets are consistent with the literature data (Giustarini et al. 2000).

Peroxynitrite forming in vascular system may cause also the oxidation, nitration, and nitrosation of platelet thiols (Crane et al. 2002). The most sensitive target in proteins is the cysteine residues. The main reaction is a two-electron oxidation leading to the formation of disulfides, being important for the peroxynitrite-induced inactivation of different enzymes. In the presence of peroxynitrite, a one-electron oxidation of thiols may also occur through formation of thiol radicals, which can link oxygen and promote an oxidative stress. Peroxynitrite (at a high concentration) also forms thionitrite and thionitrate such as *S*-nitrosoglutathione (GSNO) and *S*-nitroglutathione (GSNO$_2$; Mayer et al. 1995; Scorza and Minetti 1998). The correlation has been observed between *S*-nitrosothiol formation and inhibition of platelet aggregation indicating that *S*-nitrosothiols are probably involved in the mechanism of platelet inhibition. *S*-nitrosothiols seem to be transport intermediates or storage forms of nitric oxide. Moro et al. (1994) also observed that incubation of peroxynitrite with GSH resulted in a concentration-dependent formation of GSNO, with a maximal yield of 1–2%.

Moreover, the results of Olas et al. (2004c) suggest that resveratrol protects against changes in thiol metabolism in blood platelets induced by ONOO⁻. Arts et al. (2002) demonstrated that the tea polyphenols react with proteins, and this interaction reduces the antioxidant capacity of flavonoids. However, our earlier (Olas et al. 2004b) and the present experiments showed that the interaction of resveratrol with different thiols does not exist. Kim et al. (2002) observed that flavonoids of Inula Britannica reduced in neurons the diminution of GSH induced by receptor stimulation but did not influence the synthesis of GSH. These flavonoids may facilitate GSH redox system in glutamate-injured cortical cells through preserving the reductase GSSG and GSH peroxidase. The present study provides more information about the antioxidant activity of resveratrol analogue, *trans*-3,3',5,5'-tetrahydroxy-4'-methoxystilbene, isolated from the bark of *Y. schidigera*. We have shown that this analogue proved to be even more potent than resveratrol in vitro. The range of tested phenolics was similar to that used in studies of other authors (Brito et al. 2002; Marzocco et al. 2004).

Our earlier (Olas et al. 2006c) and present study demonstrated that *trans*-3,3',5,5'-tetrahydroxy-4'-methoxystilbene is a better antioxidant than resveratrol. We observed, for the first time, that *trans*-3,3',5,5'-tetrahydroxy-4'-methoxystilbene was more active than resveratrol in the prevention of a platelet components damage (proteins and lipids) induced by peroxynitrite (Table 1, Figs. 1 and 2). Our earlier comparative studies using in vitro tests presented that *trans*-3,3',5,5'-tetrahydroxy-4'-methoxystilbene showed also a higher inhibitory activity against the production of different reactive oxygen species in blood platelets than resveratrol (Olas et al. 2003). Moreover, this compound showed a stronger anti-platelet properties than resveratrol (Olas et al. 2002, 2005b). This ability may be caused by the presence of an additional hydroxyl group in its chemical structure. The report of Stojanovic et al. (2001) showed that the radical-scavenging activity of resveratrol and its analogues (*trans*-4-hydroxystilbene and *trans*-3,5-dihydroxystilbene) depend on the position of the hydroxyl group. The beneficial effects of resveratrol and other phenolic can be attributed to the scavenging of peroxynitrite (Zhao et al. 2003), but the reaction of

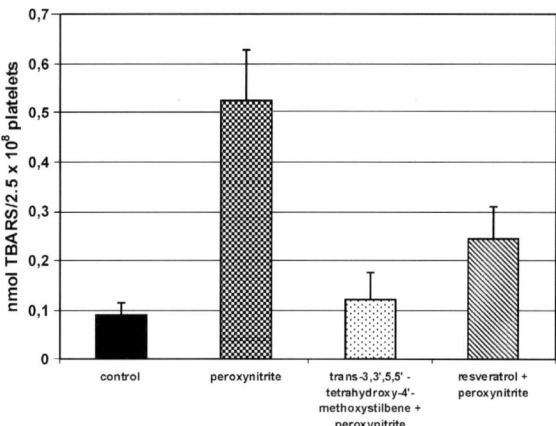

Fig. 2 The effects of *trans*-3,3',5,5'-tetrahydroxy-4'-methoxystilbene and resveratrol (0.1 mM, 30 min, 37°C) on the level of TBARS in human blood platelets treated with peroxynitrite (0.1 mM, 2 min, 37°C). The results are representative of three independent experiments and are expressed as means±SD. The presented results are three distinct paired comparisons. The effects were statistically significant according to the paired Student's *t* test, [peroxynitrite-treated blood platelets vs control ($p < 0.01$); phenolic compound (*trans*-3,3',5,5'-tetrahydroxy-4'-methoxystilbene or resveratrol) + peroxynitrite-treated blood platelets vs peroxynitrite-treated blood platelets ($p < 0.05$); *trans*-3,3',5,5'-tetrahydroxy-4'-methoxystilbene+peroxynitrite-treated blood platelets vs resveratrol+peroxynitrite-treated blood platelets ($p < 0.05$)]

ONOO⁻ with phenolics seems to be slow to play a role under physiological conditions. Probably, redox reactions take place at the aromatic B-ring of resveratrol, which contains two –OH groups. In biological systems, in the presence of CO_2, the decomposition of peroxynitrite yields 30–35% of carbonate radical (CO_3^-) and nitrogen dioxide ($^{\cdot}NO_2$), which are also strong oxidants, but natural phenols are the efficient scavengers of CO_3^- and $^{\cdot}NO_2$ (Zhao et al. 2003).

Results in the study of Marzocco et al. (2004) showed that Yucaols A–C, isolated from *Y. schidigera* bark, modulate inducible nitric oxide synthase expression via NF-κB. Results of Balestrieri et al. (2007) indicate that these phenolic compounds not only have the anti-inflammatory properties but also may inhibit cancer cell growth, migration, and platelet-activating factor synthesis in Kapasi's sarcoma cells. On the basis of our earlier (Olas et al. 2006c) and present observations, *trans*-3,3',5,5'-tetrahydroxy-4'-methoxystilbene may be a promising candidate for the future evaluations of its pharmacological activity associated with the antioxidative action, and our study provides the first evidence of the ability of *trans*-3,3',5,5'-tetrahydroxy-4'-methoxystilbene to inhibit modification of various biomolecules in blood platelets treated with peroxynitrite, which is an important factor in the pathogenesis of different diseases, including the cardiovascular and inflammatory diseases.

Acknowledgements   This study was supported by grants 505/360 from University of Lodz.

References

Ando Y, Steiner M. Sulfhydryl and disulfide groups of platelet membranes: determination of disulfide groups. Biochim Biophys Acta. 1973a;311:26–37.

Ando Y, Steiner M. Sulfhydryl and disulfide groups of platelet membranes: determination of sulfhydryl groups. Biochim Biophys Acta. 1973b;311:38–44.

Arteel GE, Briviba K, Sies H. Protection against peroxynitrite. FEBS Lett. 1999;445:226–30.

Arts MJTJ, Haenen GRMM, Wilms LC, Beetstra SAJN, Heijnen CGM, Voss HP et al. Interactions between flavonoids and proteins: effect on the total antioxidant capacity. J Agric Food Chem. 2002;50:1184–7.

Bald E, Chwatko G, Glowacki R, Kusmierek K. Analysis of plasma thiols by high-performance liquid chromatography with ultraviolet detection. J Chromatogr. 2004;1032:109–15.

Balestrieri C, Felice F, Piacente S, Pizza C, Montoro P, Oleszek W et al. Relative effects of phenolics constituents from *Yucca schidigera* Roezl. Bark on kaposi's sarcoma cell proliferation, migration, and PAF synthesis. Biochem Pharmacol. 2006;71:1479–87.

Bartosz G. Peroxynitrite: mediator of the toxic action of nitric oxide. Acta Biochim Pol. 1996;43:645–59.

Bouaziz A, Romera-Castillo C, Salido S, Linares-Palomino PJ, Alterejos J, Bartegi A et al. Cinnamtannin B-1 from bay wood exhibits antiapoptotic effects in human platelets. Apoptosis. 2007;12:489–98.

Brito O, Almeida LM, Dinis TCP. The interaction of resveratrol with ferrylmyoglobin and peroxynitrite; protection against LDL oxidation. Free Radic Res. 2002;36:621–31.

Buss H, Chan TP, Sluis KB, Domigan NM, Winterbourn CC. Protein carbonyl measurement by a sensitive ELISA method. Free Radic Biol Med. 1997;23:361–6.

Calderón AA, Zapata JM, Munoz R, Pedreno MA, Ros Barceló A. Resveratrol production as a part of the hypersensitive-like response of grapevine cells to an elicitor from *Trichoderma viride*. New Phytol. 1993;124:455–63.

Chen T, Li J, Cao J, Xu Q, Komatsu K, Namba T. A new flavanone isolated from rhizoma smilacis glabrae and the structural requirements of its derivatives for preventing immunological hepatocyte damage. Planta Med. 1999;65:56–9.

Crane MS, Ollosson R, Moore KP, Rossi AG, Megson IL. Novel role for low molecular weight plasma thiols in nitric oxide-mediated control of platelet function. J Biol Chem. 2002;277:46858–63.

Daniel O, Meier MS, Schlatter J, Schlahter J, Frischhnecht P. Selected phenolic compounds in cultivated plants: ecologic functions, health implications, and modulation by pesticides. Environ Health Perspect. 1999;17:109–14.

Dong Z. Molecular mechanism of the chemopreventive effect of resveratrol. Mutat Res. 2003;523–524:145–50.

Ducrocq C, Blanchard B, Pignatelli B, Oshima H. Peroxynitrite: an endogenous oxidizing and nitrating agent. Cell Mol Life Sci. 1999;55:1068–77.

Fernandez MI, Pedro JR, Seoane E. Two polyhydroxystilbenes from stems of *Phoenix dactylifera*. Phytochemistry. 1983;22:2819–21.

Fiala ES, Sodum RS, Bhattacharaya M, Li H. (-)-Epigallocatechin gallate, a polyphenolic tea antioxidant, inhibits peroxynitrite-mediated formation of 8-oxodeoxyguanosine and 3-nitrotyrosine. Experientia. 1996;52:922–6.

Fremont L, Belguendouz L, Delpal S. Antioxidant activity of resveratrol and alcohol-free wine polyphenols related to LDL oxidation and polyunsaturated fatty acids. Life Sci. 1999;64:2511–21.

Giustarini D, Campocia G, Fanett G, Rossi R, Giannerini F, Lusini L, Di Simplicio P. Minor thiols cysteine and cysteinylglycine regulate the competition between glutathione and protein SH groups in human platelets subjected to oxidative stress. Arch Biochem Biophys. 2000;380:1–10.

Glowacki R, Wójcik K, Bald E. Facile and sensitive method for the determination of mesna in plasma by high-performance liquid chromatography with ultraviolet detection. J Chromatogr. 2001;914:29–35.

Hakimudin F, Paliyath G, Meckling K. Selective cytotoxicity of a red grape wine flavonoid fraction against MCF-7 cells. Breast Cancer Res Treat. 2004;85:65–79.

Hata K, Baba K, Kozawa M. Chemical studies on the heartwood of *Cassia garrettina* Craib II. Nonanthraquinonic constituents. Chem Pharm Bull. 1979;27:984–9.

Ischiropoulos H, Al-Mehdi AB. Peroxynitrite-mediated oxidative protein modifications. FEBS Lett. 1995;364:279–82.

Jayatilake GS, Jayasuriya H, Lee ES, Koonchanok NM, Geahlen RL, Ashendel CL et al. Kinase inhibitors from *Polygonum cuspidatum*. J Nat Prod. 1993;56:1805–10.

Jeandet PR, Bessis M, Sbaghi M, Meunier P. Production of the phytoalexin resveratrol by grapes as a response to Botrytis attack under natural conditions. J Phytopath. 1995;143:135–9.

Kato Y, Kawakishi S, Aoki T, Itakura K, Osawa T. Oxidative modification of tryptophan residues exposed to peroxynitrite. Biochim Biophys Res Commun. 1997;234:82–4.

Khan J, Brennan DM, Bradley N, Gao B, Brukdorfer R, Jacobs M. 3-Nitrotyrosine in the proteins of human plasma determined by an ELISA method. Biochem J. 1998;330:795–801.

Kim AR, Park MJ, Lee MK, Sung SH, Park EJ, Kim J et al. Flavonoids of Inula Britanica protect cultured cortical cells from cecrotic cell death induced by glutamate. Free Rad Biol Med. 2002;32:596–604.

Kimura Y, Okuda H, Kubo M. Effects of stilbenes isolated from medicinal plants on arachidonate metabolism and degranulation in human polymorphonuclear leukocytes. J Ethnopharmacol. 1995;45:131–9.

Klotz LO, Sies H. Defenses against peroxynitrite: selenocompounds and flavonoids. Toxicol Lett. 2003;140:125–32.

Kostyuk VA, Kraemer T, Sies H, Schewe T. Myeloperoxidase/ nitrite-mediated lipid peroxidation of low-density lipoprotein as modulated by flavonoids. FEBS Lett. 2003;537:146–50.

Langcake P, Pryce RJ. The production of resveratrol by *Vitis vinifera* and other members of the Vitaceae as a response to infection and injury. Physiol Plant Pathol. 1976;9:77–86.

Lins AP, Ribeiro MN, Gottlieb OR, Gottlieb HE. Gnetins, resveratrol oligomers from *Gnetum* species. J Nat Prod. 1982;45:754–61.

Lufrano M, Balazy M. Interactions of peroxynitrite and other nitrating substances with human platelets: the role of glutathione and peroxynitrite permeability. Biochem Pharmacol. 2003;65:515–23.

Marzocco S, Piacente S, Pizza C, Oleszek W, Stochmal A, Pinto A et al. Inhibition of inducible nitric oxide synthase expression by yuccaol C from *Yucca schidigers* roezl. Life Sciences. 2004;75:1491–501.

Mayer B, Schrammel A, Klatt P, Koesling D, Schmidt K. Peroxynitrite-induced accumulation of cyclic GMP in endothelial cells and stimulated soluble guanylyl cyclase. Dependence on glutathione and possible role of S-nitrosylation. J Biol Chem. 1995;270:17355–60.

Messana I, Ferrari F, Cavalcanti MSB, Morace G. An anthraquinone and1 three naphthopyrone derivatives from *Cassia pudibunda*. Phytochemistry. 1991;30:708–10.

Mondoro TH, Shafer BC, Vostal JG. Peroxynitrite-induced tyrosine nitration and phosphorylation in human platelets. Free Rad Biol Med. 1997;22:1055–63.

Moro MA, Darley-Usmar VM, Goodwin DA, Read NG, Zamora-Pino R, Feelisch M et al. Paradoxical fate and biological action of peroxynitrite on human platelets. Proc Natl Acad Sci. 1994;91:6702–6.

Nowak P, Olas B, Bald E, Glowacki R, Wachowicz B. Peroxynitrite-induced changes of thiol groups in human blood platelets. Platelets. 2003;14:375–9.

Ogungbamila FO, Onawunmi GO, Ibewuike JC, Funmilayo KA. Antibacterial constituents of Ficus barteri fruits. Int J Pharmacogn. 1997;35:185–9.

Ohyama M, Tanaka T, Iinuma M, Goto K. Two novel resveratrol trimers, leachianols A and B, from *Sophora leachiana*. Chem Pharm Bull. 1994;42:2117–20.

Olas B, Wachowicz B. Resveratrol reduces oxidative stress induced by platinum compounds in blood platelets. Gen Physiol Biophys. 2004;23:1–12.

Olas B, Wachowicz B, Stochmal A, Oleszek W. Anti-platelet effects of different phenolic compounds from *Yucca schidigera* Roezl. Bark Platelets. 2002;13:167–73.

Olas B, Wachowicz B, Stochmal A, Oleszek W. Inhibition of oxidative stress in blood platelets by different phenolics from *Yucca schidigera* Roezl. Bark Nutrition. 2003;19:633–40.

Olas B, Wachowicz B, Bald E, Głowacki R. The protective effects of resveratrol against changes in blood platelet thiols induced by platinum compounds. J Physiol Pharmacol. 2004a;2:467–46.

Olas B, Nowak P, Kołodziejczyk J, Wachowicz B. The effects of antioxidants on peroxynitrite-induced changes in platelet proteins. Thromb Res. 2004b;113:399–406.

Olas B, Nowak P, Wachowicz B. Resveratrol protects against peroxynitrite-induced thiol oxidation in blood platelets. CMBL. 2004c;9:577–87.

Olas B, Wachowicz B, Majsterek I, Blasiak J. Resveratrol may reduce oxidative stress induced by platinum compounds in human plasma, blood platelets and lymphocytes. Anti-Cancer Drugs. 2005a;16:659–65.

Olas B, Wachowicz B, Stochmal A, Oleszek W. Inhibition of platelet adhesion and secretion by different phenolics from *Yucca schidigera* Roezl. Bark Nutr. 2005b;21:199–206.

Olas B, Nowak P, Kolodziejczyk J, Ponczek M, Wachowicz B. Protective effects of resveratrol against oxidative/nitrative modifications of plasma proteins and lipids exposed to peroxynitrite. J Nutr Biochem. 2006a;17:96–102.

Olas B, Nowak P, Ponczek M, Wachowicz B. Natural phenolic compound – resveratrol may reduce carbonylation of proteins induced by peroxynitrite in blood platelets. General Physiol Biophys. 2006b;25:215–22.

Olas B, Wachowicz B, Majsterek I, Blasiak J, Stochmal A, Oleszek W. Antioxidant properties of trans 3,3′,5,5′-tetrahydroxy-4–4′methoxystilbene against modification of different biomolecules in human cells treated with platinum compounds. Nutrition. 2006c;22:1202–9.

Oleszek W, Sitek M, Stochmal A, Piacente S, Pizza C, Cheeke P. Resveratrol and other phenolics from the bark of *Yucca schidigera* Roezl. J Agri Food Chem. 2001;49:747–52.

Orsini F, Pelizzoni F, Verotta L, Aburjai T, Rogers CB. Isolation, synthesis and antiplatelet aggregation activity of resveratrol 3-O-β-D-glucopyranoside and related compounds. J Nat Prod. 1997;60:1082–7.

Pannala AS, Rice-Evans CA, Halliwell B, Singh S. Inhibition of peroxynitrite-mediated tyrosine nitration by catechin polyphenols. Biochem Biophys Res Commun. 1997;232:164–8.

Piacente S, Pizza C, Oleszek W. Saponins and phenolics of *Yucca schidigera* Roezl: Chemistry and bioactivity. Phytochemistry Rev. 2005;4:177–90.

Powell RG, Bajaj R, McLaughlin JL. Bioactive stilbenes of *Scirpus maritimus*. J Nat Prod. 1987;50:293–6.

Pryor WA, Squadrito GL. The chemistry of peroxynitrite: a product from the reaction of nitric oxide with superoxide. Am J Physiol. 1995;268:L699–L722.

Robak J, Gryglewski RJ. Flavonoids are scavengers of superoxide anions. Biochem Pharmacol. 1988;37:837–41.

Rotondo S, Rotilio D, Cerletti CH, De Gaetano G. Red wine, aspirin and platelet function. Thromb Haemostas. 1996;76:813–21.

Sabetkar M, Low SY, Naseem KM, Bruckdorfer KR. The nitration of proteins in platelets: significance in platelet function. Free Rad Biol Med. 2002;33:728–36.

Savouret JF, Quesne M. Resveratrol and cancer: a review. Biomed Pharmacother. 2002;56:84–7.

Schroeder P, Zhang H, Klotz LO, Kalyanaraman B, Sies H. (−)-Epicatechin inhibits nitration and dimerization of tyrosine in hydrophilic as well as hydrophobic environments. Biochem Biophys Res Commun. 2001;289:1334–8.

Scorza G, Minetti M. One-electron oxidation pathway of thiols by peroxynitrite in biological fluids: bicarbonate and ascorbate promote the formation of albumin disulphide dimmers in human blood plasma. Biochem J. 1998;329:405–13.

Shin N-H, Ryu SY, Choi EJ, Kang SH, Chang IM, Min KR et al. Oxyresveratrol as the potent inhibitor of DOPA oxidase activity of mushroom tyrosinase. Biochem Biophys Res Commun. 1998;243:801–3.

Sies H. Ebselen, a selenoorganic compound as glutathione peroxidase mimic. Free Rad Biol Med. 1993;14:313–23.

Signorelli P, Ghidoni R. Resveratrol as an anticancer nutrient: molecular basis, open questions and promises. J Nutr Biochem. 2005;16:449–66.

Stojanovic S, Sprintz H, Brede O. Efficiency and mechanism of the antioxidant action of trans-resveratrol and its analogues in the radical liposome oxidation. Archiv Biochem Biophys. 2001;391:79–89.

van Acker SA, Tromp MN, Haenen GR, van der Vijgh WJ, Bast A. Flavonoids as scavengers of nitric oxide radical. Biochem Biophys Res Commun. 1995;214:755–9.

Wachowicz B. Adenine nucleotides in thrombocytes of birds. Cell Biochem Funct. 1984;2:167–70.

Walkowiak B, Michalak E, Koziołkiewicz W, Cierniewski CS. Rapid photometric method for estimation of platelet count in blood plasma or platelet suspension. Thromb Res. 1989;56:763–6.

Wippel R, Rehn M, Gorren ACF, Schmidt K, Mayer B. Interference of the polyphenol epicatechin with the biological chemistry of nitric oxide- and peroxynitrite-mediated reactions. Biochem Pharmacol. 2004;67:1285–95.

Zhao CY, Shi YM, Yao SD, Jia ZJ, Fan BT, Wang WF et al. Scavenging effects of natural phenols on oxidizing intermediates of peroxynitrite. Pharmazie. 2003;58:742–9.

Abstract

Curtiss Hunt

Originally published in the journal Cell Biology and Toxicology, Volume 24, Nos 4–5, 61–100.
DOI: 10.1007/s10565-008-9082-x © Springer Science + Business Media B.V. 2008

Trace elements in human diets, nutrition, and health: essentiality and toxicity

Preface

Curtiss D. Hunt
Chair, ISTERH/NTES/HTES'07 Planning Committee

The need to advance the field of trace element essentiality and toxicity requires high-quality, evidence-based research. The present supplement represents a compilation of review manuscripts presented at an international joint conference in Hersonissos, Crete-Greece, in October 2007 on the role of trace elements in diets, nutrition, and health in humans. The conference (ISTERH/NTES/HTES '07) constituted the VIIIth Conference of the International Society for Trace Element Research in Humans (ISTERH), the IXth Conference of the Nordic Trace Element Society (NTES), and the VIth Conference of the Hellenic Trace Element Society (HTES). The aim of the conference was to determine the current state of knowledge and gaps in experimental evidence related to the physiologic role and toxicity of trace elements.

Morbidity and mortality related to trace element deficiencies or toxicities affect more than half of the world's population. Etiologies may be related to insufficient food supply, inadequate diet quality, poor bioavailability, and physiological factors including impairments in absorption, digestion, utilization, and excretion, as well as mitigating conditions such as parasites, diseases, and inborn errors of metabolism. It is important that knowledge of trace elements is accessible to researchers, nutritionists, physicians, other health professionals, agricultural providers, and policymakers, so it can be integrated into research, and food, agriculture, and health policies. For example, although the pathogenesis and effects of iron, zinc, iodine, and selenium deficiencies are known, the difficulties in preventing the deficiencies emphasize the need for new approaches. In both transitional and affluent countries, risk of chronic diseases associated with food choices is increasing. Thus, it is imperative to understand the interrelationships of trace elements in foods and diets.

The limited understanding of the essentiality of some trace elements and incomplete knowledge of risks from environmental toxic trace elements is a major problem in trace element nutrition and toxicology. Basic knowledge of chemical mechanisms whereby trace elements affect protein structure, enzyme functions, and receptor and channel functions of membranes is essential for understanding nutritional problems and their prevention. Limited resources impede acquisition and application of new knowledge. This conference facilitated this process through face-to-face meetings of scientists who represented 41 different countries.

The conference and this supplement were sponsored by a variety of institutions, organizations, and industrial partners interested in improving human trace element nutrition and limiting trace element toxicity. The organizers of the conference wish to express appreciation for their support and encouragement in this endeavor.

An invited paper presented as the keynote address as part of ISTERH/NTES/HTES '07

Mediterranean diet, traditional foods and health: critical components and mediating mechanisms

Antonia Trichopoulou and Effie Vasilopoulou
Department of Hygiene and Epidemiology
Medical School
National and Kapodistrian University of Athens, Greece

Corresponding author:
E-mail: antonia@nut.uoa.gr

The traditional Mediterranean diet

The traditional Mediterranean diet is the dietary pattern found in the olive-growing areas of the Mediterranean region in the 1960s. Although different regions in the Mediterranean basin have their own diets, several common characteristics can be identified, most of which stem from the fact that olive oil occupies a central position in all of them. It is therefore legitimate to consider these diets as variants of a single entity, the Mediterranean diet. Olive oil is important not only because of its several beneficial properties but also because it allows the consumption of large quantities of vegetables and legumes in the form of salads and cooked foods. Mediterranean diet is characterized by high consumption of olive oil, vegetables, legumes, fruits, and unrefined cereals; moderate consumption of fish; low consumption of meat; and low to moderate intake of dairy products. It is also characterized by regular but moderate wine intake, mostly during meals, if this is accepted by religion and social norms (Trichopoulou 2007). The Greek variant of the traditional Mediterranean diet is depicted in Fig. 1 and expresses the official Greek nutritional guidelines.

Mediterranean diet and health: epidemiological evidence

The European Prospective Investigation into Cancer and Nutrition (EPIC) and the related EPIC—Elderly studies were designed to assess the impact of diet on the etiology of cancer and other chronic diseases in the adult population and in elderly Europeans, respectively. The Greek component of these studies has focused on the association between either the degree of adherence to the traditional Greek-Mediterranean diet or individual food groups and total mortality. A higher degree of adherence to the Greek version of the Mediterranean diet was associated with a significant reduction in total mortality (adjusted mortality ratio, 0.75), coronary heart disease (adjusted mortality ratio, 0.67), and cancer (adjusted mortality ratio 0.76; Trichopoulou et al. 2003). The adherence to the Mediterranean diet was further investigated in relation to survival from coronary heart disease, and a higher adherence to the Mediterranean diet was associated with a 27% reduction in overall fatality among individuals diagnosed as having coronary heart disease at enrolment (adjusted fatality ratio, 0.73). The reduced fatality was more evident and amounted to 31% (adjusted ratio, 0.69) when only cardiac deaths were considered as the relevant outcome (Trichopoulou et al. 2005a). Adherence to a modified Mediterranean diet, in which unsaturates were substituted for monounsaturates, was also associated with longer life expectancy among elderly Europeans. The reduction in overall mortality observed was more evident in Mediterranean countries (Trichopoulou et al. 2005b). The association of adherence to the modified Mediterranean diet, with survival among elderly with previous myocardial infarction was also investigated, and again, increased adherence was associated with 18% lower overall mortality rate (Trichopoulou et al. 2007). Individuals at high cardiovascular risk who improved their diet toward a traditional Mediterranean diet pattern showed significant reductions in cellular lipid levels and LDL oxidation (Fito et al. 2007)

Although the Mediterranean diet is characterised by high consumption of olive oil, no important association was found with body mass index (BMI) and W/H ratio (Trichopoulou et al. 2005c). In fact, data has suggested that the traditional Mediterranean dietary pattern could be inversely associated with BMI and obesity (Schröder et al. 2004). Compared with a low-fat diet, Mediterranean diets supplemented with olive oil or nuts have been reported to have beneficial effects on cardiovascular risk factors (Estruch et al. 2006).

Mediterranean diet and health: biochemical studies

The composition of the traditional Mediterranean diet includes several foods with antioxidant potential, but the overall diet includes other cardio-protective components, such as reduced saturated fats and greater use of unsaturated lipids, particularly from olive oil. Ongoing research aims to elucidate the role of dietary antioxidants in disease prevention. The main approach has been based on the hypothesis that the chronic disorders common in many societies are related to cumulative oxidative damage to DNA, proteins, and lipids in body tissues. Natural Mediterranean diet antioxidants, which are present in olive oil and red wine, inhibit endothelial activation, suggesting a beneficial role in homocysteine-induced vascular damage and a potential protective role on early atherogenesis prevention (Carluccio et al. 2007, 2003). In vivo effects of wine consumption (400 ml/day) on antioxidant status and oxidative stress in the circulation imply that red wine provides general oxidative protection to lipid systems in circulation via the increase in antioxidant status and decrease in oxidative stress (Micallef et al. 2007). In vivo effects of olive oil consumption (25 ml/day) imply that olive oil is more than a monosaturated fat and its phenolic content can also provide benefits against oxidative damage (Covas et al. 2006).

Traditional foods: analytical data

The traditional Mediterranean diet is associated with longer survival. This could be partly attributed to Mediterranean traditional foods that this diet contains. Rather than based on single foods or nutrients, the combination of different types of food with healthy characteristics might be necessary to express their protective potential. The diet that the Mediterranean populations developed many years ago, without any scientific input, appears to meet existing dietary recommendations (Commission of the European Communities 1993) with respect to macronutrients and certain micronutrients, such as inorganic constituents (Trichopoulou et al. 2005d), as depicted in Fig. 2. Moreover, compared to northern European and American diets, the traditional Greek menu has a higher antioxidant content (Dilis et al. 2007).

The Mediterranean diet has two basic characteristics that distinguish it from other prudent diets. The first stresses the pattern rather than individual components, and the second imposes no restriction on lipids so long as they are not saturated and are preferably in the form of olive oil (specifically, extra virgin olive oil, which is a source of polyphenols). Currently, the market offers

consumers a large variety of "functional foods," dietary supplements, and foods enriched with dietary fiber and inorganic constituents. The health claims of these products are generally based on short-term studies conducted with doses that exceed the amounts consumed in common diets, while the real effects of long-term consumption are unknown. The last three sentences can be modified to be made clearer. It is prudent to not exceed the amounts historically ingested. The natural ingredients and the processing methods used for centuries result in traditional foods with a high nutritional value, minimizing the needs for fortification. As the father of medicine, Hippocrates, wisely stated many centuries ago, "Let food be thy medicine and medicine be thy food."

Acknowledgment

The work for this review was supported by the Hellenic Health Foundation.

References

Carluccio MA, Ancora MA, Massaro M, Carluccio M, Scoditti E, Distante A, Storelli C, De Caterina R. Homocysteine induces VCAM-1 gene expression through NF-B and NAD(P)H oxidase activation: protective role of Mediterranean diet polyphenolic antioxidants. Am J Physiol Heart Circ Physiol. 2007;293:H2344–54.

Carluccio MA, Siculella L, Ancora MA, Massaro M, Massaro M, Scoditti E, Storelli C, Visioli F, Distante A, De Caterina R. Olive oil and red wine antioxidant polyphenols inhibit endothelial activation. Arterioscler Thromb Vasc Biol. 2003;23:622–9.

Commission of the European Communities: reports of the Scientific Committee for Food (thirty-first series) Office for Official Publications of the European Communities, Luxembourg. 1993; pp. 1–248.

Covas MI, Nyyssonen K, Poulsen HE, Kaikkonen J, Zunft HJF, Kiesewetter H, Gaddi A, De la Torre R, Mursu J, Baumler H, Nascetti S, Salonen JT, Fito M, Virtanen J, Marrugat J, for the Eurolive Study Group. The effect of polyphenols in olive oil on heart disease risk factors: a randomized trial. Ann Intern Med. 2006;145:333–41.

Dilis V., Vasilopoulou E. and Trichopoulou A. The flavone, flavonol and flavan-3-ol content of the Greek traditional diet. Food Chem. 105;2007:812–21.

Estruch R, Martinez-Gonzalez MA, Corella D, Salas-Salvado J, Ruiz-Gutierrez V, Covas MI, Fiol M,

Gomez-Gracia E, Lopez-Sabater MC, Vinyoles E, Aros F, Conde M, Lahoz C, Lapetra J, Saez G, Ros E, for the PREDIMED Study Investigators. Effects of a Mediterranean-style diet on cardiovascular risk factors: a randomized trial. Ann Intern Med. 2006; 145:1–11.

Fitó M, Guxens M, Corella D, Sáez G, Estruch R, de la Torre R, Francés F, Cabezas C, López-Sabater MC, Marrugat J, García-Arellano A, Arós F, Ruiz-Gutierrez V, Ros E, Salas-Salvadó J, Fiol M, Solá R, Covas MI, for the PREDIMED Study Investigators. Effect of a traditional Mediterranean diet on lipoprotein oxidation. Arch Intern Med. 2007;167:1195–203.

Micallef M, Lexis L, Lewandowski P. Red wine consumption increases antioxidant status and decreases oxidative stress in the circulation of both young and old humans. Nutr J. 2007;6:27.

Schröder H, Marrugat J, Vila J, Covas MI, Elosua R. Adherence to the traditional Mediterranean diet is inversely associated with body mass index and obesity in a Spanish population. J Nutr. 2004; 134:3355–61.

Supreme Scientific Health Council, Ministry of Health and Welfare of Greece. Dietary guidelines for adults in Greece. Archives of Hellenic Medicine. 1999;16:516–24.

Trichopoulou A. Mediterranean diet, traditional foods, and health: evidence from the Greek EPIC cohort. Food and Nutrition Bulletin—The United Nations University. 2007;28:236–40.

Trichopoulou A, Bamia C, Norat T, Overvad K, Schmidt EB, Tjønneland A, Halkjær J, Clavel-Chapelon F, Vercambre MN, Boutron-Ruault MC, Linseisen J, Rohrmann S, Boeing H, Weikert C, Benetou V, Psaltopoulou T, Orfanos P, Boffetta P, Masala G, Pala V, Panico S, Tumino R, Sacerdote C, Bueno-de-Mesquita HB, Ocke MC, Peeters PH, Van der Schouw YT, González C, Sanchez MJ, Chirlaque MD, Moreno C, Larrañaga N, Van Guelpen B, Jansson JH, Bingham S, Khaw KT, Spencer EA, Key T, Riboli E, Trichopoulos D. Modified Mediterranean diet and survival after myocardial infarction: the EPIC—Elderly study. Eur J Epidemiol. 2007;22:871–81.

Trichopoulou A, Bamia Ch, Trichopoulos D. Mediterranean diet and survival among patients with coronary heart disease in Greece. Arch Intern Med. 2005a;165:929–35.

Trichopoulou A, Orfanos P, Norat T, Bueno-de-Mesquita B, Ocke MC, Peeters PH, van der Schouw YT, Boeing H, Hoffmann K, Boffetta P, Nagel G, Masala G, Krogh V, Panico S, Tumino R, Vineis P, Bamia C, Naska A, Benetou V, Ferrari P, Slimani N, Pera G,

Martinez-Garcia C, Navarro C, Rodriguez-Barranco M, Dorronsoro M, Spencer EA, Key TJ, Bingham S, Khaw KT, Kesse E, Clavel-Chapelon F, Boutron-Ruault MC, Berglund G, Wirfalt E, Hallmans G, Johansson I, Tjonneland A, Olsen A, Overvad K, Hundborg HH, Riboli E, Trichopoulos D. Modified Mediterranean diet and survival: EPIC—Elderly prospective cohort study. BMJ. 2005b; 330:991.

Trichopoulou A, Naska A, Orfanos P, Trichopoulos D. Mediterranean diet in relation to body mass index and waist-to-hip ratio: the Greek European Prospective Investigation into Cancer and Nutrition Study. Am J Clin Nutr. 2005c;82:935–40.

Trichopoulou A, Vasilopoulou E, Georga K. Macro- and micronutrients in a traditional Greek menu. In: Elmadfa I, editor. Diet diversification and health promotion. Forum Nutr Basel Karger. 2005d; 57:135–46.

Trichopoulou A, Costacou T, Bamia Ch, Trichopoulos D. Adherence to a Mediterranean diet and survival in a Greek population. N Engl J Med. 2003;348:2599–608.

Figure captions

Fig. 1 The traditional Mediterranean diet pyramid depicting dietary guidelines for adults in Greece

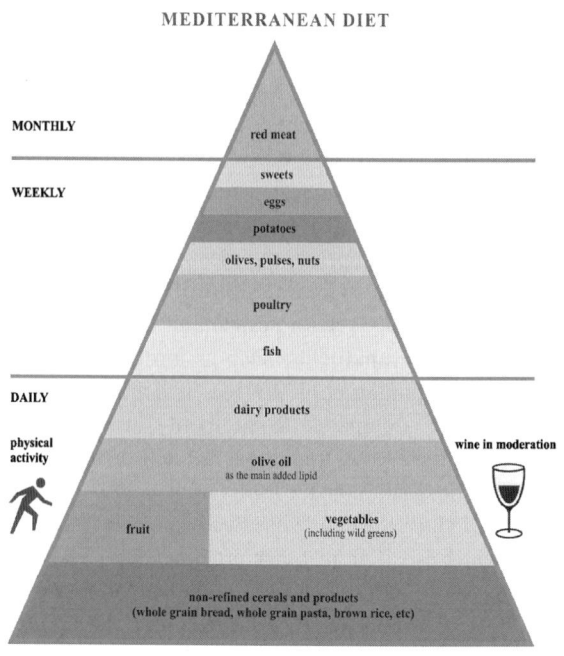

Fig. 2 Comparison of the daily intakes in inorganic constituents of a typical Mediterranean menu with existing EC daily recommendations

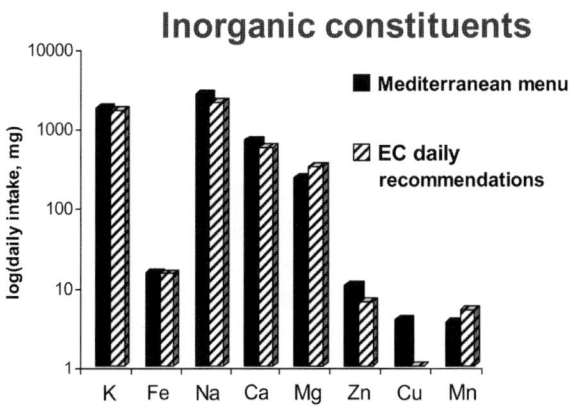

Inorganic constituents

■ Mediterranean menu

▨ EC daily recommendations

[1] Trichopoulou et al., 2005
[2] Commission of the European Communities, 1993

An invited paper presented in the plenary session "Trace Minerals: Modulators of Arterial Function"

Manganese: modulator of arterial function and metabolism

Dorothy Klimis-Zacas[1] and Anastasia Z. Kalea[2]
[1]Department of Food Science and Human Nutrition, University of Maine, Orono, ME, 04469, USA
[2]Department of Surgery, College of Physicians and Surgeons, Columbia University Medical School, NY, 10019, USA

Corresponding author:
E-mail: dorothy.klimis@umit.maine.edu

Manganese as an essential trace element

Manganese (Mn) is ubiquitous in nature; it is found in high amounts in the skeleton (25%) and exists in high concentrations in tissues rich in mitochondria. Only 3–4% of dietary manganese is absorbed, and its absorption, which is not well regulated, is independent of intake or its concentration in the body (Klimis-Tavantzis 1994). The reported clinical symptoms of experimental Mn deficiency in humans have been dermatitis (miliaria crystallina), hypocholesterolemia, depressed vitamin K-dependent clotting factors, and reddening of hair (Doisy 1972; Freidman et al. 1987). Suboptimal Mn status has been reported in epileptics (Carl et al. 1993), patients with Down's syndrome (Burlow et al. 1981), osteopo-

rosis (Freeland-Graves et al. 1988; Strause et al. 1994), congestive heart failure (Gorelic et al. 2003), atherosclerosis (Volkov et al. 1962), exocrine pancreatic insufficiency (Aggett et al. 1979), and rheumatoid arthritis (Cerhan et al. 2003). Additionally, increased consumption of processed food, refined carbohydrates, high fiber, and phytate diets and routine use of iron and calcium supplements (Temple 1983) may compromise manganese bioavailability and utilization. Manganese deficiency has also been documented in several animal models and involves skeletal deformities such as chondrodystrophy and chondrodysplasia (Leach 1971; McLaren et al. 2007), abnormal otoliths accompanied by ataxia and ultrastructural abnormalities in mitochondria (Hurley et al. 1970). Recent studies on Mn deficiency documented ocular abnormalities such as loss of photoreceptor cells in the retina (Gong and Amemiya 1996) and optic nerve changes, i.e., fewer myelinated optic nerve axons and decreased diameter and lamellae (Gong and Amemiya 1999). Additionally, Mn deficiency alters lipid and lipoprotein metabolism in animals, as it leads to a reduction in total and high-density lipoprotein (HDL) cholesterol (Klimis-Tavantzis et al. 1983; Kawano et al. 1987; Davis and Feng 1999) and alterations in HDL1 and HDL2 structure and composition (Taylor et al. 1997).

Manganese and glycosaminoglycan structure and metabolism

Manganese has been reported to influence the genesis and development of cardiovascular disease (CVD) by participating as an essential component of metalloenzymes that protect against oxidative stress, such as manganese superoxide dismutase (Greger 1998) and as a cofactor of metal-activating enzymes such as glycosyltransferases (Leach 1971) and sulfonases (Gundlach and Conrad 1985) that aid in the synthesis and maintenance of connective tissue extracellular matrix and structure.

Glycosaminoglycans (GAGs) are functionally important macromolecules of the extracellular matrix of the arterial wall. They are linear polysaccharides composed of alternating disaccharide units of hexosamine and uronic acid, and with the exception of hyaluronan, they are covalently bound to proteins forming proteoglycans (PGs). As multifunctional cell regulators, they play crucial roles as components of cell membrane receptors, influencing ligand-receptor complex function and cell signaling (Schriver et al. 2002), regulating endothelial cell permeability and migration of vascular smooth muscle cells (Koyama et al. 1998), and altering lipoprotein binding and retention (Pentikainen et al. 2000). Chondroitin sulfate (CS), heparan sulfate (HS), and dermatan sulfate (DS) are the major PGs that exist in blood vessels. Vascular endothelial cells synthesize predominantly heparan sulfate PGs, whereas vascular smooth muscle cells synthesize and secrete principally chondroitin sulfate/dermatan sulfate PGs. We now know that the degree of GAG sulfation is biosynthetically regulated and confers great structural complexity, enabling them to interact in divergent ways with biologically effective molecules, such as enzymes, cytokines, growth factors, and proteins (Turnbull et al. 2001), modulating key events in the process of atherosclerosis (Theocharis et al. 2002). We also know that the expression and distribution of HSPGs is significantly altered during disease conditions, such as vascular injury (Han et al. 1997) inflammation (Hoff and Wagner 1986), atherosclerosis and hypertension (Risler et al. 2002), thus affecting vascular response.

Manganese affects PG and GAG metabolism (Leach 1971; Yang and Klimis-Tavantzis 1998a; Yang and Klimis-Tavantzis 1998b) and is a specific activator of glycosyltransferases, enzymes that are involved in the elongation and polymerization of GAG chains in connective tissue (Leach et al. 1969). Manganese also effectively activates sulfotransferases, enzymes involved in GAG sulfation and synthesis (Gundlach and Conrad 1985). Manganese deficiency affects the biosynthesis of GAGs and decreases total and individual GAG concentrations, especially chondroitin sulfate (CS) in chick cartilage and rat skin (Leach 1969; Bolze et al. 1985; Shetlar and Shetlar 1994). We reported in the past that Mn affects arterial glycosaminoglycan (GAG) metabolism by altering the total proteoglycan (PG) content of the rat aorta and the molecular weight and sulfation pattern of CS, thus predisposing the vessel to lipid deposition, lipoprotein oxidation, and cardiovascular disease (Klimis-Tavantzis et al. 1983; Taylor et al. 1997; Yang and Klimis-Tavantzis 1998a). Additionally, suboptimal in vivo activity of arterial galactosyltransferase-I has been documented in Mn deficiency (Yang and Klimis-Tavanzis 1998b). Transmission electron microscopy of the arterial wall revealed less dense extracellular matrix surrounding smooth muscle cells, especially in the medial layers of Mn deficient rats, suggesting possible changes in the endothelial and/or vascular smooth muscle cells (Ekanayake and

Klimis-Tavantzis 1995). Recently, we examined the effect of dietary Mn on the composition and structure of rat aortic GAGs (Kalea et al. 2006a) fed a Mn-deficient (MnD), adequate (MnA), or supplemented (MnS) diet (Mn<1, 10–15, and 45–50 ppm Mn, respectively) for 15 weeks. We observed increased concentration of total GalAGs and decreased concentrations of HS and HA in the MnS aorta compared to the MnA and MnD. Aortas from animals fed the MnS diet contained higher concentration (41%) of non-sulfated units of HS chains, while tri- and di-sulfated HS units were not detectable. Overexpression of HSPGs in Mn deficiency might indicate normal endothelium repair during early stages of inflammation and wound healing, whereas oversulfated HS chains may enhance cell membrane binding and retention to a great variety of extracellular ligands including lipoprotein particles (Kaplan et al. 1998; Llorente-Cortes et al. 2002) and thus affect signal transduction pathways and functional properties of the vascular wall. The potential role of manganese in atheroprotection needs to be further investigated.

Manganese and vascular function

The vascular endothelium is crucial in regulating vasomotor tone by balancing the release of endothelium-derived contracting factors (EDCFs) such as endothelin and eicosanoids (TXA_2) and endothelium-derived relaxing factors (EDRFs) such as nitric oxide (NO), prostacyclin (PGI_2), and endothelium-derived hyperpolarizing factor (Luscher and Vanhoutte 1990). Nitric oxide induces vasodilation through the activation of the cGMP pathway (Lucas et al. 2000), while PGI_2, a product of cyclo-oxygenase (COX), acts synergistically with NO to induce vasodilation (Salvemini et al. 1996). Endothelial dysfunction is a result of an imbalance between EDRFs and EDCFs (Shimokawa 1999), and its role on the pathophysiology of vascular disease has been repeatedly documented (John and Schmieder 2000). Alterations in the biomechanical properties of the vascular system might not only affect blood flow but also platelet aggregation and vessel permeability, processes associated with early stages of atherosclerosis, hypertension, and several cardiovascular disorders (van Popele et al. 2001).

The putative role of Mn as a modulator of vascular biomechanical properties may stem from its involvement as a cofactor of enzymes such as MnSOD, arginase, CaM-dependent phosphatase, adenylate and guanylate cyclase (Korc 1993), as well as its role in receptor structure (Wedler 1994). Furthermore, Mn increases the accumulation of second messengers (cAMP, cGMP) that activate proteins for cell signaling (Korc 1993), modulates in vitro cell-surface receptor binding and adhesion (Wedler 1994), and functions as a Ca^{+2} ion channel entry blocker, affecting vascular function (Kasten et al. 1995; Yan et al. 1998). We examined the effect of dietary Mn on phenylephrine-induced vasoconstriction and acetylcholine (Ach)- and sodium nitroprusside (SNP)-induced vasodilation in rat aorta. Sprague–Dawley rats were fed either a manganese-deficient (MnD) or adequate (MnA; <1 and 10–15 ppm Mn, respectively) for 15 weeks. The maximal force (F_{max}) of contraction and relaxation, as well as vessel sensitivity (pD_2), were determined in rat intact and endothelium-disrupted aortic rings. We observed that, in the presence of endothelium, aortic rings from MnD animals developed higher vessel sensitivity (pD_2) compared to controls (MnA), an effect that was abolished when the endothelium was disrupted. Thus, manganese modifies vascular response to an a1-adrenergic receptor stimulus, which is modified by the presence of the endothelium. In other experiments we have documented (Kalea et al. 2005) that the presence of dietary manganese at 45–50 ppm affects the arterial contractile machinery by reducing maximal vessel contraction and vascular sensitivity, thus influencing signaling pathways.

We investigated ED- and endothelium-independent vasodilation (Kalea et al. 2006b) in rings precontracted with phenylephrine in the presence or absence of inhibitors of NO synthase and COX. We observed a significant decrease both in Ach-induced (endothelium-dependent) and SNP-induced (endothelium-independent) vasodilation in MnD aortas when compared to MnA (controls) but found no effect on vessel sensitivity. Inhibition of NO synthase blunted Ach-mediated vasorelaxation to the same degree for both diet groups, but inhibition of COX enhanced both Ach- and SNP-induced vasodilation of MnD rings compared to controls. Thus, Mn affects endothelium-dependent and endothelium-independent vasodilation, and seems to alter the synthesis or activity of a prostanoid-derived vasoconstrictor present at basal and stimulated levels. Furthermore, it modifies vascular response to an a1-adrenergic receptor stimulus influencing membrane-related events. Our results provide further information on the critical role of Mn on maintenance of vasomotor tone with implications on CVD.

Acknowledgment

This review was partially supported by the USDA (project no. 35483), the Maine Agriculture and Forestry Experiment Station (Scientific Contribution no. 2994), Harokopio University, Department of Nutrition and Dietetics, Athens, Greece, and the Aristidis Daskalopoulos Foundation, Athens, Greece.

References

Aggett P, Thorn J, Delves H, Harries J, Clayton B. Trace element malabsorption in exocrine pancreatic insufficiency. Monogr Paediatr. 1979;10:8–11.

Barlow P, Sylvester P, Dickerson J. Hair trace metal levels in Down syndrome patients. J Ment Defic Res. 1981;25(Pt3):161–8.

Bolze MS, Reeves RD, Lindbeck FE, Kemp SF, Elders MJ. Influence of manganese on growth, somatomedin and glycosaminoglycan metabolism. J Nutr. 1985;115(3):352–8.

Carl G, Blackwell L, Barnett F, Thompson L, Rissinger C, Olin K, et al. Manganese and epilepsy: brain glutamine synthetase and liver arginase activities in genetically epilepsy prone and chronically seizured rats. Epilepsia. 1993;34(3):441–6.

Cerhan JR, Saag KG, Merlino LA, Mikuls TR, Criswell LA. Antioxidant micronutrients and risk of rheumatoid arthritis in a cohort of older women. Am J Epidemiol. 2003;157(4):345–54.

Davis CD, Feng Y. Dietary copper, manganese and iron affect the formation of aberrant crypts in colon of rats administered 3,2′-dimethyl-4-aminobiphenyl. J Nutr. 1999;129(5):1060–7.

Doisy EA Jr. Micronutrient controls on biosynthesis of clotting proteins and cholesterol In: Hemphill D, editor. Trace substances in environmental health. Columbia, MO: University of Missouri; 1972. pp. 193–9.

Ekanayake R, Klimis-Tavantzis D. The effect of dietary manganese on the ultrastructure of aorta and liver tissues. FASEB J. 1995;9:A447.

Freeland-Graves J, Behmardi F, Bales CW, Dougherty V, Lin P-H, Crosby JB, et al. Metabolic balance of manganese in young men consuming diets containing five levels of dietary manganese. J Nutr. 1988;118:764–73.

Friedman B, Freeland-Graves J, Bales CW, Behmardi F, Shorey-Kutschke RL, Willis R, et al. Manganese balance and clinical observations in young men fed a manganese-deficient diet. J Nutr. 1987;117:133–43.

Gong H, Amemiya T. Optic nerve changes in manganese-deficient rats. Exp Eye Res. 1999;68 (3):313–20.

Gong H, Amemiya T. Ultrastructure of retina of manganese-deficient rats. Invest Ophthalmol Vis Sci. 1996;37(10):1967–74.

Gorelik O, Almoznino-Sarafian D, Feder I, Wachsman O, Alon I, Litvinjuk V, et al. Dietary intake of various nutrients in older patients with congestive heart failure. Cardiology. 2003;99(4):177–81.

Greger JL. Dietary standards for manganese: overlap between nutritional and toxicological\studies. J Nutr. 1998;128(2):368S–371S.

Gundlach M, Conrad H. Glycosyl transferases in chondroitin sulphate biosynthesis. Effect of acceptor structure on activity. Biochem J 1985;226(3):705–14.

Han RO, Ettenson DS, Koo EWY, Edelman ER. Heparin/heparan sulfate chelation inhibits control of vascular repair by tissue-engineered endothelial cells. Am J Physiol. 1997;273(6):H2586–95.

Hoff H, Wagner W. Plasma low density lipoprotein accumulation in aortas of hypercholesterolemic swine correlates with modifications in aortic glycosaminogly-can composition. Atherosclerosis. 1986;61(3):231–6.

Hurley LS, Theriault LL, Dreosti IE. Liver mitochondria from manganese-deficient and pallid mice: function and ultrastructure. Science. 1970;170 (3964):1316–8.

John S, Schmieder R. Impaired endothelial function in arterial hypertension and hypercholesterolemia: potential mechanisms and differences. J Hypertens 2000; 18:363–74.

Kalea AZ, Harris PD, Klimis-Zacas DJ. Dietary manganese suppresses a1 adrenergic receptor-mediated vascular contraction. J Nutr Biochem. 2005;16(1):44–9.

Kalea AZ, Lamari F, Theocharis A, Schuschke D, Karamanos N, Klimis-Zacas D. Dietary manganese affects the concentration, composition and sulfation pattern of heparan sulfate glycosaminoglycans in Sprague–Dawley rat aorta. BioMetals. 2006a;19 (5):535–46.

Kalea A.Z., Schuschke D, Harris P.D., Klimis-Zacas D. Cyclo-oxygenase inhibition restores the attenuated vasodilation in manganese-deficient rat aorta. J Nutr. 2006b;136:2302–7.

Kaplan M, Williams KJ, Mandel H, Aviram M. Role of macrophage glycosaminoglycans in the cellular catabolism of oxidized LDL by macrophages. Arterioscler Thromb Vasc Biol. 1998;18(4):542–53.

Kasten TP, Settle SL, Misko TP, Riley DP, Weiss RH, Currie MG, et al. Potentiation of nitric oxide-mediated vascular relaxation by SC52608, a superoxide dismutase mimic. Proc Soc Exp Biol Med. 1995;208(2):170–7.

Kawano J, Ney DM, Keen CL, Schneeman BO. Altered high density lipoprotein composition in manga-nese-deficient Sprague–Dawley and Wistar rats. J Nutr. 1987;117(5):902–6.

Klimis-Tavantzis D, editor. Manganese in health and disease. Boca Raton, FL: CRC; 1994.

Klimis-Tavantzis DJ, Leach RM Jr, Kris-Etherton PM. The effect of dietary manganese deficiency on cholesterol and lipid metabolism in the Wistar rat and in the genetically hypercholesterolemic RICO rat. J Nutr. 1983;113(2):328–36.

Korc M. Manganese as a modulator of signal tran-sduction pathways. Prog Clin Biol Res. 1993;380:235–55

Koyama N, Kinsella MG, Wight TN, Hedin U, Clowes AW. Heparan sulfate proteoglycans mediate a potent inhibitory signal for migration of vascular smooth muscle cells. Circ Res. 1998;83(3):305–13.

Leach RJ, Muenster A, Wien E. Studies on the role of manganese in bone formation. II. Effect upon chondroitin sulfate synthesis in chick epiphyseal carti-lage. Arch Biochem Biophys. 1969;133(1):22–8.

Leach RJ. Role of manganese in mucopolysaccha-ride metabolism. Fed Proc. 1971;30(3):991–4.

Llorente-Cortes V, Otero-Vinas M, Badimon L. Differential role of heparan sulfate proteoglycans on aggregated LDL uptake in human vascular smooth muscle cells and mouse embryonic fibroblasts. Arterioscler Thromb Vasc Biol. 2002;22(11):1905–11.

Lucas KA, Pitari GM, Kazerounian S, Ruiz-Stewart I, Park J, Schulz S, et al. Guanylyl cyclases and signaling by cyclic GMP. Pharmacol Rev. 2000;52 (3):375–414.

Lüscher T, Vanhoutte P. The endothelium modula-tor of cardiovascular function. Boca Raton, FL: CRC; 1990.

McLaren PJ, Cave JG, Parker EM, Slocombe RF. Chondrodysplastic calves in Northeast Victoria. Vet Pathol. 2007;44(3):342–54.

Pentikainen MO, Oorni K, Kovanen PT. Lipoprotein Lipase (LPL) strongly links native and oxidized low density lipoprotein particles to decorin-coated collagen. Roles for both dimeric and monomeric forms of LPL. J Biol Chem. 2000;275(8):5694–701.

Risler N, Castro C, Cruzado M, Gonzalez S, Miatello R. Early changes in proteoglycans production by resistance arteries smooth muscle cells of hypertensive rats. Am J Hypertens. 2002;15(5):416–21.

Salvemini D, Currie M, Mollace V. Nitric oxide-mediated cyclooxygenase activation. J Clin Invest 1996;97:2562–8.

Shetlar M, Shetlar C. The role of manganese in wound healing In: Klimis-Tavantzis D, editor. Manganese health and disease. Boca Raton, FL: CRC; 1994. pp. 146–57.

Shimokawa H. Endothelial dysfunction: a novel therapeutic target: primary endothelial dysfunction: atherosclerosis. J Mol Cell Cardiol. 1999;31:23–37.

Shriver Z, Liu D, Sasisekharan R. Emerging views of heparan sulfate glycosaminoglycan structure/activity relationships modulating dynamic biological functions. Trends Cardiovasc Med. 2002;12:71–7.

Strause L, Saltman P, Smith KT, Bracker M, Andon MB. Spinal bone loss in postmenopausal women supplemented with calcium and trace minerals. J Nutr. 1994;124(7):1060–4.

Taylor P, Patterson H, Klimis-Tavantzis D. A fluorescence double-quenching study of native lipoproteins in an animal model of manganese deficiency. Biol Trace Elem Res. 1997;60(1):69–80.

Temple N. Refined carbohydrates - a cause of suboptimal nutrient intake. Med Hypotheses. 1983;10(4): 411–24.

Theocharis A, Theocharis D, De Luca G, Hjerpe A, Karamanos N. Compositional and structural alterations of chondroitin and dermatan sulfates during the progression of atherosclerosis and aneurysmal dilatation of the human abdominal aorta. Biochimie 2002; 84(7):667–74.

Turnbull J, Powell A, Guimond S. Heparan sulfate: decoding a dynamic multifunctional cell regulator. Trends Cell Biol. 2001;11:75–82.

van Popele NM, Grobbee DE, Bots ML, Asmar R, Topouchian J, Reneman RS, et al. Association between arterial stiffness and atherosclerosis: The Rotterdam Study. Stroke. 2001;32(2):454–60.

Volkov N. The cobalt, manganese and zinc content in the blood and internal organs of atherosclerotic patients. Ter Arkh. 1962;34:52–6.

Wedler F. Biochemical and nutritional role of manganese: an overview. In: Klimis-Tavantzis D, editor. Manganese in health and disease. Boca Raton, FL: CRC; 1994. pp. 2–37.

Yan M, Lu Z, Du XJ, Han C. Effects of micromolar concentrations of Mn, Mo, and Si on alpha1-adrenoceptor-mediated contraction in porcine coronary artery. Biol Trace Elem Res. 1998;64(1–3): 75–87.

Yang P, Klimis-Tavantzis D. Effects of dietary manganese on arterial glycosaminoglycan metabolism in Sprague–Dawley rats. Biol Trace Elem Res. 1998a;64 (1):275–88.

Yang P, Klimis-Tavantzis DJ. Manganese deficiency alters arterial glycosaminoglycan structure in the Sprague–Dawley rat. J Nutr Biochem. 1998b;9(6): 324–31.

An invited paper presented in the plenary session "Trace Minerals: Modulators of Arterial Function"

The role of copper in nitric oxide-mediated vasodilation

Dale A. Schuschke
Department of Physiology and Biophysics, University of Louisville School of Medicine, Louisville, KY, USA

Corresponding author:
E-mail: daschu01@louisville.edu

Introduction

The role of copper as an essential nutrient for both structure and function in the cardiovascular system is well known. Dietary Cu deficiency in experimental animals causes a variety of vascular defects (for review, see Saari and Schuschke 1999). These defects include altered contractile responses of blood vessels. Kitano (1980) reported an increased rat aortic contraction to norepinephrine, and Allen and Saari (1994) demonstrated an augmented vasoconstriction to angiotensin II in isolated rat lungs. In addition to exaggerated constrictor responses, dilation is also altered. In separate studies, Saari (1992) and Lynch et al. (1997) reported the inhibition of nitric oxide (NO)-mediated vascular smooth muscle relaxation in aortic rings from Cu-deficient (CuD) rats. Similar inhibition was found when Cu was chelated before functional testing of rat aortic rings (Omar et al. 1991; Plane et al. 1997).

Our studies have addressed the role of dietary Cu in the vasoreactivity of microvascular arterioles.

These vessels, which have an endothelium and one or two layers of smooth muscle cells, regulate local tissue blood flow and are the primary contributors to total peripheral vascular resistance. Altered vaso-reactivity of these resistance vessels may be an important factor in the altered blood pressure that has been associated with inadequate Cu nutrition. For example, rats fed CuD diets can be either hyperten-sive (Medeiros 1987) or hypotensive (Fields et al. 1984), depending on the age when Cu restriction begins. In humans, stress-induced elevation of blood pressure occurs during short-term Cu deficiency (Lukaski et al. 1988).

Vasoreactivity in the Cu-deficient microcirculation

In initial studies, the in vivo microcirculation was examined in copper-adequate (CuA) and CuD rats. These experiments did not demonstrate a difference in the response of small arterioles (10- to 25-μm diameter) to norepinephrine-induced vasoconstriction between groups (Schuschke et al. 1995a). However, NO-mediated vasodilation was inhibited in the CuD group (Schuschke et al. 1992; 1995a). Similar results were also seen in an adult model of marginal Cu deficiency (Falcone et al. 2005). This inhibition occurred when the endothelium-dependent NO signal transduction pathway was stimulated by several different agonists including receptor-dependent ace-tylcholine (Ach) and receptor-independent calcium ionophore A23187. Vasodilation was also depressed in CuD rats when the vasculature was stimulated by the endothelium-independent NO donor, sodium nitroprusside (Schuschke et al. 1992). Similar results have been reported in aortic rings from CuD rats (Saari 1992).

Because the vasodilator response was attenuated in the CuD rat, relaxation mechanisms of the vascular smooth muscle were examined. Relaxation in response to the dibutyryl analogs of the second messengers, cGMP and cAMP, was not different between CuD and CuA groups (Schuschke et al. 1995a). Also, maximal dilation in response to the phosphodiesterase inhibitor papaverine did not differ between dietary groups in either the microcirculation (Schuschke et al. 1992) or aortic rings (Saari 1992). These results demonstrated that the ability of vascular smooth muscle to relax is not altered by dietary Cu deficiency but that the NO-mediated dilation pathway is specifically inhibited.

Possible mechanisms of attenuation

In the endothelial cell, NO is synthesized from the amino acid L-arginine in the presence of increased intracellular free calcium and the endothelial isoform of NO synthase (eNOS). The NO diffuses to the vas-cular smooth muscle and stimulates soluble guanylate cyclase (GC-S), which increases the second messenger cyclic GMP and causes relaxation. We have recently shown that arteriolar endothelium from CuD rats release significantly less NO than controls (Schuschke et al. 2007).

Cu,Zn superoxide dismutase (Cu,Zn–SOD) and solu-ble guanylate cyclase (GC–S) are two Cu-containing enzymes that are either directly or indirectly involved in the NO–cGMP signaling pathway. Cu,Zn–SOD is an antioxidant responsible for the dismutation of superoxide anion (O_2^-) to hydrogen peroxide (H_2O_2). GC–S is stimulated by NO to produce cGMP in the vascular smooth muscle cells. We hypothesized that inactivation or attenuation of these enzymes by the removal of Cu may result in the loss of NO-mediated dilation.

One possible mechanism of attenuation is the direct inactivation of NO by oxygen-derived free radicals that are by-products of cellular metabolic reactions. Dietary Cu deficiency has been shown to increase free radical activity because of the reduced activity of Cu-dependent antioxidant enzymes including Cu,Zn–SOD (Johnson and Saari 1991). Superoxide anion is known to inactivate NO and has been shown to inhibit cGMP-mediated relaxation of vascular smooth muscle in rats (Cherry et al. 1990). Superoxide dismutase (SOD) is the metabolizing enzyme of O_2^-, but because the activity of cytoplasmic Cu,Zn–SOD is reduced by restricting dietary Cu, O_2^- concentrations should be increased in CuD animals. Elevated O_2^- would lead to enhanced destruction of NO, resulting in loss of the diffusion gradient for NO between the endothelium and the underlying smooth muscle.

In the in vivo microcirculation, the dilator response of small arterioles to Ach is significantly attenuated during dietary Cu deficiency. However, this attenuation disappears when the antioxidant tempol is added to the drinking water (unpublished results) or after exposure to exogenous Cu,Zn–SOD (Schuschke et al. 1995a). These data suggest that during Cu deficiency, excess O_2^- degrades NO, directly decreasing NO dilator capability.

In addition to a direct inactivation of NO, the interaction of NO and O_2^- may indirectly inhibit the synthesis of additional NO by the endothelial cell. NO and O_2^- combine to produce peroxynitrite ($ONOO^-$), which causes oxidative damage including the inhibition of endothelial cell Ca^{2+} signaling (Elloitt 1996). We have shown in CuD rats that, when Cu,Zn–SOD activity is depressed, plasma $ONOO^-$ is increased and agonist-induced endothelial cell Ca^{2+} mobilization is decreased (Schuschke et al. 2000). These results support the hypothesis that excess O_2^- and the subsequent production of $ONOO^-$ inhibits endothelial cell Ca^{2+} signaling and causes attenuation of NO-mediated vascular dilation.

Another possible effect of Cu deficiency on NO-mediated dilation involves the interaction of NO with GC–S. Cu and Fe are transition metals that are components of this enzyme (Gerzer et al. 1981), which converts GTP to cGMP. As Cu is a functional cofactor in the NO-heme-binding site, NO may not be able to activate the GC–S when Cu concentrations are inadequate. Alternatively, iron metabolism is known to be altered in dietary Cu deficiency and may be a mechanism by which both the NO-heme binding is prevented, and the NO activation of GC-S is depressed in CuD animals.

Aside from the effects on NO binding, Cu depletion may also depress the activity of the GC–S enzyme independently of heme content. H_2O_2, which activates GC–S by a NO-independent mechanism, was used to test the activity of the GC–S during Cu deficiency (Schuschke et al. 1995a). In these studies, the microvessel dilation to H_2O_2 was not different between the CuD and the CuA groups. These data suggest that the general activity of the GC–S is not affected by dietary Cu deficiency. Therefore, our results indicate that, if Cu is a functional component of GC–S, its role is likely at the NO-binding site, but it is not a requisite for the basal activity of the enzyme. However, because the administration of Cu,Zn–SOD restored the dilation to Ach (Schuschke et al. 1995a), it is unlikely that altered NO-heme binding is the primary mechanism for the depressed vasodilation.

Other studies have examined the generation of NO in endothelial cells. Western blot analysis of eNOS did not demonstrate a difference between CuD and CuA groups, and pretreatment with the eNOS substrate L-arginine did not alter the attenuated dilation to Ach in CuD arterioles (Schuschke et al. 2000). Therefore, inactivation of Cu,Zn–SOD by inadequate Cu intake appears to be the primary mechanism by which NO-mediated dilation is reduced.

Compensatory mechanisms

While the attenuation of NO-dependent vasodilation is consistent among models of Cu deficiency, the effect on blood pressure is less predictable. As noted in the introduction, Cu deficiency may cause either hypertension or hypotension. However, other studies report no difference in blood pressure associated with dietary Cu restriction (Schuschke et al. 1997). The lack of an effect on blood pressure when NO-mediated vascular relaxation is decreased in resistance vessels suggests that compensatory mechanisms are involved. This idea is supported by recent data showing that inhibition of NO synthesis has less of an effect on blood pressure in normotensive CuD rats than in CuA controls (Saari 2002).

One possible compensatory mechanism is the up-regulation of the inducible isoform of NO-synthase (iNOS) during Cu deficiency. Although eNOS is the prevailing isoform of NOS in the vascular system, Saari and Bode (1999) report that iNOS and NO production are elevated in hearts of CuD rats. These results suggest that iNOS is up-regulated at a time when endothelial-derived NO may be inhibited.

Another compensatory mechanism may involve the up-regulation of the prostacyclin (PGI_2)–cAMP vasodilation pathway. We have shown that the sensitivity to carbacyclin (a stable analog of PGI_2) is increased in the in vivo microcirculation of CuD rats when NO-mediated dilation is depressed (Schuschke et al. 1997). This change in sensitivity may indicate an up-regulation of receptors on the vascular smooth muscle that maintains vasodilator input.

Cu requirement

The relationship between dietary Cu concentration and NO-mediated vasorelaxation was studied to determine the minimal dietary Cu intake necessary to prevent attenuation of the signaling pathway. By using Ach as the NO-dependent agonist, we have shown that the dilator response decreases when liver Cu concentration is less than 5 μg/g dry weight (Schuschke et al. 1999). The sensitivity of this dilation pathway to dietary Cu restriction is similar to that reported previously in a study on the role of Cu in hemostatic mechanisms (Schuschke et al. 1995b). Based on a study by Klevay and Saari (1993), dietary Cu intakes of greater than 1 μg/g diet are required to maintain liver Cu concentration above 5 μg/g in rats.

Conclusions

Several groups using various models of Cu deficiency have demonstrated that NO-mediated vasodilation is Cu-dependent. These data suggest that inactivation of cytosolic Cu,Zn–SOD by Cu restriction or chelation results in the depression of NO.

We have proposed that this depression of the NO response is caused by the buildup of O_2^- in the microcirculation, which then inhibits the NO pathway by direct and indirect mechanisms. O_2^- reacts with NO to produce $ONOO^-$, which reduces the NO available to diffuse to the smooth muscle. The $ONOO^-$ also reduces the requisite increase in intracellular Ca^{2+} for the further synthesis of NO from L-arginine. This hypothesis is supported by data showing that $ONOO^-$ is increased and agonist-stimulated endothelial Ca^{2+} mobilization is depressed in the vasculature of Cu deficient rats.

Acknowledgment

This work was supported in part by NIH DK55030.

References

Allen CB, Saari JT. Pulmonary vascular responses are exaggerated in isolated lungs from copper-deficient rats. Med Sci Res. 1994;22:815.

Cherry PD, Omar HA, Farrell KA, Stuart JS, Wolin MS. Superoxide anion inhibits cGMP-associated bovine pulmonary arterial relaxation. Am J Physiol 1990;259:H1056–62.

Elliott SJ. Peroxynitrite modulates receptor-activated Ca^{2+} signaling in vascular endothelial cells. Am J Physiol. 1996;270:L954–61.

Falcone JC, Saari JT, Kang YJ, Schuschke DA. Vasoreactivity in an adult rat model of marginal copper deficiency. Nutr. Res. 2005;25:177–86.

Fields M, Ferretti RJ, Smith JC, Reiser S. Effect of dietary carbohydrates and copper status on blood pressure of rats. Life Sci. 1984;34:763–9.

Gerzer R, Böhne E, Hofmann F, Schultz G. Soluble guanylate cyclase purified from bovine lung contains heme and copper. FEBS Lett. 1981;132:71–4.

Johnson WT, Saari JT. Temporal changes in heart size, hematocrit and erythrocyte membrane protein in copper-deficient rats. Nutr Res. 1991;11:1403–14.

Kitano, S. Membrane and contractile properties of rat vascular tissue in copper-deficient conditions. Circ Res. 1980;46:681.

Klevay LM, Saari JT. Comparative responses of rats to different copper intakes and modes of supplementation. Proc Soc Exp Biol Med. 1993;203:214–20.

Lukaski HC, Klevay LM, Milne DB. Effects of dietary copper on human autonomic cardiovascular function. Eur J Appl Physiol. 1988;58:74–80.

Lynch SM, Frei B, Morrow JD, Roberts LJ, Xu A, Jackson T, Reyna R, Klevay LM, Vita JA, Kearney JF. Vascular superoxide dismutase deficiency impairs endothelial vasodilator function through direct inactivation of nitric oxide and increased lipid peroxidation. Arteriosclerosis Thromb Vasc Biol. 1997;17:2975–81.

Medeiros DM. Hypertension in the Wistar–Kyoto rat as a result of post-weaning copper restrictions. Nutr Res. 1987;7:231–5.

Omar HA, Cherry PD, Mortelli MP, Burke-Wolin T, Wolin MS. Inhibition of coronary artery superoxide dismutase attenuates endothelium-dependent and -independent nitrovasodilator relaxation. Circ Res. 1991;69:601–8.

Plane F, Wigmore S, Angelini GD, Jeremy JY. Effect of copper on nitric oxide synthase and guanylyl cyclase activity in the rat isolated aorta. Br J Pharmacol. 1997;121:345–50.

Saari JT. Dietary copper deficiency and endothelium-dependent relaxation of rat aorta. Proc Soc Exp Biol Med. 1992;200:19–24.

Saari JT, Schuschke DA. Cardiovascular effects of dietary copper deficiency. BioFactors. 1999;10:359–75.

Saari JT, Bode AM. Expression of inducible nitric oxide synthase is elevated in hearts of copper-deficient rats. FASEB J. 1999;13:A371.

Saari JT. Dietary copper deficiency reduces the elevation of blood pressure caused by nitric oxide synthase inhibition in rats. Pharmacol. 2002;65:141–4.

Schuschke, DA, Reed MWR, Saari JT, Miller FN. Copper deficiency alters vasodilation in the rat cremaster muscle microcirculation. J Nutr. 1992;122:1547–52.

Schuschke DA, Saari JT, Miller FN. A role for dietary copper in nitric oxide-mediated vasodilation. Microcirculation. 1995a;2:371–6.

Schuschke LA, Saari JT, Miller FN, Schuschke DA. Hemostatic mechanisms in marginally copper-deficient rats. J Lab Clin Med. 1995b;125:748–53.

Schuschke DA, Saari JT, Miller FN. Arteriolar dilation to endotoxin is increased in copper-deficient rats. Inflammation. 1997;21:45–53.

Schuschke DA, Percival SS, Saari JT, Miller FN. Relationship between dietary copper concentration and acetylcholine-induced vasodilation in the microcirculation of rats. BioFactors. 1999;10:321–7.

Schuschke DA, Falcone JC, Saari JT, Fleming JT, Percival SS, Young SA, Pass JM, Miller FN. Endothelial cell calcium mobilization to acetylcholine is attenuated in copper-deficient rats. Endothelium. 2000;7: 83–92.

Schuschke DA, Cox J, Johnson WT, Falcone JC. Copper deficiency attenuates endothelial nitric oxide release. FASEB J. 2007;A721.

An invited paper presented in the plenary session "Trace Minerals: Modulators of Arterial Function"

Selenium status and regulation of vascular homeostasis

Lorraine M. Sordillo
College of Veterinary Medicine, Michigan State University, East Lansing, MI, 48824, USA

This review was partially supported by a grant from USDA 2007-35200-18235.

Corresponding author:
Email: sordillo@msu.edu

Introduction

Evidence suggests that there may be an inverse relationship between selenium (Se) nutrition and cardiovascular disorders. Several intervention studies are currently underway to assess the benefits of Se supplementation to control a wide variety of condition in which oxidant stress and inflammation are the predominant pathological features, including atherosclerosis. Earlier epidemiological and ecological studies that examined the potential benefit of Se administration to prevent or treat cardiovascular disease however have proven to be inconclusive (Alissa et al. 2003; Huttunen 1997; May 2002). An underlying factor to explain some of the equivocal finding from these prospective studies includes the inability to accurately assess Se status within different tissue microenvironments. The metabolism of Se in mammals is determined largely by the dietary sources, and it is known that the level of bioavailability will vary considerably in the body (Stadtman 2000). Therefore, to design diets that will maximize the benefits of Se on human health, it will be necessary to not only identify the specific cellular processes that are affected by Se status but also determine the specific Se-dependent bioactive components that are responsible for the desired response in targeted cellular environments.

The importance of Se to human health may be related to selenoprotein activities, such as glutathione peroxidase and thioredoxin reductase, that have diverse biological roles. These enzymes can function as potent antioxidants by directly reducing pro-atherogenic reactive oxygen species (ROS) and fatty acid hydroperoxides (FAHP) to less reactive water and alcohols, respectively. However, more recent evidence suggests that certain selenoproteins also are capable of modifying cellular responses to oxidant challenge by controlling the balanced expression of cytoprotective, apoptotic, and pro-inflammatory factors. This paper will describe some of the regulatory roles of individual selenoproteins in orchestrating vascular homeostasis during oxidant stress. The long-term implications for this area of research will be the ability to identify foods that can provide the optimal amount of specific biological active selenoproteins needed to control the development of atherosclerosis and other cardiovascular disorders.

Selenoproteins and endothelial anti-oxidant defense

Since the recent discovery of selenocysteine as the 21st amino acid in proteins, the field of Se biology has expanded rapidly. Indeed, many of the beneficial effects of this micronutrient are thought to be mediated by selenoproteins, which have selenocysteine residues incorporated into their active sites. There are at least 25 mammalian selenoproteins that have been identified, and some have important enzymatic functions (Papp et al. 2007). Recent studies showed that cytosolic glutathione peroxidases (GPX1), phospholipid hydroperoxide GPX (GPX4), and thioredoxin reductase 1 (TrxR1) are the major selenoproteins expressed by endothelial cells (Brigelius-Flohe et al. 2003; Hara et al. 2001). An important regulatory phenomenon that may be of particular importance to the development of cardiovascular disease is the antioxidant capabilities of these selenoproteins. Antioxidant potential is catalyzed either directly or indirectly by these selenoproteins based upon their ability to reduce many different forms of hydro-peroxides, including H2O2 and FAHP, to less reactive water and alcohols. For example, 15-hydroperoxyeico-satetraenoic acid (15HPETE) is a FAHP that represents the immediate oxygenated product formed from arachidonic acid metabolism via the 15-lipoxygenase (15LOX1) pathway. Several studies have documented the significance of this FAHP in vascular dysfunction (Cornicelli and Trivedi 1999; Cyrus et al. 2001). Indeed, research from our laboratory suggests that 15HPETE can directly affect vascular homeostasis by inducing apoptosis and enhancing the expression of pro-inflammatory mediators (Sordillo et al. 2008; Sordillo et al. 2005). Both GPX1 and TrxR1 have the capacity to reduce 15HPETE to a less toxic form, 15-hydroxyeico-satetraenoic acid. Therefore, selenoproteins clearly can help maintain cellular integrity by combating the accumulation of toxic hydroperoxides and reducing the oxidative modification of membrane lipids in artery walls that is associated with cardiovascular disease (Neve 2002).

Selenoproteins and eicosanoid biosynthesis

By controlling the accumulation of hydroperoxides within endothelial cells, selenoproteins also play a role in regulating the activities of enzymes involved in eicosanoid metabolism. Both prostaglandins and leukotrienes are essential for the regulation of vascular tone. For example, prostacyclin (PGI_2) causes vasodilation and inhibits platelet aggregation, while thromboxane A_2 (TXA_2) promotes aggregation and vasoconstriction. The peroxide tone of endothelial cells can directly affect the activity of enzymes involved in arachidonic acid metabolism such as cyclooxygenase, prostacyclin synthatase, and the lipoxygenases (Cao et al. 2000). Recent research showed that high peroxide levels resulting from the accumulation of the primary 15LOX product, 15HPETE, can reduce PGI2 production by the inactivation of prostacyclin synthase while having no effect on thromboxane synthase activity (Mayer et al. 1986; Weaver et al. 2001). As both PGI2 and TXA2 are derived from the same cyclooxygenase product (prostaglandin G2), the end result of elevated peroxide tone is reduced PGI2 synthesis and increased TXA2 levels during oxidant stress (Schilling and Elliott 1992). Therefore, the ability of selenoproteins to control the accumulation of intracellular lipid hydroperoxides can impact eicosanoid biosynthesis and vascular health.

Selenoproteins and cell signaling

Beyond the well-characterized hydroperoxide scavenging role, selenoproteins also can impact the activities of several enzymes involved in cell signaling cascade by controlling the intracellular redox environment (Brigelius-Flohe et al. 2003; McKenzie et al. 2002). Cellular redox state is a consequence of the balance between oxidizing and reducing equivalents, the levels of which can be controlled by both thioredoxin (Trx)/TrxR1 and glutathione (GSH)/GPX redox couples. There is a growing body of evidence to suggest that hydroperoxides can influence endothelial cell signaling cascades by redox modification of various protein kinases, protein phosphatases, and transcription factor activities. For example, the mitogen-activated protein kinase (MAPK) are a family of serine/threonine kinases that can control cellular physiologic responses through several redox-sensitive pathways including the extracellular signal-regulated kinase (ERK1/2), cJun N-terminal kinase (JNK), and p38. Previous studies showed that hydroperoxide-induced apoptosis of EC occurs through activation of the apoptosis signal-regulating kinase 1 (ASK1) and its downstream molecules JNK and p38 (Griendling et al. 2000). However, phosphorylation of the ERK1/2 pathway protects endothelial cells from oxidant stress. Treatment of cells with Se can suppress hydroperoxide-induced apoptosis by inhibiting ASK1 activation of JNK and p38 through a thiol-dependent mechanism. It was shown that ASK1 is inactivated when complexed with reduced Trx. Exposure to hydroperoxides can oxidizes Trx and results in its dissociated from ASK1, thereby enabling ASK1 to become active to promote the apoptotic process (Sarker et al. 2003; Yoon et al. 2002a; Yoon et al. 2002b). As TrxR1 can regenerate reduced Trx, the Trx/TrxR1 system can effectively modulate cell death by regulating the intensity of signaling cascades.

Further downstream in the signaling cascade, there are several transcription factors that are modified during oxidant stress including AP1 and NFκB (Papp et al. 2007). These redox-sensitive transcription factors are thought to control vascular homeostasis by modifying the expression of genes that are under the control of antioxidant-responsive elements. Se was shown to regulate some of these transcription factors by several different mechanisms. One mechanism involves the modification of the binding strength of transcription factors to DNA that involves a redox-sensitive regulator,

Ref1. For example, the transcription factor AP1 is a dimer complex composed of either Jun family (c-jun, JunB, and JunD) homodimers or c-jun/Fos family (c-fos, fosB, Fra-1, and Fra-2) heterodimers. These proteins are joined by a leucine zipper domain that utilizes a conserved cysteine to bind DNA and are therefore subject to redox control. Studies have shown that Trx can increase AP1 activity indirectly by its ability to translocate to the nucleus and bind Ref1. The Trx-bound Ref1 then associates transiently with AP1 and reduces the conserved cysteines in Fos and Jun family members, thus enhancing their binding activity (Hirota et al. 1999).

Another mechanism by which Se can regulate transcription factor activity is by changing the activation state of transcription factor regulatory subunits. For example, the NFκB/IκB complex resides in the cytoplasm and requires the release of phosphorylated IκB from this core complex for activation of NFκB subunits (p50 and p65). Considerable evidence suggests that addition of Se to cells in culture or overexpression of GPX1 and GPX4 can decrease NFκB activation by blocking IκB phosphorylation (Brigelius-Flohe et al. 2003; Brigelius-Flohe et al. 1997). This would prevent the migration of NFκB subunits to the nucleus where they can bind to DNA (Barchowsky et al. 1995). The impact of Se or selenoproteins on NF_kB activation was suggested to be from the breakdown of excess hydroperoxides that are responsible for oxidant-induced phosphorylation of IκB (Brigelius-Flohe et al. 2003). Through the actions of selenoproteins, Se can regulate intracellular signaling and transcription factor activation during oxidant stress. Therefore, it follows that this micronutrient also may impact the repertoire of gene expression that determines whether a cell is able to return to a state of homeostasis after oxidant challenge.

Conclusions

Considerable evidence suggests that low Se intake can cause adverse health effects while supra-nutritional levels may provide added protection from disease. Despite the clear relationship between Se status and optimal health, the mechanisms responsible for the beneficial effects remain elusive. Se is thought to mediate many of its beneficial effects through the antioxidant capabilities of selenoproteins. The ability of selenoproteins to control the redox environment of the cell also is likely to have an impact on the expression of genes that will determine the survival of endothelial cells during oxidant stress. It is not known whether the optimal health benefits of Se depends upon maximization of one or more of the selenoproteins within a localized tissue area. Further characterization of the role of selenoproteins in endothelial cell metabolism may provide new insights as to how Se may function as a nutraceutical and produce specific health benefits in combating cardiovascular disease.

Acknowledgment

The project was supported by the National Research Initiative of the USDA Cooperative State Research, Education and Extension Service, grant 2006-35200-17190. This review was partially supported by a grant from USDA 2007-35200-18235.

References

Alissa EM, Bahijri SM, Ferns GA. The controversy surrounding selenium and cardiovascular disease: a review of the evidence. Med Sci Monit. 2003;9(1): RA9–18.

Barchowsky A, Munro SR, Morana SJ, Vincenti MP, Treadwell M. Oxidant-sensitive and phosphorylation-dependent activation of NF-kappa B and AP-1 in endothelial cells. Am J Physiol. 1995;269(6 Pt 1): L829–36.

Brigelius-Flohe R, Banning A, Schnurr K. Selenium-dependent enzymes in endothelial cell function. Antioxid Redox Signal. 2003;5(2):205–15.

Brigelius-Flohe R, Friedrichs B, Maurer S, Schultz M, Streicher R. Interleukin-1-induced nuclear factor kappa B activation is inhibited by overexpression of phospholipid hydroperoxide glutathione peroxidase in a human endothelial cell line. Biochem J. 1997;328 (Pt 1):199–203.

Cao YZ, Reddy CC, Sordillo LM. Altered eicosanoid biosynthesis in selenium-deficient endothelial cells. Free Radic Biol Med. 2000;28(3):381–9.

Cornicelli JA, Trivedi BK. 15-Lipoxygenase and its inhibition: a novel therapeutic target for vascular disease. Curr Pharm Des. 1999;5(1):11–20.

Cyrus T, Pratico D, Zhao L, Witztum JL, Rader DJ, Rokach J, FitzGerald GA, Funk CD. Absence of 12/15-lipoxygenase expression decreases lipid peroxidation and atherogenesis in apolipoprotein e-deficient mice. Circulation. 2001;103(18):2277–82.

Griendling KK, Sorescu D, Lassegue B, Ushio-Fukai M. Modulation of protein kinase activity and gene expression by reactive oxygen specieis and their role in vascular physiology and pathophysiology. Arterioscler Thromb Vasc Biol. 2000;20:2175–83.

Hara S, Shoji Y, Sakurai A, Yuasa K, Himeno S, Imura N. Effects of selenium deficiency on expression of selenoproteins in bovine arterial endothelial cells. Biol Pharm Bull. 2001;24(7):754–9.

Hirota K, Nishiyama A, Yodoi J. Reactive oxygen intermediates, thioredoxin, and Ref-1 as effector molecules in cellular signal transduction. Tanpakushitsu Kakusan Koso. 1999;44(15 Suppl):2414–9.

Huttunen JK. Selenium and cardiovascular diseases—an update. Biomed Environ Sci. 1997;10(2–3):220–6.

May SW. Selenium-based pharmacological agents: an update. Expert Opin Investig Drugs. 2002;11(9): 1261–9.

Mayer B, Moser R, Gleispach H, Kukovetz WR. Possible inhibitory function of endogenous 15-hydroperoxyeicosatetraenoic acid on prostacyclin formation in bovine aortic endothelial cells. Biochim Biophys Acta. 1986 Feb 28;875(3):641–53.

McKenzie RC, Arthur JR, Beckett GJ. Selenium and the regulation of cell signaling, growth, and survival: molecular and mechanistic aspects. Antioxid Redox Signal. 2002;4(2):339–51.

Neve J. Selenium as a 'nutraceutical': how to conciliate physiological and supra-nutritional effects for an essential trace element. Curr Opin Clin Nutr Metab Care. 2002;5(6):659–63.

Papp LV, Lu J, Holmgren A, Khanna KK. From selenium to selenoproteins: synthesis, identity, and their role in human health. Antioxid Redox Signal. 2007;9 (7):775–806.

Sarker KP, Biswas KK, Rosales JL, Yamaji K, Hashiguchi T, Lee KY, Maruyama I. Ebselen inhibits NO-induced apoptosis of differentiated PC12 cells via inhibition of ASK1-p38 MAPK-p53 and JNK signaling and activation of p44/42 MAPK and Bcl-2. J Neurochem. 2003;87(6):1345–53.

Schilling WP, Elliott SJ. Ca2+ signaling mechanisms of vascular endothelial cells and their role in oxidant-induced endothelial cell dysfunction. Am J Physiol. 1992;262(6 Pt 2):H1617–30.

Sordillo LM, Streicher KL, Mullarky IK, Gandy JC, Trigona W, Corl CM. Selenium inhibits 15-hydroperoxyoctadecadienoic acid-induced intracellular adhesion molecule expression in aortic endothelial cells. Free Radic Biol Med. 2008 Jan 1;44(1):34–43.

Sordillo LM, Weaver JA, Cao YZ, Corl C, Sylte MJ, Mullarky IK. Enhanced 15-HPETE production during oxidant stress induces apoptosis of endothelial cells. Prostaglandins Other Lipid Mediat. 2005 May;76(1–4): 19–34.

Stadtman TC. Selenium biochemistry. Mammalian selenoenzymes. Ann N Y Acad Sci. 2000;899:399–402.

Weaver JA, Maddox JF, Cao YZ, Mullarky IK, Sordillo LM. Increased 15-HPETE production decreases prostacyclin synthase activity during oxidant stress in aortic endothelial cells. Free Radic Biol Med. 2001;30 (3):299–308.

Yoon SO, Kim MM, Park SJ, Kim D, Chung J, Chung AS. Selenite suppresses hydrogen peroxide-induced cell apoptosis through inhibition of ASK1/JNK and activation of PI3-K/Akt pathways. FASEB J. 2002a;16(1):111–3.

Yoon SO, Yun CH, Chung AS. Dose effect of oxidative stress on signal transduction in aging. Mech Ageing Dev. 2002b;123(12):1597–604.

An invited paper presented as the Raulin Award Lecture as part of ISTERH/NTES/HTES '07'

The ISTERH Raulin Award lecture: zinc nutriture and the fetal origins of disease

Harold H. Sandstead
Preventive Medicine and Community Health, University of Texas Medical Branch, Galveston, TX, 77555-1109, USA

Corresponding author:
E-mail: hsandste@utmb.edu

Adverse effects of gestational malnutrition on progeny have long been known (Ebbs et al. 1941; Smith 1916). In recent times, birth weight was shown to be inversely and linearly related to risk of coronary heart disease (Barker et al. 1989), type-2 diabetes mellitus, and hypertension (Osmond and Barker 2000), and gestational malnutrition was discovered to increase the risk of adult diseases, such as atherosclerotic cardiovascular disease and schizophrenia, in progeny of Dutch women who conceived during the famine of 1944–1945 (Roseboom et al. 2006; Susser et al. 1998).

Current theory suggests that malnutrition affects risk of later diseases through epigenetic mechanisms that covalently modify DNA and core histones so as to affect genome function without altering the DNA nucleotide sequence (Ozanne and Constancia 2007). Results of animal experiments implicate deficiencies of micronutrients that affect the synthesis of *S*-adenosylmethionine and the activity of methyl transferases (Duerre and Wallwork 1986; Wallwork and Duerre 1985; Waterland and Jirtle 2003; Wolff et al. 1998). Consideration of the above in light of the estimated 20.5% prevalence of Zn deficiency (Wuehler et al. 2005), prompted the thesis of this discussion: "Gestational Zn deficiency is a common cause of changes in epigenetic function that increase the risk of diseases of metabolism in later life."

Zinc deficiency is common in populations that infrequently eat flesh foods and subsist on foods prepared from unrefined cereals and legumes, foods that are rich in indigestible Zn-binding ligands such as phytic acid, certain dietary fibers, lignin, and products of non-enzymatic Maillard browning (Sandstead 2000). Thus, the poor and others who choose not to eat flesh are at high risk of Zn deficiency. Because diets that cause Zn deficiency also cause iron (Fe) deficiency (Sandstead 2000), we suspect the prevalence of Zn and Fe deficiencies are similar. Consistent with this idea, we found, through measurements of Zn kinetics, that premenopausal women with serum ferritin concentrations <20 ng/ml were highly likely to have a low rapidly exchangeable tissue Zn pool that is consistent with Zn deficiency (Yokoi et al. 2007). In this regard, it is notable that a large national survey, NHANES-II, found that more than 25% of premenopausal US women have serum ferritin concentrations <20 ng/ml (Pilch and Senti 1984).

Severe consequences of developmental Zn deficiency were first observed in experimental animals (Sandstead et al. 2000). Chicks and rats displayed malformations (Blamberg et al. 1960; Hurley and Swenerton 1966). Embryo DNA synthesis was suppressed (Swenerton and Hurley 1968), and morphology of preimplantation embryos was highly abnormal (Hurley and Shrader 1975). Abnormal development of cerebellar Purkinje cells was evident in rat progeny that were deprived of Zn from birth to weaning (Dvergsten et al. 1984). Residual later sequellae in rat progeny after Zn deficiency during the latter half of gestation or from birth to weaning included poor learning and memory, and increased aggression (Sandstead 1985). Relatively mild Zn deprivation from conception through weaning also impaired

memory and learning in adult progeny (Halas et al. 1986), and resulted in abnormal histological findings including dark staining of cytoplasm and nuclei of hippocampal neurons by toluidine blue in specimens from progeny >200 days of age (Hunt 1984).

Maternal Zn deficiency in humans is associated with increased risk of neural tube defects and other malformations (Velie et al. 1999), fetal stunting (Goldenberg et al. 1995; Scholl et al. 1993), prematurity (Scholl et al. 1993), newborn respiratory distress (Cherry et al. 1989), and decreased neonatal attention and motor skills at 6 months of age (Kirksey et al. 1994). Effect on risk of disease in later life is unknown.

Chemically, Zn nutriture affects gene expression through synthesis of nucleic acids (Dreosti et al. 1972; Sandstead and Rinaldi 1969; Terhune and Sandstead 1972) and proteins (Duerre et al. 1977; Hicks and Wallwork 1987); DNA repair (Ho and Ames 2002); formation and function of microtubules (Mackenzie and Oteiza 2007) through a host of Zn-finger protein transcription factors such as the Zic family Zn finger transcription factors that mediate development of the neural crest, cerebellum, and other neural tissues; somite development; and left–right axis patterning (Merzdorf 2007), and as Zn–ATP that is essential for activity of pyridoxal kinase and flavokinase, which respectively mediate synthesis of pyridoxal-5-phosphate (PLP) and FMN, the precursor of FAD (McCormick 2003). PLP and FAD affect specific steps in the folate pathway: PLP is the coenzyme for serine hydroxymethyltransferase, and FAD is the coenzyme for N5, N10–methylene tetrahydrofolate reductase.

Zinc also affects several steps in the methionine cycle/transsulfuration pathway (Maret and Sandstead 2008). While requirements for folate, pyridoxine, riboflavin, cobalamine, and choline/betaine in this pathway are well known, the role of Zn is less appreciated. Zinc is a catalytic metal ion for certain enzymes and a structural metal ion for certain transcription factors. Betaine-homocysteine methyltransferase is a Zn enzyme. Based on homology, methionine synthase is believed to be a Zn enzyme. Both of these enzymes synthesize methionine from homocysteine and thus provide *S*-adenosylmethionine for methylation reactions. At the transcriptional level, cystathionine β-synthase that makes cystathionine from homocysteine (with the help of coenzyme PLP) is under control of Sp1, a Zn-dependent transcription factor. The transcription of serine hydroxymethyltransferase (which requires coenzyme PLP) is regulated by two Zn-dependent transcription factors, Sp1 and MTF-1. Finally, at the level of the epigenome, Zn affects gene expression through its essentiality for the activity of methyl transferases that methylate DNA and histone proteins and through its essentiality for the function of enzymes that deacetylate histone proteins.

In summary, malnutrition during early developmental increases the risk for abnormal function and disease later in life, a phenomenon observed in experimental animals and humans. The timing of malnutrition, relative to the phase of development, affects later outcomes. Current theory attributes the increased risks for abnormal function and diseases in later life to effects of malnutrition on the epigenome that alter gene expression.

Zinc alone or in concert with other micronutrients affects gene expression through its essentiality for synthesis, structure, and function of transcription factors and enzymes that control DNA replication, repair, and fidelity. In addition but less appreciated, Zn nutriture affects epigenetic processes that result in methylation of DNA and histone proteins. Therefore, Zn deficiency should be included in the list of adverse factors that can impair the epigenome. Given the current 20.5% estimated prevalence of Zn deficiency, this suggestion has important health implications. Public health measures for maintenance of function and prevention of diseases in later life must include experimental-research-based optimization of nutrition, including Zn and other micronutrients, in girls and women who are potentially future mothers, before and during pregnancy.

Acknowledgment

I thank my colleague Wolfgang Maret for many informative conversations.

References

Barker D, Winter P, Osmond C, Margetts B, Simmonds S. Weight in infancy and death from ischemic heart disease. The Lancet, 1989;ii:577–80.

Blamberg DL, Blackwood UB, Supplee WC, Combs GF. Effect of zinc deficiency in hens on hatchability and embryonic development. Proc Soc Exp Biol Med. 1960; 104:217–20.

Cherry FF, Sandstead HH, Rojas P, Johnson LK, Batson HK, Wang XB. Adolescent pregnancy: associations among body weight, zinc nutriture, and pregnancy outcome. Am J Clin Nutr. 1989;50:945–54.

Dreosti IE, Grey PC, Wilkins PJ. Deoxyribonucleic acid synthesis, protein synthesis and teratogenesis in zinc-deficient rats. S Afr Med J. 1972;46:1585–8.

Duerre JA, Ford KM, Sandstead HH. Effect of zinc deficiency on protein synthesis in brain and liver of suckling rats. J Nutr. 1977;107:1082–93.

Duerre JA, Wallwork JC. Methionine metabolism in isolated perfused livers from rats fed on zinc-deficient and restricted diets. Br J Nutr. 1986;56:395–405.

Dvergsten CL, Fosmire GJ, Ollerich DA, Sandstead HH. Alterations in the postnatal development of the cerebellar cortex due to zinc deficiency. II. Impaired maturation of Purkinje cells. Brain Res. 1984;318:11–20.

Ebbs J, Tisdall F, Scott W. The influence of prenatal diet on the mother and child. J Nutr. 1941;22:515–26.

Goldenberg RL, Tamura T, Neggers Y, Copper RL, Johnston KE, DuBard MB, Hauth JC. The effect of zinc supplementation on pregnancy outcome. JAMA. 1995;27:463–8.

Halas ES, Hunt CD, Eberhardt MJ. Learning and memory disabilities in young adult rats from mildly zinc deficient dams. Physiol Behav. 1986;37:451–8.

Hicks SE, Wallwork JC. Effect of dietary zinc deficiency on protein synthesis in cell-free systems isolated from rat liver. J Nutr. 1987;117:1234–40.

Ho E, Ames BN. Low intracellular zinc induces oxidative DNA damage, disrupts p53, NFkappa B, and AP1 DNA binding, and affects DNA repair in a rat glioma cell line. Proc Natl Acad Sci U S A. 2002;99: 16770–5.

Hunt C. Mild zinc deficiency affects hippocampal morphology and behavior. Fed Proc. 1984;43:382A.

Hurley LS, Shrader RE. Abnormal development of preimplantation rat eggs after three days of maternal dietary zinc deficiency. Nature. 1975;254:427–9.

Hurley LS, Swenerton H. Congenital malformations resulting from zinc deficiency in rats. Proc Soc Exp Biol Med. 1966;123:692–6.

Kirksey A, Wachs TD, Yunis F, Srinath U, Rahmanifar A, McCabe GP, Galal OM, Harrison GG, Jerome NW. Relation of maternal zinc nutriture to pregnancy outcome and infant development in an Egyptian village. Am J Clin Nutr. 1994;60:782–92.

Mackenzie GG, Oteiza PI. Zinc and the cytoskeleton in the neuronal modulation of transcription factor NFAT. J Cell Physiol. 2007;210:246–56.

Maret W, Sandstead H. Possible roles of zinc nutriture in the fetal origins of disease. Exp Gerontology. 2008; 43:378–81.

McCormick DB. Metabolism of vitamins in microbes and mammals. Biochem Biophys Res Commun. 2003; 312:97–101.

Merzdorf C. Emerging roles for *zic* genes in early development. Dev Dyn. 2007;236:922–40.

Osmond C, Barker DJ. Fetal, infant, and childhood growth are predictors of coronary heart disease, diabetes, and hypertension in adult men and women. Environ Health Perspect. 2000;108(Suppl 3):545–53.

Ozanne SE, Constancia M. Mechanisms of disease: the developmental origins of disease and the role of the epigenotype. Nat Clin Pract Endocrinol Metab. 2007;3:539–46.

Pilch S, Senti F. Assessment of the iron nutritional status of the US population based on data collected in the second National Health and Nutrition Examination Survey, 1976–1980. Bethesda, MD: Life Sciences Research Office, Federation of American Societies for Experimental Biology; 1984.

Roseboom T, de Rooij S, Painter R. The Dutch famine and its long-term consequences for adult health. Early Hum Dev. 2006;82:485–91.

Sandstead HH. W.O. Atwater memorial lecture. Zinc: essentiality for brain development and function. Nutr Rev. 1985;43:129–37.

Anonymous. Causes of iron and zinc deficiencies and their effects on brain. J Nutr. 2000;130:347S–9S. Sandstead HH, Frederickson CJ, Penland JG. History of zinc as related to brain function. J Nutr. 2000;130: 496S–502S.

Sandstead HH, Rinaldi RA. Impairment of deoxy-ribonucleic acid synthesis by dietary zinc deficiency in the rat. J Cell Physiol. 1969;73:81–3.

Scholl TO, Hediger ML, Schall JI, Fischer RL, Khoo CS. Low zinc intake during pregnancy: its association with preterm and very preterm delivery. Am J Epidemiol. 1993;137:1115–24.

Smith G. An investigation into some of the effect of the state of nutrition of the mother during pregnancy and labor on the condition of the child a birth and for the first few days of life. Lancet. 1916;188:54–6.

Susser E, Hoek HW, Brown A. Neurodevelopmental disorders after prenatal famine: the story of the Dutch Famine Study. Am J Epidemiol. 1998;147:213–6.

Swenerton H, Hurley LS. Severe zinc deficiency in male and female rats. J Nutr. 1968;95:8–18.

Terhune MW, Sandstead HH. Decreased RNA polymerase activity in mammalian zinc deficiency. Science. 1972;177:68–9.

Velie EM, Block G, Shaw GM, Samuels SJ, Schaffer DM, Kulldorff M. Maternal supplemental and dietary zinc intake and the occurrence of neural tube defects in California. Am J Epidemiol. 1999;150:605–16.

Wallwork JC, Duerre JA. Effect of zinc deficiency on methionine metabolism, methylation reactions and protein synthesis in isolated perfused rat liver. J Nutr. 1985;115:252–62.

Waterland RA, Jirtle RL. Transposable elements: targets for early nutritional effects on epigenetic gene regulation. Mol Cell Biol. 2003;23:5293–300.

Wolff GL, Kodell RL, Moore SR, Cooney CA. Maternal epigenetics and methyl supplements affect agouti gene expression in Avy/a mice. FASEB J. 1998;12:949–57.

Wuehler SE, Peerson JM, Brown KH. Use of national food balance data to estimate the adequacy of zinc in national food supplies: methodology and regional estimates. Public Health Nutr. 2005;8:812–9.

Yokoi K, Sandstead HH, Egger NG, Alcock NW. Sadagopa Ramanujam VM., Dayal HH, Penland JG. Association between zinc pool sizes and iron stores in premenopausal women without anaemia. Br J Nutr. 2007;98:1214–23.

An invited paper presented in the plenary session "Trace element nutrition and dietary recommendations"

The relevance of trace element nutrition in human health

S. Ermidou-Pollet and S. Pollet
Department of Biochemistry, Medical School, University of Athens, Greece

Corresponding author:
E-mail: sermid@med.uoa.gr

Introduction

Trace elements are defined as "important constituents of the human body that are required in very small amounts in the diet of a living organism" (Ashworth 1991). Physiologists have studied their constitutive and functional roles in the functioning of cells as well as of various organs and tissues. Toxicologists have performed research into their harmful properties. Nutritional sciences have discovered that a wide range of common pathologies are caused by a lack of them. The relevance of trace element nutrition in human health is obvious.

Trace element nutrition during pregnancy

Proper trace element nutrition during pregnancy is important for maternal health and fetal growth and development. Inadequate stores or intake of trace elements may have adverse effects to the mother (hypertension, anemia, and complications of labor) and the fetus (congenital malformations, pre-term delivery, and intrauterine growth retardation). The effect of improper nutrition is influenced by gestational age and/or severity of deficiency (Lorenzo Alonso et al. 2005). Climate, geographical, ecological, socio-economical, and traditional factors also may play an important role (Jiang 2005). On the other hand, obesity may be associated with alterations in maternal–fetal disposition of some essential trace elements and antioxidant enzyme status. These alterations may pose a potential health risk for the mother, as well as the fetus (Al-Saleh 2006).

Nutritional deficiencies during pregnancy might be difficult to detect. While some micronutrients have been studied extensively (iron, zinc, and iodine), much less is known about others. It has been shown that multiple micronutrient deficiencies rather than single deficiencies are common (Kontic-Vucinic et al. 2006). The role of the interactions between trace elements in improving pregnancy outcome need to be investigated more precisely (Kontic-Vucinic et al. 2006).

Supplementation of certain trace elements and minerals could prevent some of the most severe adverse pregnancy outcomes by improving antioxidant defense (Laskowska-Klita et al. 2005). Although sometimes it is unnecessary (Arkkola et al. 2006), its potential benefits may outweigh any potential adverse reaction that can be attributed to nutrient consumption (Kontic-Vucinic et al. 2006).

Trace element nutrition during infancy

Infants and, especially, newborns grow rapidly. Since they double their body weight within 5 months, they require more trace elements per kilogram body mass than adults. Human milk is regarded as the best and complete nourishment for a neonate. It is not a uniform body fluid but a secretion of the mammary gland of changing composition. Variations in milk composition occur due to various factors such as maternal trace element intake and status, maternal age, parity, residing area, family income, length of gestation, and infant weight (Arnaud and Favier 1995; Kwapulinski et al. 1997). Yet, the content of milk component varies greatly between infants and the duration of lactation (Yamawaki et al. 2005).

Physiologic changes in milk and the infants' status determine the dependence of the infant on complementary foods, in addition to human milk, when meeting trace element requirement (Krebs and Hambidge 2007). Moreover, maternal milk may sometimes contain chemical contaminants, which could have adverse effects on neonates. Occupational chemicals and hazardous persistent environmental chemicals are factors limiting breast-feeding in some cases (Tripathi et al. 1999). Therefore, trace element supplementation with infant formulae is recommended. The infant's organs and the rapidly developing brain (Georgieff 2007) are particularly vulnerable to trace element deficiencies. These may develop in very low birth weight infants (<1,500 g) as a result of rapid growth, low body stores, and low content of these substances in human milk (Loui 2004). Suboptimal intake may cause growth retardation, immune imbalance, and/or impaired organ functions.

Trace element nutrition during childhood and adolescence

Most health-damaging behaviors, including eating behaviors, are learned during childhood and adolescence (Pratt and Tsitsika 2007; Stockman et al. 2005). This period of intense physiological change needs adequate nutrition to achieve normal adult size and reproductive capacity (Seidenfeld 2004).

Adequacy of nutrient intake has been studied considerably in children and adolescents across Europe (Prentice et al. 2004; Lambert et al. 2004; Vicente-Rodriguez et al. 2007). Trace element deficiencies have been observed (Arvanitidou et al. 2007; Choi and Kim 2005; Rossipal 2001). However, it seems that there are insufficient data for drawing any conclusions (Vicente-Rodriguez et al. 2007). Nutritional risks may be associated with socio-economic and educational variables of the family, and some lifestyle factors including physical activity and the quality of the breakfast meal (Serra-Majem et al. 2002).

Trace element nutrition and adults

Due to the continuous turnover of mineral elements in adult organism, there is a necessity of an appropriate daily intake of these elements. However, in the last decades, lifestyle changes, chemical use in agriculture, and proliferation of scientific results concerning food components and additives as factors for the etiology and pathogenesis of some diseases have led to a decrease in the population with an adequate diet. In order to avoid risk from uncontrolled intake of trace elements, a "Recommended Dietary Allowance" was established for humans and dietary reference intakes are continuously brought up to date (Schumann 2006).

Deficiencies of trace elements can have profound effects on the development, health, and well-being of human subjects. They have various etiologies: inadequate dietary intake, inherited genetic disorders, malabsorption due to intestinal pathology or reduced bioavailability, total parenteral nutrition with inadequate feeding solution, and excessive urinary and/or fecal excretion. The World Health Organization has estimated that over 2 billion people around the globe suffer from diseases caused by trace element deficiency (Abdulla et al. 2005). Diagnosis of deficiency and the monitoring of individuals receiving treatment require the knowledge of both the trace element status of these individuals before treatment and, in case of deficiency, the trace element requirements needed for restoring an adequate trace element status.

Trace element supplementation is difficult to perform. Interactions with other minerals or dietary constituents need consideration in the evaluation. There is growing concern that balance studies may be inappropriate for estimating the requirements for minerals (Ermidou-Pollet et al. 2005). On the other hand, as several elements interact metabolically, the understanding of the concurrent metal levels and their interrelationship pattern is very essential for clinical correlations. More than an individual metal, the comprehensive metal homeostasis and its interrelationships are known to play a significant role in biological systems.

Trace element nutrition in elderly people

Ageing is associated with reduced energy intake and loss of appetite. Living and eating alone further diminishes food consumption and dietary quality. Older adults are at greater risk for nutritional deficiencies than are younger adults due to physiologic changes associated with aging, acute and chronic illnesses, prescription and over-the-counter medications, financial and social status, and functional decline. Consequently, trace element deficiencies, mainly Fe, Zn, Cr, and Cu are often observed in the elderly (Marniemi et al. 2005; Andriollo-Sanchez et al. 2005; Roussel et al. 2007; Latheef et al. 2006).

There is little specific information regarding micronutrient requirements for the elderly. One reason for this is the difficulty in conducting reliable and valid studies due to the heterogeneity of older adults and their unique rate of aging associated with their health status, limited income, disability, and living situation (Chernoff 2005).

Conclusions

The knowledge of the trace element contents of human diets is a prerequisite for a correct appraisal of their conformity to the existing hygienic and sanitary recommendations and of their potential health hazards. Deficiencies of trace elements can have profound effects on the development, health, and well-being of human subjects. However, trace element supplementation for meeting the requirement is not so easy to perform. More interdisciplinary work is necessary to further the understanding of the role of trace element nutrition in human health.

References

Abdulla M, Chazot G, Gamon S, Bost M. Are trace elements a health problem in developing countries? In: Ermidou-Pollet S, Pollet S, editors. Abstracts of the 5th International Symposium on Trace Elements in Human: New Perspectives, Athens, 2005, p. 7.

Al-Saleh E, Nandakumaran M, Al-Harmi J, Sadan T, Al-Enezi H. Maternal–fetal status of copper, iron, molybdenum, selenium, and zinc in obese pregnant women in late gestation. Biol. Trace Elem. Res. 2006;113(2): 113–23.

Andriollo-Sanchez M, Hininger-Favier I, Meunier N, Toti E, Zaccaria M. Brandolini-Bunlon M, Polito A, O'Connor JM, Ferry M, Coudray C, Roussel AM. Zinc intake and status in middle-aged and older European subjects: the zenith study. Eur J Clin Nutr. 2005;59 Suppl. 2:S37–41.

Arkkola T, Uusitalo U, Pietikainen M, Metsala J, Kronberg-Kippila C, Erkkola M, Veijola R, Knip M,

Virtanen SM, Ovaskainen ML. Dietary intake and use of dietary supplements in relation to demographic variables among pregnant Finnish women. Br J Nutr. 2006;96(5):913–20.

Arnaud J, Favier A. Copper, iron, manganese and zinc contents in human colostrum and transitory milk of French women. Sci Total Environ. 1995;159:9–15.

Arvanitidou V, Voskaki I, Tripsianis G, Athanasopoulou H, Tsalkidis A, Filippidis S, Schulpis K, Androulakis I. Serum copper and zinc concentrations in healthy children aged 3–14 years in Greece. Biol Trace Elem Res. 2007;115(1):1–12.

Ashworth W. The Encyclopedia of Environmental studies. Facts on File, New York, 1991, p. 397.

Chernoff R.. Micronutrient requirements in older women. Am J Clin Nutr. 2005; 81(5):S1240–5.

Choi JW, Kim SK. Relationships of lead, copper, zinc, and cadmium levels versus hematopoiesis and iron parameters in healthy adolescents. Ann Clin Lab Sci. 2005;35(4):428–34.

Ermidou-Pollet S, Szilágyi M, Pollet S. Problems associated with the determination of trace element status and trace element requirements. A mini-review. Trace Elem Electrolytes. 2005;22(2):105–13.

Georgieff MK. Nutrition and the developing brain: nutrient priorities and measurement. Am J Clin Nutr. 2007;85(2):S614–20.

Jiang T, Christian P, Khatry SK, Wu L, West KP. Micronutrient deficiencies in early pregnancy are common, concurrent, and vary by season among rural Nepali pregnant women. J Nutr. 2005;135(5):1106–12.

Kontic-Vucinic O, Sulovic N, Radunovic N. Micronutrients in women's reproductive health: II. Minerals and trace elements. Int J Fertil Women's Med. 2006;51 (3):116–24.

Krebs NF, Hambidge KM. Complementary feeding: clinically relevant factors affecting timing and composition. Am J Clin Nutr. 2007;85(2):S639–45.

Kwapulinski J, Gsrka P, Wiechuta D, Matera L, Nogaj E. Heavy metals in women milk living in industrial region. In: Ermidou-Pollet S, Pollet S, editors. Abstracts of the International Symposium on Trace Elements in Human: New Perspectives, Athens, 1997, p. 57.

Lambert J, Agostoni C, Elmadfa I, Hulshof K, Krause E, Livingstone B, Socha P, Pannemans D, Samartin S. Dietary intake and nutritional status of children and adolescents in Europe. Br J Nutr. 2004;92 Suppl. 2:S147–211.

Laskowska-Klita T, Chelchowska M, Kubik P. Zinc, copper, selenium and activities of superoxide dismutase (SOD) and glutathione peroxidase (GPx) in blood of pregnant women after mineral supplementation. In: Ermidou-Pollet S, Pollet S, editors. Abstracts of the 5th International Symposium: "Trace Elements in Human: New Perspectives, Athens, 2005, pp. 26–7.

Latheef SAA, Subramanyam G, Reddy KN. Association of serum copper and coronary artery disease in elderly population of South India. Trace Elem Electrolytes. 2006;23(1):29–36.

Lorenzo Alonso, MJ, Bermejo BA, Cocho de Juan JA, Fraga Bermúdez JM, Bermejo Barrera P. Selenium levels in related biological samples: human placenta, maternal and umbilical cord blood, hair and nails. J Trace Elem Med Biol. 2005;19(1):49–55.

Loui A, Raab A, Wagner M, Weigel T, Gruters-Kieslich T, Bratter P, Obladen M. Nutrition of very low birth weight infants fed human milk with or without supplemental trace elements: a randomized controlled trial. J. Pediatr. Gastroenterol Nutr. 2004;39(4):346–53.

Marniemi J, Alanen E, Impivaara O, Seppänen R, Hakala P, Rajala T, Rönnemaa T. Dietary and serum vitamins and minerals as predictors of myocardial infarction and stroke in elderly subjects. Nutr. Metab. Cardiovasc. 2005;15(3):188–97.

Pratt HD, Tsitsika AK. Fetal, childhood, and adolescence interventions leading to adult disease prevention. Primary Care. 2007;34(2):203–17.

Prentice A, Branca F, Decsi T, Michaelsen KF, Fletcher RJ, Guesry P, Manz F, Vidailhet M, Pannemans D, Samartin S. Energy and nutrient dietary reference values for children in Europe: methodological approaches and current nutritional recommendations. Br J Nutr. 2004;92 (Suppl. 2):S83–146.

Rossipal E. Are there evidence based data for a possible marginal selenium deficiency in healthy infants, children or adolescents living in the South East of Europe? In: Ermidou-Pollet S, Pollet S, editors. Proceedings of the 3rd International Symposium: "Trace Elements in Human: New Perspectives," Athens, 2001, 449–56.

Roussel AM, Andriollo-Sanchez M, Ferry M, Bryden NA, Anderson RA. Food chromium content, dietary chromium intake and related biological variables in French free-living elderly. Br J Nutr. 2007;98(2):326–31.

Schümann K. Dietary reference intakes for trace elements revisited. J Trace Elem Med Biol. 2006;20 (1):59–61.

Seidenfeld MEK, Sosin E, Rickert VI. Nutrition and eating disorders in adolescents. Mt. Sinai J Med. 2004;71(3):155–61.

Serra-Majem L, Ribas L, Perez-Rodrigo C, Garcia-Closas R, Pena-Quintana L, Aranceta J. Determinants of nutrient intake among children and adolescents: results from the enKid study. Ann Nutr Metab. 2002;46 (Suppl. 1): 31–38.

Stockman NKA, Schenkel TC, Brown JN, Duncan AM. Comparison of energy and nutrient intakes among meals and snacks of adolescent males. Prev Med. 2005;41(1):203–10.

Tripathi RM, Ragunath R, Sastry VN, Krishnamoothy TM. Daily intake of heavy metals by infants through milk and milk products. Sci Total Environ. 1999;227: 229–39.

Vicente-Rodriguez G, Libersa C, Mesana MI, Beghin L, Iliescu C, Aznar LAM, Dallongeville J, Gottrand F. Healthy lifestyle by nutrition in adolescence (HELENA). A new EU funded project. Therapie. 2007;62(3):259–70.

Yamawaki N, Yamada M, Kan-No T, Kojima T, Kaneko T, Yonekubo A. Macronutrient, mineral and trace element composition of breast milk from Japanese women. J Trace Elem Med Biol. 2005;19(2–3):171–81.

An invited paper presented in the plenary session "Trace element nutrition and dietary recommendations"

International dietary standards for trace elements

Jeanne H. Freeland-Graves and Jodi M. Cahill
Division of Nutrition, The University of Texas at Austin, Austin, TX, 78712, USA

Corresponding author:
E-mail: jfg@mail.utexas.edu

Status of trace element dietary standards

The essentiality and toxicity of trace elements in the human diet have been estimated to be related to mortality and morbidity in over half the world's population (Welch and Graham 2005). This impact of microminerals on health and society necessitates the formulation of recommendations for dietary standards that can be disseminated to health professionals, consumers, researchers, agricultural and government agencies, and policy makers. As the world is now so interconnected through technology of rapid communications, one would assume that dietary standards are coordinated throughout the world. Thus, the purpose of this paper was to review the status of dietary standards for trace elements on a global basis.

Unfortunately, dietary standards are not uniform or harmonized throughout the world. Vast differences exist in terminology, values, and methodologies used to derive reference intakes in developed, transitional, and developing countries. The nations may vary significantly in geographical locations, ability to produce a safe and sustainable food supply, and environmental factors such as contamination, parasites, and economic situations. In addition, cultural and societal norms greatly impact the type, quantity, and preparation of foods (Wahlqvist 2003). This enormous diversity of countries, terrain, populations, and diets across the planet makes it difficult to identify the most appropriate values for each segment. Priorities among regions may vary, from elimination of hunger, malnutrition, and maintenance of biological functions to prevention of chronic diseases via optimal intakes.

Assessment of trace element status

Trace element status is influenced by metabolism (absorption, digestion, transport, utilization, and excretion), chemical form, interactions of dietary components, immunocompetence, infection, and consequences of diseases and chronic health conditions (Mertz et al. 1994). However, dietary standards have been set only for "healthy" populations, so that risks of chronic disease are not a consideration.

Yet, even in healthy populations, a multitude of other factors affect dietary requirements. These include age, gender, physical activity, exposure to sun (vitamin D), host factors, diet patterns, food processing, and socio-economic status (Gibson 2007; King et al. 2007; Yates 2007). Variations due to genetic determinants, body composition, stages of life (growth, timing of puberty, and type of feeding), and lifestyle may further complicate issues (Atkinson and Koletzko 2007; Stover 2007). Finally, politics and environmental events can produce adverse consequences on nutrient adequacy. Despite the huge food surplus in developed countries such as the USA, political situations in other areas of the world can limit food distribution and create malnutrition and hunger. Environmental events such as pollution and natural disasters also affect health status. For instance, pollution from a zinc smelter may adversely influence copper status and contribute to cadmium toxicity (Spierenburg et al. 1988).

The most common approaches to assess trace element status have included clinical consequences, depletion/

repletion studies, nutrient balance, animal studies, functional indicators (biomarkers), epidemiological observations, and population-based assessments of nutrient intakes associated with good health (Institute of Medicine 2000, 2002; Yates 2007). Clinical consequences are the most crude assessment of status, as these represent the endpoint of a continuum from nutrient deficiency, biochemical alterations, metabolic response and/or failure, and ultimately, physical symptoms. Nutrient balance studies that utilize the factorial approach determine negligible losses from diets almost absent in the nutrient. A factor for availability is added to the level required for a very slight positive balance (Freeland-Graves 1994). However, in this method, the size of the metabolic storage pool is a determinant of the quantity required to maintain balance; also, the small sample size reduces the ability to extrapolate the data to larger populations. Animal studies yield controlled data, but the results may not always be applicable for humans.

Functional indicators (biomarkers such as an enzyme or stable isotopes in the blood or urine) are considered the "gold standard" of status if a consistent, statistical relationship can be shown between dietary intake and metabolic response. Their use in depletion/repletion studies provides valuable information. Yet accurate biomarkers are lacking for many nutrients, necessitating the use of population-based assessments of dietary levels associated with good health. In this technological age, it is surprising to find that something as simple as dietary levels related to health are the basis for the USA DRIs for manganese, chromium, and fluoride (Institute of Medicine 1997, 2002).

Diversity of dietary standards in the world

With the multiplicity of differences in the world's environment, populations, and culture, it is exceedingly difficult to find commonality in the diversity of global dietary standards. Table 1 compares dietary standards from some major countries and communities.

Some obvious illustrations of the differences above are that (1) a lower reference intake is not part of the recommendations for Japan, USA/Canada, and WHO/FAO; (2) only DACH, EC, and USA/Canada have the category of safe intake; and (3) the EC does not have an upper level of safe intake. Also, names for key terms, methods for determining requirements, and concepts of expressing recommendations vary considerably. Physical activity, for example, is included only in the Nordic recommendations.

The Expert Group on the Methodological Approaches and Current Nutritional Recommendations in Children and Adolescents evaluated the current guidelines in 29 countries of Europe (Prentice et al. 2004). Huge disparities in values for nutrient recommendations were found. Remarkably, reference intakes for zinc in young children varied threefold, ranging from 3 to 10 mg. The same magnitude of discrepancy was true for copper; iron varied only twofold. Although some heterogeneity could be attributed to environment and physiology, much of the differences were due to philosophical and methodological

Table 1 List of gill lesions and their stage from Poleksić and Mitrović-Tutundžić,1984

Group/ country	Title of recommendations	Average requirement	Recommended intake level	Lower reference intake	Safe intake	Upper level of safe intake
DACH	Reference values		Recommendations	Guiding values	Estimated values	Guiding values
EC	European recommended dietary allowances	Average requirement	Population reference intake	Lowest threshold intake	Acceptable ranges	
Japan	Recommended dietary allowances	Estimated average requirement	Recommended dietary allowance			Tolerable upper intake level
Nordic Council[a]	Nordic nutrition recommendations	Average requirement	Recommended intake	Lower limit of intake		Upper intake levels
USA/ Canada	Dietary reference intakes	Estimated average requirement	Recommended dietary allowance		Adequate intake	Tolerable upper intake level
WHO/ FAO		Estimated average requirement	Recommended nutrient intake			Tolerable upper intake level

[a] Nordic Council = Denmark, Iceland, Norway, and Sweden

approaches. Pavlovic et al. (2007) observed that some countries do not separate recommendations according to gender at certain ages or use age groups that differ in children. It is clear that confusion exists in the terminology and interpretation of dietary standards across the world.

Harmonization of dietary standards

The United Nations University's Food and Nutrition Programme recognized this problem of a lack of global uniformity for reference intakes. In conjunction with the FAO/WHO/UNICEF, a committee was created to harmonize the approaches for establishing nutrient intake values throughout the world. This concept of coordination of standards internationally is not new, as it was the basis of the Codex Alimentarius created by the WHO/FAO for food standards (Orriss 1998).

A significant body of work was produced and published by this committee chaired by Janet King and Culberto Garza (2007) to address the lack of harmonization. Table 2 shows the key terms related to nutrients recommended by this United Nations committee.

Table 2 Terms and definitions for the proposed harmonization of nutrient recommendations (derived from King et al. 2007)

Concept	Key terms	Acronym	Definition
Overall name	Nutrient intake value	NIV	Set of nutrient recommendations based on primary data
Average requirement	Average nutrient requirement	ANR	Median requirement estimated from a statistical distribution related to a specific outcome in healthy persons
Upper level of safe intake	Upper nutrient level	UNL	Highest level of daily nutrient intake that is likely to pose no risk of adverse health effects for almost all individuals in a specified life-stage group
Recommended intake level	Individual nutrient level	INL_x	Recommended nutrient level for all healthy individuals computed by adding a factor (x) to the ANR in order to meet the individual needs of a specified percentage of the population

The umbrella name for the recommendations of nutrients is the nutrient intake value (NIV). This term replaces the DACH RV, USA/Canada DRI, the United Kingdom DRV, and others. The term NIV is neutral and broad, as it does not use the specific wording of any country. Rather, NIV is an amalgamation of the numerous terms in current use. The plan was that, once the NIV is developed for a nutrient, then each country could modify the base value according to its regional differences in foods, host factors, genetics, and health status (King and Garza 2007).

Only two key terms were established, the ANR and the UNL, because all other terms would be derived from these. An RDA, RNI, or RI was not included, as this could be calculated from the ANR by adding two standard deviations to the mean. The concept of lower levels of reference intakes was not utilized because it is thought to be derived from the NIV and had limited usefulness. Safe intakes also were excluded due to subjectivity, with the exception of targets for infants. To meet the needs of individuals, the INL_x was designed to be computed from the ANR by a factor that corresponds to a specified percentage of the population. A factor (x) of 80 would represent an individual nutrient level that would be adequate for 80% of the population. Further details are presented in the excellent report by King and Garza (2007).

If the proposed harmonization of key terms of dietary recommendation developed by this committee were adopted, it would simplify comparisons of nutrient intakes on a global basis and further understanding of how standards are created. These common terms could be utilized for the development of consistent methods to create food-based dietary guidelines and formulate all aspects of nutrient-related policies (Vorster et al. 2007). Also, harmonization of nutrient-based dietary standards could result in consistent nutrient labeling that would promote international trade and development (Ramaswamy and Viswanathan 2007).

Harmonization is a theme that also has captured attention in Mesoamerica (Central Mexico to Panama). Solomons et al. (2004) proposed consistency in nutrient recommendations that fit within the ecological niche of the population. These standards must be achievable via available and culturally appropriate foods. Yet, criticism exists for harmonization. These new standards would lead to more regulations from the developed countries that would have to be met by developing countries. If nutritional labeling was standardized according to these harmonized terms, it might negatively impact populations whose occupation is based on agriculture and food trade (Ramaswamy and Viswanathan 2007).

Given the benefits versus risks of harmonization for the world, one might think that these new terms would be readily accepted by communities and governments that formulate dietary recommendations. However, it appears that nations and communities will persist in setting their own standards, based on their national, social, cultural, and ethnic differences. For example, a European Micronutrient Recommendations Aligned (EURRECA) Network of Excellence has been created by the European Commission by 34 partners in 17 countries (EURRECA 2007). Its purpose is to develop quality assured and aligned recommendations for micronutrients for varying population groups across Europe, including immigrants and low-income individuals. However, these standards will once again not match those of most of the countries on Earth. Thus, the "tower of Babel" that exists throughout the world regarding nutrient recommendations seems destined to continue.

Acknowledgment

This review was partially supported by grants from NIH 1R13DK080637-01, USDA 2007-35200-18235, and the Bess Heflin Centennial Professorship.

References

Atkinson A, Koletzko B. Determining life-stage groups and extrapolating nutrient intake values (NIVs). Food Nutr Bull. 2007;28:S61–76.

EURRECA—European Recommendations Aligned Network of Excellence. http://www.eurreca.org/everyone/2976. Accessed February 4, 2008.

Freeland-Graves J. Derivation manganese estimated safe and adequate daily dietary intakes. In: Mertz W, Abernathy C, Olin S. Risk assessment of essential elements. Washington, DC: ILSI, 1994:237–52.

Gibson R. The role of diet- and host-related factors in nutrient bioavailability and thus nutrient-based dietary requirement estimates. Food Nutr Bull. 2007;28:S77–100.

Institute of Medicine Panel on Micronutrients. Dietary reference intakes: vitamin A, vitamin K, arsenic, boron, chromium, copper, iodine, iron, manganese, molybdenum, nickel, silicon, vanadium, and zinc. Washington, DC: National Academy Press, 2002.

Institute of Medicine. Dietary reference intakes for calcium, phosphorus, magnesium, vitamin D, and fluoride. Washington, DC: National Academy Press; 1997. pp. 46–7.

Institute of Medicine. Dietary reference intakes: applications in dietary assessment. Washington, DC: National Academy Press; 2000.

King J, Garza C. International harmonization of approaches for developing nutrient-based dietary standards. Food Nutr Bull. 2007;28:S1–53.

King J, Vorster H, Tome D. Nutrient intake values (NIVs): a recommended terminology and framework for the derivation of values. Food Nutr Bull. 2007;28:S16–26.

Mertz W, Abernathy C, Olin S. Risk assessment of essential elements. Washington, DC: ILSI Press; 1994:237–52.

Orriss GD. Food fortification: safety and legislation. Food Nutr Bull. 1998;19:109–15.

Pavlovic M, Prentice A, Thorsdottir I, Wolfram G, Branca F. Challenges in harmonizing energy and nutrient recommendations in Europe. Ann Nutr Metab. 2007;51108–14.

Prentice A, Branca F, Decsi T, Michaelsen K, Fletcher R, Guesry P, Manz F, Vidailhet M, Pannemans D, Samartin S. Energy and nutrient dietary reference values for children in Europe: Methodological approaches and current nutritional recommendations. Br J Nutr. 2004;92:S83–146.

Ramaswamy S, Viswanathan B. Trade development, and regulatory issues in food. Food Nutr Bull. 2007;28:S123–40.

Solomons NW, Kaufer-Horwitz M, Bermudez OI. Harmonization for mesoamerican nutrient-based recommendations: regional unification or national specification? Arch Latinoam Nutr. 2004;54:363–73.

Spierenburg TJ, De Graaf GN, Baars AJ, Brus DHJ, Tielen MJM, Arts BJ. Cadmium, zinc, lead and copper in livers and kidneys of cattle in the neighbourhood of zinc refineries. Environ Monit Assess. 1988;11:107–14.

Stover P. Human nutrition and genetic variation. Food Nutr Bull. 2007;28:S101–15.

Wahlqvist M. Regional food diversity and human health. Asia Pac J Clin Nutr. 2003;12:304–8.

Welch R, Graham R. Agriculture: the real nexus for enhancing bioavailable micronutrients in food crops. J Trace Elem Med Biol. 2005;18:299–307.

Vorster HH, Murphy SP, Allen LH, King JC. Application of nutrient intake values (NIVs). Food Nutr Bull. 2007;28:S116–22.

Yates A. Using criteria to establish nutrient intake values (NIVs). Food Nutr Bull. 2007;28:S38–48.

An invited paper presented in the plenary session "Trace Element Speciation"

Salivary arsenic as a biomarker for arsenic exposure

Kristi Lew[1], Chungang Yuan[1,2], Jason P. Acker[1,3], and X. Chris Le[1*]

[1]Department of Laboratory Medicine and Pathology, Faculty of Medicine and Dentistry, 10–102 Clinical Sciences Building, University of Alberta, Edmonton, Alberta, T6G 2G3, Canada Telephone: +1-780-4926416 Fax: +1-780-4927800
[2]School of Environmental Sciences and Engineering, North China Electric Power University, Baoding, 071003, Hebei Province, People's Republic of China
[3]Research and Development, Canadian Blood Services, 8249 114 Street, Edmonton, Alberta, T6G 2R8, Canada

Corresponding author:
E-mail: xc.le@ualberta.ca

Speciation of arsenic in human biological samples

Traditionally, human exposure to arsenic has been assessed in biological samples such as blood, urine, hair, and nails (Buchet et al. 1981; Das et al. 1996; Engstrom et al. 2007; Hopenhayn-Rich C et al. 1996; Le et al. 1994, 2000; Ma and Le 1998; Mandal et al. 2004; Tanaka et al. 1996; Todorov et al. 2005; Van Hulle et al. 2004; Zhang et al. 1995). Blood and urine are currently used for determining recent exposure to arsenic. Urine is the more commonly used sample for this purpose as arsenic has a longer half-life in urine than in blood. Conversely, hair and nail samples are used to measure past and long-term exposure to arsenic. Other biological samples tested for the measurement of arsenic in humans include stomach contents, breast milk, and bile (Gregus et al. 2000; Samanta et al. 2007; Tanaka et al. 1996).

A relatively new sample type for the measurement of arsenic concentrations is saliva (Yuan et al. 2008). There are several advantages to the use of saliva for determining arsenic concentrations: The collection procedure is non-invasive and saliva is easier to collect than urine, especially from young children, and there is high blood flow to the salivary glands, which allows for the excretion of drugs and other compounds (Hold et al. 1996). Saliva is similar to other body fluids in that it contains the same electrolytes. Its osmolality is also similar to that of plasma.

The current understanding of arsenic metabolism is that, as inorganic arsenic is absorbed, it is metabolized though a series of methylations (Cullen and Reimer 1989; Hayakawa et al. 2005). By performing arsenic analysis on saliva, the understanding of arsenic metabolism and excretion in humans can be enhanced. It was unknown what arsenic species are present in saliva, as there have been no data published on arsenic analysis in saliva. Our laboratory has been examining the use of saliva for the detection of arsenic biomarkers. The objectives consisted of developing a method for the detection of arsenic in saliva and identifying each species present. With these objectives achieved, we can demonstrate the potential use of salivary arsenic as a biomarker of arsenic exposure.

As the concentrations of analytes in human saliva are normally quite low, the method used for the detection of arsenic in saliva must be sensitive. We used high-performance liquid chromatography (HPLC) for separation of the arsenic species, coupled with inductively coupled plasma mass spectrometry (ICPMS) for detection. We confirmed the identity of each arsenic species using electrospray ionization tandem mass spectrometry (ESI–MS/MS) in the multiple reaction monitoring (MRM) mode.

For arsenic speciation, the samples were first diluted three times in distilled deionized water, ultrasonicated, and centrifuged. The supernatant was then filtered through 0.45-μm nylon membrane filters into HPLC vials for analysis. Chromatographic separation was performed using a reversed-phase and an anion exchange column. The identity of each arsenic species was confirmed using ESI–MS/MS in the negative ionization mode for inorganic trivalent arsenite (iAs(III)) and inorganic pentavalent arsenate [iAs(V)]. The positive ionization mode was used for the detection of dimethylarsinic acid (DMA(V)) and monomethylarsonic acid [MMA(V)].

With the techniques for the speciation and quantification of arsenic in saliva in place, we then performed an arsenic speciation study (Yuan et al. 2008). Saliva samples were collected from 32 volunteers from Edmonton, Alberta, Canada, who had been exposed to background levels of arsenic (less than 5 μg/l in drinking water). Figure 1 shows typical chromatograms from the HPLC–ICPMS analyses of a standard solution containing iAs(III), DMA(V), MMA(V), and iAs(V) and a saliva sample. The results show that iAs(III), DMA(V), and iAs(V) were detectable in this saliva sample. From the 32 volunteers, the mean value of the sum of arsenic species was 0.8 µg/l.

Saliva samples were then collected from 301 residents of Ba Men, Inner Mongolia, China. They were exposed to arsenic concentrations up to 826 µg/l in their drinking water. The species detected in these samples were similar to the ones found in the Edmonton residents with the exception of the presence of an unknown species. The mean sum of species in these samples was 11.9 µg/l. There is a good correlation between the arsenic concentration in drinking water and in saliva (r=0.610), as well as between the arsenic concentration in drinking water and in urine (r=0.644). This demonstrates that salivary arsenic can be used as a biomarker for assessing arsenic exposure.

Environmental exposure to arsenic

Industrial uses of arsenic compounds include their functions as a pesticide, a drug, an animal feed additive, and a wood preservative. As a wood preservative, it has been used for decades in the form of chromated copper arsenate (CCA). This compound is injected into wood through a process that uses high pressure to saturate the wood. CCA protects wood products from the deteriorative effects of fungi, molds, and termites. As of 2004, pesticide manufacturers have voluntarily phased out CCA use in Canada and the USA for wood products around the home [Health Canada Pest Management Regulatory Agency (HCPMR) 2005; United States Environmental Protection Agency (US EPA) 2008]. Because of the toxic effects of various arsenic compounds, public concerns arise over children's exposure to arsenic as a result of contact with CCA-treated wood in playground structures.

There are numerous studies on arsenic dislodging and leaching from CCA-treated wood onto the surrounding sand and soil (De Miguel et al. 2007; Nico et al. 2006; Shalat et al. 2006). Models have also been used to estimate children's exposure to arsenic based on the average child's hand surface area, activity patterns in playgrounds, and types of soil (Hemond and Solo-Gabriele 2004; US EPA 2003a, 2003b). The knowledge gap was a lack of direct measurements of the arsenic levels on the hands of children. Thus, we determined the quantitative amounts of arsenic and chromium on the hands of children playing on CCA-treated wood structures and in the sand surrounding the playgrounds (Kwon et al. 2004; Hamula et al. 2006).

We chose eight playgrounds constructed with CCA-treated wood and eight playgrounds that did not contain CCA-treated wood in the city of Edmonton. These represented several geographic locations and were similar in age and manufacturer. After children completed their play period on these playgrounds, their hands were washed in 150 ml of deionized water in a plastic bag for 1 min. The samples were taken to the laboratory, filtered, and stored at 4°C until analysis. Sand and soil samples from the surrounding playgrounds were also collected for arsenic analysis. The total arsenic quantification was performed using ICP–MS. The first measurement included the analysis of soluble arsenic on the children's hands; that is, the arsenic present in the filtrate after the original hand wash sample was filtered. Children playing on CCA-treated playgrounds had approximately five times as much arsenic in the filtrate as in the children playing on the non-CCA playgrounds. The difference in the amount of arsenic between the two types of playgrounds was statistically significant ($p<0.001$). The arsenic concentrations in the sand of these two types of playgrounds were not statistically significant ($p=0.07$). The amount of sand on the children's hands between the CCA and non-CCA playgrounds was also similar ($p=0.23$). The total arsenic on the children's hands is the sum of the insoluble arsenic on the filter plus the water soluble arsenic in the filtrate. The mean arsenic load in the samples from children playing on CCA playgrounds was 934 ng and in children playing on playgrounds not constructed from CCA-treated wood was 265 ng. There is also a significant difference between these values ($p<0.001$).

These results are useful in that it provides a direct measurement of arsenic on the children's hands following play on CCA-treated wood. The transfer of arsenic onto the children's hands was a result of direct contact with the sand and treated wood. As young children display a high hand-to-mouth frequency, they have the potential to ingest the arsenic on their hands. Children less than 24 months of age display hand-to-mouth contacts between 13 and 18 times per hour, whereas children over 24 months may place their hands in or near their mouths anywhere from 11 to 16 times per hour (AuYeung et al. 2004; Tulve et al. 2002). The main concern is with ingestion as the main route of arsenic exposure, as any dermal absorption would be minimal.

Arsenic biomonitoring in children playing on CCA and non-CCA playgrounds

Although the higher amounts of arsenic on the hands of children playing on CCA-treated playgrounds could potentially result in higher exposure to arsenic, it is not known whether this exposure is substantially higher than the daily exposure to arsenic from other sources, such as food and water. To address this concern, we designed an arsenic biomonitoring study that determined children's overall internal arsenic exposure levels. We performed quantification and speciation of arsenic in urine and saliva samples of children playing on CCA and non-CCA playgrounds. From our previous study, the maximum amount of arsenic collected from a child's hands was 4.7 µg. In Canada, the average daily intake of arsenic from food is 38 µg for adults and 15 µg in children between 1 and 4 years of age (Dabeka et al. 1993). Even if the maximum level of 4.7 µg of arsenic were ingested, this would be minor in comparison to what is ingested through the diet. Thus, we hypothesize that there will be no significant difference in the concentration and speciation patterns of arsenic in the urine and saliva samples of children playing on CCA and non-CCA playgrounds.

This work uses the methods previously developed and optimized by our laboratory for the speciation and quantification of arsenic in urine and saliva samples. We collected 56 urine samples and 78 saliva samples from children playing on CCA playgrounds. From the children playing on non-CCA playgrounds, we collected 45 urine samples and 47 saliva samples. The mean urinary arsenic concentrations in children playing on CCA playgrounds was 15 ± 28 µg/l and on non-CCA playgrounds was 12 ± 23 µg/l ($p=0.60$). The mean arsenic concentrations in the saliva of children playing on CCA playgrounds was 1.1 ± 2.1 µg/l and on non-CCA playgrounds was 1.4 ± 1.1 µg/l ($p=0.32$). These findings demonstrate that there were no significant differences in the arsenic concentrations in the urine and saliva samples of children playing on CCA and non-CCA playgrounds. We conclude that playing on CCA-treated wood playgrounds does not considerably contribute to children's total ingested arsenic.

Acknowledgment

We thank V. Charoensuk, A. Goulko, C. Hamula, U. Idiong, A. LeBlanc, X. Lu, and N. Oro for their help in this study. We also thank the children who participated in this study, along with their parents for their cooperation and help with the sample collection. This work was supported by Alberta Health and Wellness, the Metals in the Human Environment Strategic Network, the Canadian Water Network, and the City of Edmonton.

References

AuYeung W, Canales RA, Beamer P, Ferguson AC, Leckie JO. Young children's mouthing behavior: an observational study via videotaping in a primarily outdoor residential setting. J Child Health. 2004;2(3):271–95.

Buchet JP, Lauwerys R, Roels H. Urinary excretion of inorganic arsenic and its metabolites after repeated ingestion of sodium metaarsenite by volunteers. Int Arch Occup Environ Health. 1981;48:111–8.

Cullen WR, Reimer KJ. Arsenic speciation in the environment. Chem Rev. 1989;89(4):713–64.

Dabeka RW, McKenzie AD, Lacroix GM, Cleroux C, Bowe S, Graham RA, Conacher HP, Verdier P. Survey of arsenic in total diet food composites and estimation of the dietary intake of arsenic by Canadian adults and children. J Assoc Off Anal Chem Internat. 1993;76:14–25.

Das AK, Chakraborty R, Cervera ML, delaGuardia M. Metal speciation in biological fluids—a review. Mikrochim Acta. 1996;122(3–4):209–46.

De Miguel E, Iribarren I, Chacon E, Ordonez A, Charlesworth S. Risk-based evaluation of the exposure of children to trace elements in playgrounds in Madrid (Spain). Chemosphere. 2007;66(3):505–13.

Engstrom KS, Broberg K, Concha G, Nermell B, Warholm M, Vahter M. Genetic polymorphisms influencing arsenic metabolism: evidence from Argentina. Environ Health Perspect. 2007;115(4):599–605.

Gregus Z, Gyurasics A, Csanaky I. Biliary and urinary excretion of inorganic arsenic: monomethylarsonous acid as a major biliary metabolite in rats. Toxicol Sci. 2000;56(1):18–25.

Hamula CA. Wang Z, Zhang H, Kwon E, Gabos S, Li XF, Le XC. Chromium on the hands of children after playing in playgrounds built from chromated copper arsenate (CCA)-treated wood. Environ Health Perspect. 2006;114:460–5.

Hayakawa T, Kobayashi Y, Cui X, Hirano S. A new metabolic pathway of arsenite: arsenic-glutathione complexes are substrates for human arsenic methyltransferase Cyt19. Arch Toxicol. 2005;79:183–91.

HCPMR. Fact sheet on chromated copper arsenate (CCA) treated wood. Ottawa, ON, Canada: Health Canada Pest Management Regulatory Agency; 2005. http://www.pmra-arla.gc.ca/english/pdf/fact/fs_cca-e.pdf. Accessed 22 January 2007.

Hemond HF, Solo-Gabriele HM. Children's exposure to arsenic from CCA-treated wooden decks and playground structures. Risk Anal. 2004;24(1):51–64.

Hold K, de Boer D, Zuidema J, Maes R. Saliva as an analytical tool in toxicology. Int J Drug Testing. 1996;1(1):1–36.

Hopenhayn-Rich C, Biggs ML, Smith AH, Kalman D, Moore LE. Methylation study in a population environmentally exposed to high arsenic water. Environ Health Perspect 1996;104:620–8.

Kwon E, Zhang HQ, Wang ZW, Jhangri GS, Lu XF, Fok N, et al. Arsenic on the hands of children after playing in playgrounds. Environ Health Perspect. 2004;112(14):1375–80.

Le XC, Cullen WR, Reimer KJ. Human urinary arsenic excretion after one-time ingestion of seaweed, crab, and shrimp. Clin Chem. 1994;40(4):617–24.

Le XC, Lu XF, Ma MS, Cullen WR, Aposhian HV, Zheng BS. Speciation of key arsenic metabolic intermediates in human urine. Anal Chem. 2000;72(21):5172–7.

Ma MS, Le XC. Effect of arsenosugar ingestion on urinary arsenic speciation. Clin Chem. 1998;44(3):539–50.

Mandal BK, Ogra Y, Anzai K, Suzuki KT. Speciation of arsenic in biological samples. Toxicol Appl Pharmacol. 2004;198(3):307–18.

Nico PS, Ruby MV, Lowney YW, Holm SE. Chemical speciation and bioaccessibility of arsenic and chromium in chromated copper arsenate-treated wood and soils. Environ Sci Technol. 2006;40(1):402–8.

Samanta G, Das D, Mandal BK, Chowdhury TR, Chakraborti D, Pal A, et al. Arsenic in the breast milk of lactating women in arsenic-affected areas of West Bengal, India and its effect on infants. J Environ Sci Health Part A Toxic/Hazard Subst Environ Eng. 2007;42(12):1815–25.

Shalat SL, Solo-Gabriele HM, Fleming LE, Buckley BT, Black K, Jimenez M, et al. A pilot study of children's exposure to CCA-treated wood from playground equipment. Sci Total Environ. 2006;367(1):80–8.

Tanaka T, Hara K, Tanimoto A, Kasai K, Kita T, Tanaka N, et al. Determination of arsenic in blood and stomach contents by inductively coupled plasma/mass spectrometry (ICP/MS). Forensic Sci Int. 1996;81(1):43–50.

Todorov TI, Ejnik JW, Mullick FG, Centeno JA. Arsenic speciation in urine and blood reference materials. Microchim Acta. 2005;151(3–4):263–8.

Tulve NS, Suggs JC, McCurdy T, Hubal EAC, Moya J. Frequency of mouthing behavior in young children. J Expo Anal Environ Epidemiol. 2002;12(4):259–64.

US EPA. A probabilistic risk assessment for children who contact CCA-treated playsets and decks. Draft preliminary report. Washington, DC: Office of Pesticide Programs, Antimicrobial Division, US Environmental Protection Agency; 2003a.

US EPA. A probabilistic exposure assessment for children who contact CCA-treated playsets and decks using the stochastic human exposure and dose simulation model for the wood preservative exposure scenario (SHEDS–Wood). Draft preliminary report. Washington, DC: Office of Research and Development and Office of Pesticide Program, US Environmental Protection Agency; 2003b.

US EPA. Chromated copper arsenate (CCA)—fact sheets. http://www.epa.gov/oppad001/reregistration/cca/. Accessed on March 7, 2008.

Van Hulle M, Zhang C, Schotte B, Mees L, Vanhaecke F, Vanholder R, et al. Identification of some arsenic species in human urine and blood after ingestion of Chinese seaweed Laminaria. J Anal Atom Spectrom. 2004;19(1):58–64.

Yuan CG, Lu XF, Oro N, Wang ZW, Xia YJ, Wade TJ, Le XC. Arsenic speciation analysis in human saliva. Clin Chem. 2008;54(1):163–71.

Zhang X, Cornelis R, Dekimpe J, Mees L, Vanderbiesen V, Vanholder R. Determination of total arsenic in serum and packed cells of patients with renal insufficiency. Fresenius J Anal Chem. 1995;353(2):143–7.

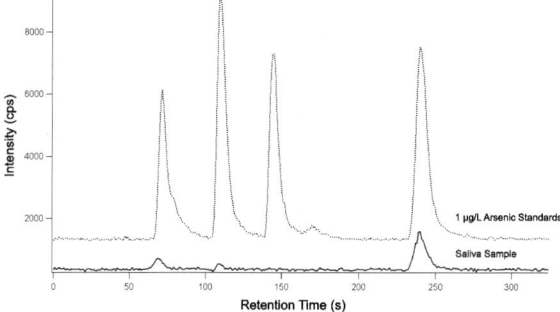

Fig. 1 Typical chromatograms displaying the separation of arsenic species in a saliva sample and a standard solution. A reverse phase column (ODS-3, 150×4.6 mm, 3-μm particle size; Phenomenex, Torrance, CA, USA) was used to separate the species. The mobile phase contained 5 mmol/l tetrabutylammonium hydroxide and 3 mmol/l malonic acid in 5% methanol, with the pH adjusted to 5.85. The flow rate was 1.2 ml/min. The ICP–MS monitored arsenic oxide (*m/z* 91). *Dotted line* 1 μg/l standards of iAs(III) (tR =75 s), DMA(V) (tR=115 s), MMA(V) (tR=148 s), and iAs(V) (tR=245 s). *Solid line* Saliva sample of an individual exposed to background levels of arsenic in drinking water (<5 μg/l).

An invited paper presented in the plenary session "Health consequences of trace element deficiencies"

Studies on the placental and mammary gland transfer of trace elements: Impact of possible trace element deficiencies in infancy

Erich Rossipal[1] and Michael Krachler[2]

[1]Department of Pediatrics, Medical School, University of Graz, Austria

[2]Institute of Environmental Geochemistry, University of Heidelberg, Germany

Corresponding author:
E-mail: krachler@ugc.uni-heidelberg.de
http://www.uni-heidelberg.de/institute/fak12/ugc/mkrachler/krachler.htm

Introduction

By the design of nature, the placenta has to secure the optimal flow of nutrients to the foetus and also has the function to eliminate foetal catabolic products. If these responsibilities are not disturbed, normal growth of the foetus during intrauterine life and its healthy development during the neonatal period is secured. Disturbances of this foetoplacental circulatory system inevitably lead to an intrauterine growth restriction. From the therapeutic point of view, only very little can be done about it, except by preventive measures like asking pregnant women very distinctly to refrain from smoking and to take an adequate diet.

After birth the design to nourish a newborn or infant up to the fifth month of age is breast-feeding. If this is not possible, we do have the therapeutic possibility of formula feeding. In any case, the foetoplacental circulatory system and mothers' milk have to be considered as gold standards to guarantee normal growth of the foetus, the mature newborn, and infants up to the fifth month of age.

Placenta

To increase our knowledge about the barrier function of the placenta at the end of gestation, we investigated the transfer of 17 selected trace elements in 29 maternal sera and corresponding umbilical cord sera. The mothers were healthy women, and the mature newborns were born between the 38th and the 40th week of gestation. We examined sera—instead of whole blood or plasma—to avoid the addition of an anticoagulant to the blood samples and hence potential contamination with trace elements. All trace elemental were determined using inductively coupled plasma-mass spectrometry (ICP–MS), applying suitable quality control measures (Krachler et al. 1999a).

Our investigations revealed significantly higher concentration of several essential trace elements in umbilical cord sera compared to that in corresponding maternal sera. Manganese, for example, showed an increase of 150% (*p*<0.005), Zn one of 148% (*p*< 0.0001), and Mg a value of 105% of the maternal serum content, i.e., 100% (Krachler et al. 1999b; Rossipal et al. 2000). These results indicate that the placenta activates the transfer of selected elements, yet the placenta can also show an inhibitory effect on the trace element transfer. The most pronounced effect that could be found concerned Cu. In umbilical cord serum (UCS), the Cu content was only 20% of that of maternal sera. But also the transfer of Se is inhibited (Rossipal et al. 2000). In UCS, the Se content was only 55% of the maternal serum. Concentrations of Co were only 60% and that of Sn 85% of the maternal value. Two toxic elements, namely Pb and Cd proved to have UCS concentrations of 50% and of 66% of the maternal sera, respectively. For the trace elements Li and Sr, the concentration gradient seems to be the decisive factor for the placental transfer. Correlation coefficients for the elemental distributions between the two compartments UCS and maternal sera were 0.98 and 0.96, respectively.

By evaluating the trace element concentration in UCS, we were aware of the fact that one is doing a measurement on a mixture of arterial and venous umbilical cord serum. What we wanted to find out was to determine the concentration difference between venous and arterial UCS. This investigation would allow figuring out which amount of different trace elements the foetus is incorporating at the end of gestation. To this end, small polyethylene catheters and syringes were used for sampling venous and arterial UCS. With this method, nine pairs of venous and arterial UCS of mature newborns were collected.

The investigations on these nine pairs of UCS samples revealed that, at the end of pregnancy, the baby is incorporating essential trace elements at a range of 2.5% to 16.7% (Rossipal et al. 2000). Our findings indicate—expressed as the median—an uptake of 2.5% of the Ca of the content of venous UCS. For Zn, the uptake amounts to 3.7%; for Mg, to 5.7%; and for Cu, to 11.4%. The highest absorption was found for Mn (16.2%) and Mo (16.7%), respectively. For Sn, no detectable uptake rates could be established.

Our studies also indicate that the foetus possibly excretes trace elements via the arterial UCS. This assumption holds especially true for Li and Sr (Rossipal et al. 2000). For Li, in six out of nine samples, there was excretion via arterial UCS; and for Sr, in two out of nine samples (Rossipal et al. 2000). The essential trace element Cu is also tentatively excreted via arterial UCS. In three out of nine samples investigated, the concentrations of Cu in arterial UCS were 2.1%, 4.0% and 7.6% higher than in venous UCS. This seems to be a mechanism maintaining homeostasis of Cu. Copper as

well as Zn is bound intercellularly to metallothionein. As there is an interchange between the Cu metallothionein pool and the caerulaplasmin pool, a surplus of Cu can be excreted by the latter pool via arterial UCS and placenta (Barrow and Tanner 1988; Bremner 1987; Ettinger et al. 1986; Weiss and Lindner 1985).

Concerning Zn, in one out of nine samples, the concentration in arterial UCS was 2.5% higher than in venous UCS. This finding points to a possible excretion mechanism via placenta comparable to that of Cu (Rossipal et al. 2000). Such a mechanism does not seem to exist for Ca and Mn (Rossipal et al. 2000).

Another important factor that may have an essential impact on uptake and excretion of trace elements is the absolute amount of blood that passes the umbilical cord. Ultrasound examinations with colour and pulsed waves Doppler modes, which were applied during recent years yielded valuable information in this respect (Bellotti et al. 2004). These studies highlighted that the blood flow in the umbilical vein approaches its maximum with 130 ml/min per kg foetal weight at the 27th week of gestation. It decreases to 70 ml/min per kg foetal weight at the 38th week of gestation. Both figures are values of the 50th percentile. As the hematocrit is increasing at the same time with a median value of 42% at the 27th week of gestation to a mean value of 51% at the 38th week, the flow of plasma is much more reduced. Compared with the total blood flow, the reduction in plasma flow amounts from 75 ml/min per kg foetal weight in the 27th week of gestation to 34 ml/min per kg foetal weight in the 38th week of gestation.

In this context, we would like to emphasise that the gain in weight of the foetus up to the 27th week of gestation is almost exclusively caused by the increase in weight of the tissue of the different organs. There is very little fat in the body apart from essential lipids in the nervous tissue at that time. From the 28th week of gestation on, fat begins to be deposited in the adipose tissue cells. At the 30th week of gestation, the fat accounts for 6.2% and, at birth, 13–15% of the weight of the baby. The relation of the increase of weight of the foetus from the 30th to the 40th week of gestation for lean body mass and fat is 40% to 60%. This change in metabolism could be caused by (1) an aging placenta, which no longer is able to keep up with the ever increasing demands of the foetus or (2) a change in aims and pattern of the metabolism of the foetus. The healthy newborn continues to lay down fat to an even greater extent. At the age of 4 months, fat is at its peak, making up about 25% of the weight of the infant. These facts are indicative for the latter mentioned cause of the change of the metabolism of the fetus (Widdowson and Spray 1951; Widdowson and Dickerson 1964; Widdowson 1985).

Mammary gland

The impact on trace element transfer by the tubulo alveolar mammary gland can be determined by investigating the concentrations of trace elements in maternal sera and in colostrum samples. We have evaluated the barrier function of the mammary gland, analysing 27 pairs of maternal sera and corresponding colostrums samples for nine essential trace elements. The transfer of the elements Ca, Co, Cu, Mg, Mn, Mo, Se, Sn, and Zn from maternal serum across the barrier of the epithelia of the mammary gland into colostrums did not reveal a homogenous pattern. The inequality of the transfer of the different trace elements can be demonstrated by setting the median (ng/l) of the maternal sera trace element concentrations—as a reference value—to 100% and comparing them with the median of the corresponding concentration in colostrum (Krachler et al. 1999b). The results of this investigation showed quite clearly that the mammary gland activates the transport of Zn, Mn, Sn, Ca, and Mg. The concentration of Zn was 1470%, of Mn 275%, of Ca 222%, of Sn 228% and of Mg 146% that of the maternal sera. In contrast, transfer of the three essential trace elements, Co, Se and Cu, is strongly inhibited by the mammary gland. Concentrations of Li and Sr were comparable in all pairs of maternal sera and corresponding colostrum samples. Therefore, solely a concentration gradient influence on the transfer between the two compartments maternal sera and colostrums could be established for these three trace elements.

During the course of lactation, there is a change of the pattern of transfer of trace elements by the mammary gland into human milk. We have investigated 18 samples of transitional milk (*T*, days 4–17), eight samples of mature milk M1 (days 42–60), eight samples of mature milk M2 (days 66–90) and eight samples of mature milk M3 (days 97–293) from healthy mothers on an adequate diet. The change in the transfer pattern of essential trace elements by the mammary gland can be highlighted by setting the median (ng/l) of the colostrum trace element concentrations to 100% and comparing them with the median of *T*, M1, M2 and

M3 human milk samples. Zinc and Co interestingly revealed increasing concentrations during the first 2 weeks of gestation, whereas Cu, Mn, and Mo showed a slight but distinct decrease at the same time. During the periods of mature milk production, there was a similar slight decrease in the concentrations of the trace elements Zn, Cu and Mo. Only Mn concentrations in mature milk remained quite stable (Krachler et al. 1998).

Among the trace elements investigated, Co showed a different behaviour. The concentration of Co increased during the course of lactation. The highest concentration of Co was found in the milk of mothers who breast-fed their babies for a period of 92–293 days. Our speculation on this data is that Co, as it is linked to antibody synthesis and phagocytic activity of neutrophils and macrophages, could be of great importance in the neonatal period and early infancy. At this time, babies have to build up there own immunological defence mechanisms.

Conclusions

Our findings indicate that the placenta can exhibit an activation or inhibition on the transfer of essential trace elements as well as a gradient mode of action for several other trace elements. Our results highlight that the placenta acts as an organ of excretion to maintain homeostasis between Cu and Zn, for example. There is a great demand for Zn during the period of about the 27th–28th up to the 38th–40th week of gestation. The total Zn content of the foetus at the 27th–28th week of gestation is about 18 mg. At term (38th–40th week of gestation), the baby has a total Zn content of about 58 mg. Premature babies lack this optimal Zn supply via the placenta and hence may show Zn deficiency in infancy.

The gestational period before the 28th week is devoted to the formation of organs, and the gain in weight is almost exclusively caused by the lean body mass enlargement. After that period, some organs, such as the liver, start to take up their functions. The liver serves as a blood and protein-forming organ, just to mention two of its functions. From the 28th week of gestation on, there is obviously a change in aims and pattern of the metabolism of the foetus. The gain in weight from that time on is caused by 40% by lean body mass and 60% of deposition of fat.

Concerning the human mammary gland, we could show that it may exert an activating, inhibiting, or gradient mode of action on the transfer of trace elements. The pattern of transfer for essential trace elements is changing during the course of lactation. In general, the transfer of trace elements is reduced. Interestingly, the trace element Co is an exception revealing increasing concentrations during the course of lactation. Our speculation of this data is that Co seems to be an important essential trace element in the neonatal period and in infancy because it is linked to immunological processes and to erythropoesis. Therefore, mothers' milk seems to keep up the high Co serum concentration of infants that is five times higher than in healthy adults.

Interestingly, there is also an increase of vitamin B_{12} concentration during the course of lactation. In colostrums, the concentration is ~0.06 µg/l and, in mature milk, ~0.34 µg/l (Wissenschaftliche Tabellen Geigy 1979). These findings also support to our speculation on the importance of Co in early infancy.

References

Barrow L, Tanner MS. Copper distribution among serum proteins in paediatric liver disorders and malignancies. Eur J Clin Invest. 1988;18:555–60.

Belotti M, Pennati G, De Gasperi C, Bozzo M, Battaglia FC, Ferrazzi E. Simultaneous measurements of umbilical veneous, fetal hepatic, and ductus venosus blood flow in growth-restricted human fetuses. Am J Obst Gynecol. 2004;190:1347–58.

Bremner I. Involvement of metallothionein to the hepatic metabolism of copper. J Nutr. 1987;117:19–29.

Ettinger MJ, Darwish HM, Schmitt RC. Mechanism of copper transport from plasma to hepatocytes. Fed Proc. 1986;45:2800–4.

Krachler M, Shi Li F, Rossipal E, Irgolic KJ. Changes in the concentration of trace elements in human milk during lactation. J Trace Elem Med Biol. 1998;12:159–76.

Krachler M, Rossipal E, Micetic-Turk D. Concentrations of trace elements in arterial and venous umbilical cord sera. Trace Elem Electrolytes. 1999a;16:46–52.

Krachler M, Rossipal E, Micetic-Turk D. Trace element transfer from the mother to the newborn: investigation on triplets of colostrum, maternal and umbilical cord sera. Eur J Clin Nutr. 1999b;53:486–94.

Rossipal E, Krachler M, Li F, Micetic-Turk D. Investigation of the transport of trace elements across barriers in humans: studies of placental and mammary transfer. Acta Paediatr. 2000;89:1190–5.

Weiss KC, Lindner MC. Copper transport in rats involving a new plasma protein. Am J Physiol. 1985;249: E77–88.

Widdowson EM, Spray CM. Chemical development in utero. Arch Dis Child. 1951;26:205–14.

Widdowson EM, Dickerson JWT. Chemical composition of the body. In: Comar U, Bronner F, editors. Mineral metabolism, vol. 2A. New York: Academic; 1964. pp. 1–247.

Widdowson EM. Growth and body composition in childhood. In: Clinical nutrition of the young child. Nestle Nutrition. New York: Ravens; 1985. pp. 1–14.

Wissenschaftliche Tabellen Geigy, Teilband Hämatologie und Humangenetik, 8th edition, Basel, Switzerland; 1979.

An invited paper presented in the plenary session "Health consequences of trace element deficiencies"

An adaptation of the in vitro digestion methodology employed in the prediction of iron bioavailability meets new challenges

Konstantina Argyri[1], Aggeliki Birba[1], Dennis D. Miller[2], Michael Komaitis[1] and Maria Kapsokefalou[1]

[1]Department of Food Science and Technology, Agricultural University of Athens, Iera Odos 75, Athens, 11634, Greece [2]Department of Food Science, Cornell University, Ithaca, NY, 14853, USA

Corresponding author:
kapsok@aua.gr

Iron bioavailability

Bioavailability, defined as the proportion of ingested iron that is available for use in metabolic processes or deposition in storage compounds, is a key concept in iron nutrition. Low bioavailability rather than the food iron content is the main reason that iron deficiency is one of the most common deficiencies worldwide. It is therefore crucial to be able to evaluate the bioavailability of iron from foods.

Iron bioavailability has been systematically studied in the past years and a great volume of information has been gathered. In general, plant foods have been shown to provide iron of low bioavailability, while foods that contain animal tissue provide iron of high bioavailability. Moreover, a variety of dietary factors that enhance or inhibit iron bioavailability have been identified. Meat and ascorbic acid are potent enhancers of iron bioavailability, while dietary fiber, protein sources other than meat, calcium, and tannins are inhibitors of iron bioavailability (Cook and Monsen 1976; Hallberg et al. 1986).

Despite the knowledge obtained so far, there is a continuous need for measuring or predicting iron bioavailability to meet new challenges in nutrition and in food technology. For example, new or novel food ingredients such as sterols, β-glucan, and prebiotics have been employed in the development of functional foods; new fortified foods (e.g. milk products and gluten-free bread) have been introduced into the market frequently formulated using new iron compounds as fortificants; local, ethnic, and traditional foods have attracted new interest in nutrition research because it appears that they contribute significantly in dietary intake of iron. Therefore, improved protocols for measuring iron bioavailability are demanded.

In vitro methodology for the prediction of iron bioavailability

Human studies provide ultimate answers in questions concerning nutrition issues, including iron bioavailability. However, in vitro methods can be rapid and inexpensive; therefore, they are attractive for screening purposes or as a first step in assessing iron bioavailability in a food or meal in humans. Therefore, results interpreted from in vitro methods may provide valuable contribution in setting up solutions regarding iron in our diets, provided that limitations are recognized and considered.

The in vitro digestion protocol as described by Kapsokefalou and Miller (1991)

An in vitro procedure for predicting the bioavailability of iron was proposed by Miller, Schricker, Rasmussen, and Van Campen in 1981, and was subsequently modified by Kapsokefalou and Miller (1991). This dialyzability method has been employed as a means for the prediction of iron bioavailability by many researchers (Chiplonkar et al. 1999; Drago and Valencia 2004; Forbes et al. 1989; Hazell and Johnson 1987; Kapsokefalou et al. 2005; Kloots et al. 2004; Whittaker et al. 1989). The index employed for the prediction of iron bioavailability is dialyzable iron.

Briefly, samples of 20 ml pH adjusted to 2.8 with concentrated HCl were transferred in 120 ml screw cap vials and placed in a shaking water bath maintained at 37°C. The samples are incubated for 2 h in the presence of 1 ml pepsin suspension added to each sample. At the end of this incubation, the pH of the samples is adjusted gradually from 2.8 to 6 with the aid of a dialysis sac filled with 20 ml of PIPES buffer, pH 6.3. The dialysis sac is immersed into the incubating samples. After 30 min, 5 ml of a pancreatin–bile salt mixture is added to the samples, and the incubation continues for another 2 h. At the end of this incubation period, the dialysis sac is removed. The dialysate, containing soluble compounds of low molecular weight, and the retentate, containing insoluble compounds and high-molecular-weight soluble compounds are collected. The pHs of the retentate and dialysate are recorded. Dialysates and retentates are centrifuged at $10,000 \times g$ for 20 min, and the supernatants are transferred for measurements of the iron concentration, spectrophotometrically, using ferrozin.

An adaptation of the in vitro digestion methodology

The in vitro procedure of Kapsokefalou and Miller (1991) as proposed so far has some practical limitations: Because of the relative large volume of the vials and space limitations in the water bath, only a small number of samples can be screened in one experiment (usually eight to ten samples in triplicate). Also, because of the large sample volume required (20 ml) to hold the dialysis bag immersed, it is difficult to test the effect of dietary components isolated in small amounts (e.g., fractions eluted from gel chromatography) or expensive compounds (e.g. phenol compounds or some proteins or peptides). Consequently, the in vitro method of Kapsokefalou and Miller (1991) was adapted to decrease the sample volume required, to allow greater sample through-put, and to lower the costs of materials and reagents employed.

A new approach to the in vitro procedure

The pH of samples is adjusted to 2.8 with 6 M HCl, and 2 ml aliquots are transferred to wells in a six-well plate. A 0.1-ml pepsin suspension is added to each well, and the plates are covered with a plastic lid. The plates are placed in a shaking incubator maintained at 37°C and are incubated for 2 h. At the end of this period, a cylindrical insert to the well plate, with a piece of dialysis membrane fastened to one end with an elastic band, is placed on top of each well in such a way that the membrane is in contact with the digest in the well (Fig. 1) as in Glahn et al. (1998). The insert is filled with 2 ml PIPES buffer, pH 6.3.

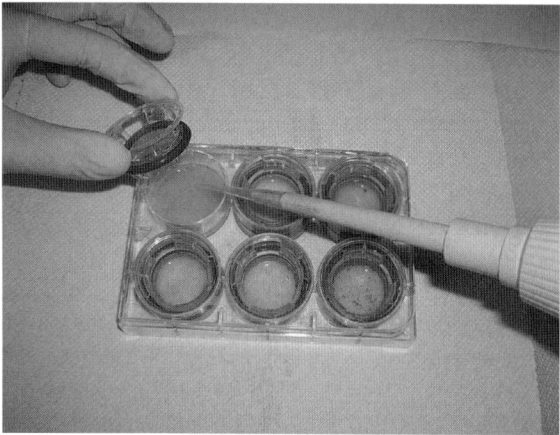

Fig. 1 In the proposed adaptation, the digestion procedure is performed in a six-well plate. The dialysis membrane is secured with an elastic band on a ring insert. Buffer digestive enzymes and bile salts are added as in the in vitro procedure described in the past by Kapsokefalou and Miller (1991).

The buffer diffuses through the membrane, thereby gradually adjusting the pH of the samples from 2.8 to 6. After 30 min, the insert is slightly lifted, a 0.5-ml of a pancreatin–bile salt mixture is added to the samples, the insert is replaced, and the incubation is continued for another 2 h. At the end of this incubation period, the insert holding the dialysis membrane is removed. The dialysate, containing soluble compounds of low molecular weight, and the retentate, containing insoluble compounds and high-molecular-weight soluble compounds are transferred to centrifuge tubes. The pHs of the retentate and dialysate are recorded. Dialysates and retentates are centrifuged at $10,000 \times g$ for 20 min, and the iron concentration is measured in the supernatants, spectrophotometrically in a microplate reader using ferrozin.

Evaluation of the newly proposed adaptation

The adaptation proposed herein was compared with the protocol of the dialyzability method previously proposed, the rational being that, if there are no differences in the results obtained with the two protocols, then the one introduced herein may be used as an alternative for the dialyzability method. A series of solutions (water, ascorbic acid, and phytate), liquid foods (fresh and condensed milk), and solid foods (meat and bread meal, and corn flakes) were tested in the presence of added

iron. These three categories have different physicochemical characteristics and consequently present different challenges in applying the procedure. The important finding of this study was that the convenient adaptation proposed herein produces results that are in good agreement with those obtained with the in vitro approach previously proposed (Fig. 2).

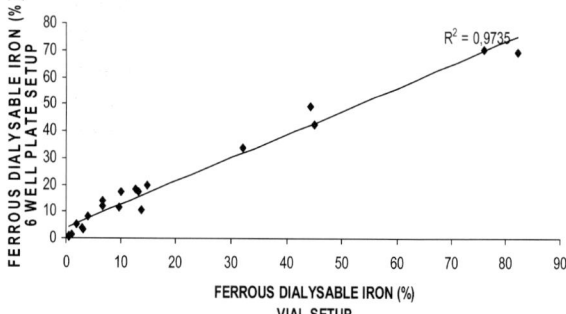

Fig. 2 Correlation of results obtained from the two protocols employed for the in vitro digestion procedure ("vial," for the method of Kapsokefalou and Miller 1991 and "six-well plate," for the adaptation proposed herein).

The adaptation proposed offers two important advantages. One is that it allows the parallel screening of a large number of samples, in comparison with the previously developed protocol. The option of stacking six-well plates in an incubator, instead of inserting vials in a space limiting water bath, facilitates the simultaneous, simple, and well-organized testing of many samples. Therefore, it reduces the time and the cost of the analysis. At the same time, it improves the ability to perform comparisons among samples because all would have been digested under the same conditions. The use of a microplate reader for the spectroscopic determination of iron that follows the in vitro digestion, although optional, further increases the efficiency of the system, as it enables the simultaneous analysis of up to 96 samples. This is very important for ferrous iron determination, which is time-dependent. Therefore, the combination of the in vitro system proposed with the plate reader as a tool for the iron analysis, provides accurate measurements in a large number of samples and in relatively little time.

Another advantage is that a smaller volume of sample (2 ml) is required for the digestion process in relation to the volume used in the previous protocol (20 ml). Therefore, it is feasible to test samples obtained in small volumes. This is an important advantage because some factors that need to be tested for their effect on iron dialyzability are available in small amounts. Examples include samples that are eluted through liquid chromatography or condensed extracts or expensive isolated compounds (e.g., phenol compounds or selected proteins or peptides). Testing these compounds is now possible to perform.

In conclusion, the adaptation proposed herein allows the rapid and efficient application of the dialyzability method. This adaptation was evaluated for its applicability and was compared with the one proposed in the past for the dialyzability method. The results from the two protocols were well correlated. These findings signify that the adaptation proposed herein produces comparable results with the protocol used until today for the application of the dialyzability method.

References

Chiplonkar SA, Agte VV, Tarwadi KV, Kavadia R. In vitro dialyzability using meal approach as an index for zinc and iron absorption in humans. Biol Trace Elem Res. 1999;67(3):249–56.

Cook JD, Monsen ER. Food iron absorption in human subjects. III. Comparison of the effect of animal proteins on nonheme iron absorption. Am J Clin Nutr. 1976; 29:859–67.

Drago SR, Valencia ME. Influence of components of infant formulas on in vitro iron, zinc, and calcium availability. J Agric Food Chem. 2004;52(10):3202–7.

Forbes AL, Adams CE, Arnaud MJ, Chichester CO, Cook JD, Harrison MN, Hurrell RF, Kahn SG, Morris ER, Tanner JT, Whittaker P. Comparison of in vitro, animal, and clinical determinations of iron bioavailability: international and nutritional anemia consultative group task force report on iron bioavailability. Am J Clin Nutr. 1989;49:225–38.

Glahn RP, Lee OA, Yeung A, Goldman MI, Miller DD. Caco-2 cell ferritin formation predicts nonradiolabeled food iron availability in an in vitro digestion/ Caco-2 cell culture model. J Nutr. 1998;128:1555–61.

Hallberg L, Brune M, Rossander L. Effect of ascorbic acid on iron absorption from different types of meals. Studies with ascorbic-acid-rich foods and synthetic ascorbic acid given in different amounts with different meals. Hum Nutr Appl Nutr. 1986;40(2):97–113.

Hazell T, Johnson IT. In vitro estimation of iron bioavailability from a range of plant foods: influence of phytate, ascorbate and citrate. Br J Nutr. 1987;57:223–33.

Kapsokefalou M, Miller DD. Effects of meat and selected food components on the valence of nonheme iron during in vitro digestion. J Food Sci. 1991;56(2):352–8.

Kapsokefalou M, Alexandropoulou I, Komaitis M, Politis I. In vitro evaluation of iron solubility and dialyzability of various iron fortificants and of iron-fortified milk products targeted for infants and toddlers. Int J Food Sci Nutr. 2005;56(4):293–302.

Kloots W, Op den Kamp D, Abrahamse L. In vitro iron availability from iron-fortified whole-grain wheat flour. J Agric Food Chem. 2004;52(26):8132–6.

Miller DD, Schricker BR, Rasmussen RR, Van Campen D. An in vitro method for estimation of iron availability from meals. Am J Clin Nutr. 1981; 34(10): 2248–56.

Whittaker P, Spivey Fox MR, Forbes AL. In vitro prediction of iron bioavailability for food fortification. Nutr Rep Int. 1989;39:1205–10.

An invited paper presented in the plenary session "Health consequences of trace element deficiencies"

Iodine intake, balance and normative requirement of man in Central Europe

Manfred Anke, Bernd Groppel and Ulrich Schäfer
Institute of Nutrition and Environment, Friedrich Schiller University of Jena, Jena, Germany

Corresponding author:
Manfred Anke, Am Steiger 12, 07743, Jena, Germany

In the past, Germany and Central Europe as a whole, was an iodine-deficiency region. In Germany, iodine deficiency developed in animals and man after World War II to varied degrees. In East Germany, no iodine deficiency existed until the late 1970s due to the importation of fish meal for farm animals. However, after the cessation of fish meal imports from Peru and substitution of rapeseed-extracted meal for this protein source, iodine deficiency appeared in the form of struma connata (piglets, calves, birds, dogs, and babies). After 1985, the feed for ruminants and later for hens and pigs was supplemented with mineral mixtures containing 10 or 5 mg I/kg (iodide in the beginning, iodate later). Together with the iodization of common salt with 20 mg I/kg, this increased the daily iodine intake by omnivorous people from <30 µg to approximately 50 and 60 µg for women and men, respectively.

The aim of our study was an analysis of the iodine intake, excretion, and apparent absorption by women and men with mixed and ovolactovegetarian diets in Central Europe and Mexico as a function of gender, time, age, body weight, season, region, and performance (breast-feeding), as well as the specification of the normative iodine intake and the limit for a beginning iodine overload. The determination of iodine intake by the duplicate portion technique was to provide new information about the influence of the changeover from local food production in the GDR to global trade and supermarket purchasing habits on the iodine consumption in Central Europe and far-away Mexico.

Iodine intake in Central Europe and Mexico by omnivorous and ovolactovegetarian adults

Following the reunification of German in 1990, iodine intake stagnated but then increased again in the following years to ultimately 80 µg per day in omnivorous women and 110 µg per day in men. The iodine consumption of ovolactovegetarians corresponded to that of omnivores. Milk and eggs deliver equal amounts of iodine to the food consumed by adults with both forms of nutrition (Table 1).

Mexican adults from rural regions of different geologies took in significantly higher amounts of iodine. The reason for the different iodine intake was iodination of industrially used salt, as in the USA. In Germany, it is expected that, during the period from 2005 to 2010, the daily iodine intakes of German male and female adults, respectively, also reach 150 and 200 µg/day on the average of a week. Meanwhile, Germany has allowed the iodination of industrially used salt and increased the iodine concentration of preserved vegetables, bread, rolls, and sausage dramatically. Actually, the iodination of industrially used salt was not necessary for satisfying the iodine requirement of 1 µg/kg body weight or 50 to 80 µg/day in women and 60 to 100 µg/day in men, which, on average, was already covered in 1996.

The significantly higher iodine intake by men compared with women is a result of their 24% higher dietary dry matter consumption and their preference for animal food compared with women, who favor vegetables. Regardless of the increasing iodine intake, Germans took in insufficient amounts of iodine at the end of the last century. The normative iodine requirement is similar to the iodine amount that is a component of thyroxine (T_4); in the case of women and men, this is ~65 µg I and ~75 µg I per day, respectively. Amazingly, the iodine intake by adults varies with habitat,

time, season, age, and body weight. Besides gender, the habitat has a significant influence on iodine intake.

Table 1 Daily iodine intake (µg) by German and Mexican women (W) and men (M) with omnivorous and ovolactovegetarian diets, varying with time and gender (n=1750)

Diet	Germany (G) or Mexico (M)	Year (for W, for M)	n	Women SD[c]	Women Mean[d]	Men Mean	Men SD	p value[a]	Percent[b]
Omnivores	G	1988	196, 196	36	51	57	35	<0.001	112
	G	1992	294, 294	30	47	66	52	<0.001	140
	G	1996	217, 217	47	83	113	59	<0.001	136
	M	1996	98, 98	118	150	195	134	<0.001	130
Vegetarians, %		1996	70, 70	52	80	123	80	<0.001	154
	G	1988: 1996			163	198			
	G: M	1996			181	173		-	
	MD: V	1996			96	109			

[a] p, significance level, Student's t test
[b] Women=100%, men=x%
[c] SD, standard deviation
[d] Arithmetic mean

From 1988 (consumption of locally produced food in East Germany) to 2007 (consumption of globally traded food), the iodine intake by both genders increased significantly. The WHO recommended a daily iodine intake of 200 µg by pregnant and nursing women. In Germany, pregnant and nursing women without iodine supplementation by iodine-containing tablets took in 150–210 µg per day between the seventh month of pregnancy and the 35th day of nursing. Approximately 10% to 20% of the tested women ingested <100 µg I per day. Amazingly, iodine intake by omnivorous adults varies with the season. In winter, women and men consumed 40% more iodine than in summer, the reason being a higher intake of fruits and beverages during summer than in winter.

In 1996, 29% and 26% of German women and men, respectively, took in <1.0 µg I/kg body weight, while on the whole, omnivorous women and men typically consumed 1.3 and 1.5 µg I per day, respectively, and ovolactovegetarian women and men took in 1.4 and

1.8 µg I/kg body weight and day, respectively. The normative requirement of adult men was found to be 1 µg/kg body weight and day, while the iodine intake recommended by the World Health Organisation (WHO) is 2 µg per day and kilogram body weight over a week. In contrast to these data for Europe, women and men in Mexico consumed 2.5 and 2.6 µg I/kg body weight and day, which satisfy the recommend iodine level. It is anticipated that this intake will be reached in Germany before 2010.

Iodine apparent absorption, excretion, and balance of omnivorous and ovolactovegetarian adults

In the past, iodine intake was equated to renal iodine excretion, with fecal excretion of iodine being neglected. In two test populations with daily iodine intakes of 34 µg in women and 48 µg in men, renal excretion was found to be 21 and 28 µg per day, and fecal excretion 15 and 18 µg per day, respectively. Under these experimental conditions, 42% and 39%, respectively, of the iodine intake was excreted fecally (Table 2). Generally, feces seem to contain a relatively constant amount of iodine. The iodine in the digestive tract of humans originates from the bile (<10 µg per day) and is composed primarily of organic materials. Very little inorganic iodine is found in the feces. At an iodine intake of 30 to 100 µg per day by humans, average daily fecal excretion amounted to 15 µg.

The main excretory routes for iodine are the kidneys and the breast or udder, which compete with the thyroid for plasma iodine. Kidneys and mamma lack a mechanism to conserve iodine. The levels of iodine excretion via urine and milk correlate well with plasma iodine concentrations and iodine intake. The iodine contents of urine and milk are very good indicators of iodine status and intake if fecal iodine excretion by humans (and animals) is taken into consideration. On average, the apparent iodine absorption rate in men amounted to 83%. Breastfeeding women with 146 µg I/day had an apparent absorption rate of 93%, and nursing woman with 312 µg I/day reached only 74%. Women and men with poor iodine content in the thyroid accumulate more iodine in the thyroid and have a high apparent absorption rate and a high positive balance of iodine. On average, women and men had an iodine balance varying between −15 and

+27%, or +7% on average. The balance demonstrated the normal iodine intake, which allows normal thyroxin production.

Table 2 Intake, excretion, apparent absorption, and balance of omnivores and ovolactovegetarians (97 women, 69 men; n=2,338)

Parameter	Women						Men	
	Omnivores					Ovolacto-vegetarian	Omni-vores	Ovolacto vegetarian
	Breast feeding		Not breast-feeding					
	1	2	1	2	3			
Intake (µg/day)	146	75	64	103	251	80	123	90
Excretion Milk µg/day	66	163	–	–	–	–	–	–
Urine µg/day	62	81	51	72	159	76	93	70
Feces µg/day	10	24	16	20	23	16	17	16
Excretion Milk %	48	51	–	–	–	–	–	–
Urine %	45	25	76	78	87	83	85	81
Feces %	7	74	24	22	13	17	15	19
Apparent absorption rate, %[a]	93	74	75	81	91	80	86	82
Balance µg/day	+8	−7	−3	+11	+68	−12	+13	+4
Percent	+5	−2	−4	+11	+27	−15	+11	+4

[a]Apparent absorption = [consumed iodine − (fecal iodine excretion × 100)]/consumed iodine

Iodine deficiency in humans

The only known metabolic role of iodine is the synthesis of the thyroid hormones thyroxine (T_4) and triiodothyroxine (T_3). The thyroid of adult humans must trap about 60–65 µg I per day to provide adequate amounts to humans. The normal human adult thyroid contains about 70–80% of the total iodine stored in the body (14–20 mg). The follicular cells of the thyroid extract iodine from the blood, with iodine trapping being dependent on thyroid stimulating hormone (TSH) produced in the anterior pituitary gland. In several steps, the iodine trapped is converted into T_4, T_3, and a small amount of 3,5,3'-triiodothyronine (reserve T_3). Now, it is known that T_4, which is produced in man at a daily rate of 110 mmol, is deiodinated to T_3 and reserve T_3 by deiodinase in a wide range of tissues. There is also evidence that the T_3 form is more potent than the T_4 form. Deiodination of T_4 is catalyzed by three different deiodinases, which are selenium-depen-dent. In an endemic iodine- and selenium-deficient region of Germany (Thuringia), the iodine intake by nursing women on the 35th day after birth was nor-malized by iodinated salt, and a normal serum T_4 content developed, but it was not possible to normalize the f T_3 level in the blood serum (Table 9; f = free; Table 3).

Table 3 Iodine and selenium intake by nursing women, and iodine, thyroxine, and free triiodothyronine contents of the blood ($n=14$)

Parameter	Placebo SD	Mean	Preparation Mean	SD	p value	Percent[a]
Intake I (μg day^{-1})	88	146	312	127	<0.001	214
Se (μg l^{-1})	6.2	14	69	4.6	<0.001	493
Serum I (μg l^{-1})	6	63	59	28	>0.05	94
T_4 (nmol l^{-1})	13	98	92	10	>.005	94
f T_3 (pmol l^{-1})	0.3	2.0	4.7	0.5	<0.001	235

[a]Placebo = 100%, preparation = x%

The glutathione peroxidase activity (GSH–Px) of the women's blood serum (170 U/L) and their TSH concentration (2.0–2.5 mEqL) were normal. Supple-mentation with 50 μg Se and 100 μg I per day from the end of the seventh month of pregnancy to the 35th day of nursing normalized the serum f T3 level. Serum GSH–Px activity was not effected by the application of 50 μg Se per day. Selenium supplementation clearly increased the iodothyronine 5′-deiodinase activity and normalised the f T3 concentration. A normalization of iodine metabolism is only given if both the iodine and selenium requirements are met. The normative iodine

and selenium requirements of adult humans amount to 1 μg I/kg body weight or 50 to 90 μg I/day and 0.4 μg Se/kg body weight or 20 to 25 μg Se/day. The recom-mended iodine and selenium intakes are 2 μg I and 0.6 μg Se/kg body weight or 100 to 180 μg I/day and 30 to 50 μg Se/day.

The use of iodinated mineral mixtures for farm animals and the iodination of kitchen salt and salt used in the manufacturing of processed foods were found to satisfy the iodine requirement of humans (Anke 2007). The consumption of iodinated salt in iodine deficiency is correlated with the appearance of an iodine-induced hyperthyreosis in a limited number of elderly people. This iodine-induced hyperthyreosis is also common in Germany, Europe, and worldwide, affecting ~5% of the population. For that reason, the "working group" re-commended to limit the iodine intake to 500 μg/day. The normative requirement of adults is 1 μg/kg body weight, which is satisfied to >95%. The consumption of 2 μg I/kg body weight is recommended. To attain an intake of 500 μg I/day, it is necessary to consume 7 μg I/kg body weight (70 kg; Anke 2004).

References

Anke M. Iodine. In: Merian E, Anke M, Ihnat M, Stoeppler M, editors. Elements and their compounds in the environment. Weinheim: Wiley–VCH; 2004. pp. 1457–95.

Anke M. Iod. In: Dunkelberg H, Gebel T, Hartwig, editors. Handbuch der Lebensmitteltoxikologie. Weinheim: Wiley–VCH; 2007. pp. 2317–79.

Cell motility assays

Angela Hague · Gareth E Jones

Originally published in the journal Cell Biology and Toxicology, Volume 24, Nos 4–5, 101–109.
DOI: 10.1007/s10565-007-9049-3 © Springer Science + Business Media B.V. 2007

Abstract This report summarises practical aspects to measuring cell motility in culture. The methods described here were discussed at a 1-day European Tissue Culture Society (ETCS-UK) workshop organised by John Masters and Gareth E Jones that was held at University College London on 19th April 2007.

Keywords Migration · Motility · Invasion · Protocols

Cell attachment assays

Cell attachment assays are important measures of integrin-mediated adhesion. To assess the involvement of particular integrins, adhesion can be measured using cells pre-incubated with specific integrin-blocking antibodies or using cells deficient in specific integrin

A. Hague (✉)
Department of Oral and Dental Science,
University of Bristol,
Lower Maudlin Street,
Bristol BS12LY, UK
e-mail: a.hague@bristol.ac.uk

G. E. Jones
Randall Division of Cell and Molecular Biophysics,
King's College London,
New Hunt's House, Guy's Campus,
London SE1 1UL, UK

subunits. The specific combination of alpha and beta integrin subunits verifies ligand specificity. For example, integrin $\alpha 3\beta 1$ is the main receptor for an extracellular component, laminin, and is highly expressed on keratinocytes during wound healing (Hodivala-Dilke et al. 1998). At the meeting, Kairbaan Hodivala-Dilke (CRUK Laboratories, Bart's and the London) creatively illustrated how integrins alter conformation when they become activated using members of the audience to enact the process! (see Hodivala-Dilke et al. 2003). Cell attachment assays are important because they tell us about the function of integrins, rather than just their expression. Kairbaan described methods for measuring attachment of cells to a substrate in detail. These methods involve either counting whole cells or colorimetric assays.

For the whole cell assays, she described how these can be carried out on bacteriological 96-well plate lids, which have a raised ring of plastic which acts as a very nice boundary for coating with different matrices and seeding out cells. Note that when doing matrix coating, the thawing of matrices is critical to the success of the assay – laminin 1 is thawed slowly on ice, while fibronectin and collagen VI are thawed quickly at 37°C and then placed on ice. A matrix concentration that is suboptimal for the specific cell type should be selected (typically 1–10μg/ml). The protein synthesis inhibitor cycloheximide can be used to prevent cells from producing their own matrix if necessary. Once the matrices have polymerised excess liquid is carefully sucked off (avoiding cross-contamination between the wells), and the plates are washed briefly with phosphate-buffered saline (PBS). The lids are immersed in a blocking solution of 0.1% heat-inactivated bovine serum albumin (BSA) in PBS for 2h at 37°C in a humidified chamber. Tryspinised cells are washed twice in OPTIMEM and plated at 3×10^4 per circle in 80μl. For this, a multichannel pipette is essential. They are left to adhere for 45min at 37°C in a humidified chamber. The adherence time depends on the cell type – 30–60min is typical. Non-adherent cells are gently washed off with PBS. If washing plates manually, a "dip and flick" method should be used, turning the plate around during washing such that it is flicked in two directions. The remaining adherent cells are fixed using 4% paraformaldehyde for 20min at room temperature. To stain the cells, lids are immersed in 0.1% methylene blue solution for 2–24h before washing with distilled water. Stained cells are counted under the microscope for four to six fields going across the well in a methodical fashion – not randomly because the seeding is never random – there are always edge effects. The results are given as mean number of adherent cells per field. For functional blocking studies, cells are incubated for 20min on ice with the blocking antibody before plating. One of the advantages of the whole-cell counting method is that it is also possible to score the number of cells that are still rounded and the number that have spread and flattened.

For colorimetric adhesion assays, the 96-well plate is used in the usual way, coating the wells in a humidified chamber. After PBS washing, the plates are blocked for 1h at 37°C with 50μl 2% BSA in PBS. Three empty wells are also blocked for each cell line or antibody combination to give an indication of background binding. Wells are washed once with 100μl PBS. Cells are seeded into the wells at 1×10^4 per well in 50μl OPTIMEM and are left to adhere for 30–40min at 37°C in a humidified chamber. Wells are washed three times with 100μl PBS to remove non-adherent cells. Kairbaan then uses a substrate buffer of 7.5mM *p*-nitrophenyl *N*-acetyl-beta-D-glucosami-dem (NPAG) and 0.1M sodium citrate, pH5.0 mixed 1:1 with 0.5% Triton-X-100 to lyse and stain the cells. Of this substrate buffer, 50μl is added to each well and incubated overnight at 37°C. Stop buffer of 50mM glycine, pH10.4 with 5mM EDTA is added 75μl per well, and the optical density is measured on a plate reader at 405nm.

Video tracking of cells

Time-lapse acquisitions permit the observation and investigation of fast (milliseconds) or slow (hours, days) cellular motility events. Video tracking involves measuring the position of objects of interest (wound edges; whole cells; intracellular vesicles) in these sequences at each time point. One consideration when choosing an assay is how these objects are to be tracked post-acquisition. Deborah Aubyn (London Research Institute) described two main modes of tracking software available for digital sequences, Automatic and Interactive. Each mode has advantages and disadvantages, which Deborah illustrated by using random walk assays. For these, she showed how a homemade chamber slide can be used. This consisted of a slide with holes drilled into it, sealed with a large coverslip on the bottom and a round coverslip on the top. A key consideration here is avoidance of evaporation and stable CO_2 provision or use of Hanks or Hepes to buffer pH. Automatic tracking software can produce a large amount of quantitative data fairly quickly for statistical analysis, if the size, intensity and shapes to be tracked are consistent. Deborah suggested that Volocity or Meta-morph software can be used in combination: Meta-morph morphological filters can be used to emphasise objects, then Volocity can be used to make the measurements. Interactive tracking software is slower in generating quantitative data as it is more labour intensive for the user and, therefore, generates less data. However, interactive tracking has the advantages of being able to resolve the fine detail of motility and being applicable to all digital sequences. Tracking can either be done with the mouse, which requires a steady hand, or using clicked points, clicking the position of a cell on each frame. Track data can be translated into speed values over time for statistical analysis using Mathematica software.

Rolling adhesion assays for leukocytes

The passage of leukocytes from the bloodstream into surrounding tissues is a fundamental aspect of immune surveillance and inflammation. Cell-to-cell contact between leukocytes and endothelial cells that line blood vessel walls involves a large number of cell adhesion molecules derived from both cell types, which collectively contribute to the well-characterised "multistep adhesion cascade". The parallel plate flow chamber is used to mimic leukocyte endothelial cell interactions *in vitro* and enables individual steps of the adhesion cascade to be studied in isolation – for example, tethering, rolling, firm adhesion and transmigration. Aleksandar Ivetic (Imperial College, London) discussed some common uses for the parallel plate flow chamber and showed us some remarkable video of rolling leukocytes moving across a surface of endothelial cells, with occasional cells showing transient tethering – a brief "sticking and stopping" of the flowing cells. Leukocytes sense pro-inflammatory clues such as chemoattractants on the endothelial cell surface. They have rolling receptors on the tips of microvilli on the leukocyte surface that interact with glycoproteins on the endothelial cells. The leukocytes can be fluorescently labelled, for example, with CellTracker Green (Molecular Probes), which allows them to be imaged through the cultured sheet of endothelial cells. In other experiments, empty ligand-coated slides can be used. For example, L-selectin is a leukocyte cell adhesion molecule that mediates the initial capture (tethering) and subsequent rolling of leukocytes along ligands normally expressed on endothelial cells; the parallel plate flow chamber has been used to illustrate that L-selectin mutants that cannot bind ERM proteins have reduced tethering to the L-selectin ligand P-selectin glycoprotein ligand-1, but that their rolling velocity on P-selectin glycoprotein ligand-1 is not affected (Ivetic et al. 2004). In the chamber, a shear stress is created such that the liquid flows over the slide, and the moving leukocytes (at about 3×10^5/ml) are video-imaged. To measure the transient tethering of leukocytes to the endothelial cells, "Cell Motion" software is used. This indicates that rolling cells travel at between 3 and 200µm/s. Arrested cells travel at less than 3µm/s. The software is critical for quantification, as tethering is transient, and there are typically 30 cells in a field at a given time. This cell system represents a true triumph in cell culture modelling of *in vivo* processes.

Method of quantifying transendothelial migration

Transendothelial migration (TEM) is the process by which leukocytes exit the bloodstream, traversing the walls of blood vessels to infiltrate the underlying tissues. Under normal conditions, the number of transmigrating cells is small; however, it increases dramatically during inflammation and contributes significantly to the pathogenesis of inflammatory diseases such as rheumatoid arthritis as well as non-inflammatory diseases such as atherosclerosis and cancer. TEM is a multistage process, and efforts to design new disease treatments require assessment of leukocytes numbers at each step. Inflammatory cytokines induce expression of E- and P-selectins on the surface of endothelial cells lining blood vessels, which allow leukocytes to be captured from the bloodstream. Captured leukocytes form a firm attachment by binding adhesion receptors ICAM-1 and VCAM-1 and, subsequently, migrate across the surface of the endothelium in search of a suitable transmigration site. TEM occurs either by disruption of, and transit between, endothelial junctions (paracellular TEM), or directly through endothelial cells by inducing formation of transcellular channels (transcellular TEM). Rob Cain (King's College, London) showed us how this can be modelled *in vitro* using cultured endothelial cells and leukocytes. Many TEM quantification methods exist, which draw on multiple techniques, including confocal and time-lapse microscopy and use of Boyden chambers. HUVEC cells are grown on a collagen gel support in a transwell insert to form a sheet of cells through which movement of CellTracker-labelled leukocytes towards a chemoattractant can be measured. Leukocyte TEM can also be examined under flow conditions in a parallel-plate flow chamber (Millán et al. 2006).

The Dunn Chemotaxis chamber

Cell chemotaxis is conventionally defined as the migratory response of cells to a gradient of diffusible reagent. The most commonly used method for assaying cell chemotaxis is the Boyden chamber or its many variants, based upon scoring cells that have migrated through a filter membrane towards a source of chemotactic factor. Although it is useful for screening potential chemoattractants, it has limitations for studying the mechanisms that underlie the chemotactic responses of cells. Unequivocal confirmation of chemotaxis requires direct observation of the cells, together with knowledge of the direction and magnitude of the concentration gradient of the diffusing factor. The chemotaxis Dunn chamber was developed to address these issues. It has proved to be immensely successful and, from early beginnings some 15 years ago, has become one of the major tools for chemotaxis workers.

Gareth Jones (King's College, London), spoke about how his group have used the Dunn chamber to analyse the chemotactic responses of a variety of cell types (Jones et al. 2000; Kellie et al. 2004). This allows direct visualisation of cells under conventional phase contrast optics as they move under the influence of a linear gradient of diffusing chemo-attractant. The device is simple in concept, and resembles a modified Helber bacteria counting chamber with two concentric circular wells and an optical bridge between them. It can be purchased from Hawklsey (http://www.hawksley.co.uk/cell-count_glassware/05c_spec-chambers/index.shtml). Cells grown on a coverslip can be inverted onto the chamber, which will contain the chemoattractant in the outer ring and the inner ring acting as a sink. Initially, both concentric wells of the chemotaxis chamber are filled with medium, and the coverslip seeded with cells is inverted over the chamber in an offset position to leave a narrow slit at one edge for access to the outer well. This is sealed in place using hot wax mixture (vaseline:paraffin:beeswax – 1:1:1) around all the edges except for the filling slit. To set up a chemotactic gradient, the medium is drained from the outer well via a fine-bore syringe needle and replaced with medium containing chemoattractant (100–200μl). The Dunn chamber must be pre-warmed and pre-gassed, with an air bubble in the outer well to act as a sink for carbon dioxide. Then, the filling slit is sealed with the hot wax mixture. A diffusion gradient is formed, the slope of which depends on the cubed root of the molecular weight of the chemo-attractant. For example, a 36-kD protein would form a stable gradient after 30min. Horizon plots can be calculated using in-house software (available upon request) that quantify not only the number of cells that migrate beyond a selected distance from their origin, but also provide a statistical test of unidirectional migration (Jones et al. 2000; Fig. 1).

Wound healing and scattering assays

During embryogenesis, metastasis and regeneration, normally sedentary cells become migratory. Claire

Wells (King's College London) described here two *in vitro assays,* the wound-healing assay and the cell scattering assay, which seek to model stimulated cell migration. In a wound-healing assay, cells in a confluent monolayer are stimulated to migrate by the creation of an artificial wound. Cells either move as individuals as or as part of a group to close the wound, enabling the researcher to study cell–cell interactions, directed migration into the wound and single cell migration. This technique has been used to study the migration of epithelial and mesenchymal cells. In a cell-scattering assay, agents are used to stimulate the dissociation and dispersion of epithelial cells from small clusters (or colonies). This method allows the study of cell–cell dissociation and initiation of single-cell migration, a process often referred to as epithelial–mesenchymal transition.

During wound healing, considerable cell proliferation occurs. Proliferating cells at a wound edge find substrate to adhere to and, hence, push the leading edge of the wound forward. Inhibiting proliferation inhibits migration in wound healing assays. In *in vitro* wound healing assays or "scratch assays", a confluent monolayer is scratched with a yellow Gilson tip, and wound closure is measured. Clare referred us to Denker and Barber (2002) for wound healing assay protocols. The density of the confluent monolayer is important in determining how fast the wound closes; therefore, it is critical to keep to the same cell density each time and to be consistent in methodology between experiments. Seeding cells onto gridded coverslips helps to quantify wound closure, particularly if time lapse movies are being used. These allow the same area of the coverslip and, hence, of the scratch, to be measured over time. High-power views also give information on why cells do not close a wound or how cells are behaving during wound closure – for example, information on proliferation and motility can be obtained by time lapse microscopy. The localisation of the Golgi apparatus in moving cells is informative, as the Golgi orientates towards the wound.

To illustrate scatter assays, Clare used the example of DU145 human prostate cells. Small colonies that are clearly separated are required for this assay. In response to hepatocyte growth factor, these cells show a ruffling response at 5min, followed by peripheralisation of actin at 4h and scattering by 24h (Wells et al. 2005). This process can be quantified by measuring the relative spread area or the percentage of cells with elongated morphology. As cells scatter and divide within the colony, cell migratory speed is difficult to measure. On low-power time lapse images, colonies can be categorised into (1) tight colonies; (2) attempted (partial) scattered colonies; (3) scattered colonies. Using immunocytochemistry, it is possible to score, for example, E-cadherin-positive adhesions and paxillin-positive focal complexes.

Transwell migration and chemotaxis assays

Quantitative measurement of migration is essential to understand the molecular pathways controlling this behaviour in normal (wound healing) and transformed (cancer) cell behaviour. Similarly, reliable migration assays are required to screen for drugs that may modulate this process. When considering the role of the matrix in motility, scratch assays have the disadvantage that it is not possible to control how much matrix is scratched off. A modified Boyden chamber is used for transwell assays, in which cells migrate through pores in a semipermeable membrane from the top of the chamber to the bottom. John Marshall (Bart's and the London) beautifully illustrated, using scanning electron microscopy, how cells adhere to the upper surface of this semipermeable membrane and spread themselves over it. The thickness of this membrane is only 10μm and typically for 10–20μm diameter cells, an 8-μm pore size is used. Therefore, to migrate through the pores of the membrane, cells must receive a stimulus to do so, and they must physically "squash" themselves through. In chemotaxis assays, a chemokine is placed in the lower well, beneath the insert with the semipermeable membrane (Fig. 2a). Cells will move towards the higher concentration of chemoattractant, but the gradient will only be maintained for a few hours. Therefore, the usefulness of this type of assay will depend on the speed of migration relative to the speed of diffusion. In haptotaxis assays, an extracellular matrix is used to coat the base of the inserts, depending on the integrin heterodimer-mediating cell movement (Fig. 2b). For example, the $\alpha_v\beta_6$ integrin mediates keratinocyte migration on fibronectin, vitronectin and transforming growth factor ß (TGF-ß) latency-associated peptide (LAP; Ramsay et al. 2007). The base of the insert is coated with extracellular

matrix protein solution, typically for 15–60min. The protein not only coats the base, but also enters some of the pores in the membrane. The inserts are blocked in BSA for 30min. For 24-well plates, 500μl serum-free medium is placed in the bottom well, and 100μl of cell suspension (5×10^4 cells per insert) in serum-free medium is placed inside the insert. Harvesting is usually after 8–24h, when, the number of cells that have migrated to the bottom of the insert is measured. The cells do not fall off into the wells, but remain adherent to the underside of the semipermeable membrane. The cells can be trypsinised off from both the upper and lower chambers for as long as 1h and counted using an accurate automatic cell counter such as a Casy counter. Alternatively, cells on the top and bottom of the membrane can be stained using crystal violet, and a colorimetric approach taken. The stained cells from the upper side of the insert are removed using a cotton wool bud, and it usually takes two cotton wool buds to get the inside of the insert completely clean. The crystal violet is solubilised in 10% acetic acid, and the intensity of stain is measured using a spectrophotometer at 560nm. A further method is to use fluorescently stained cells and to measure the proportion moving through the membrane of a FluoroBlock transwell system. These plates have fluorescence opaque blocking microporous membranes in the inserts, and the wells have opaque sides, such that fluorescence from cells in the top chamber of the insert is blocked from detection of cells on the underside of the insert, and fluorescence from one well is not picked up in the next.

Gel invasion

In vivo, most cells move within three-dimensional (3D) environments that are significantly different from the two-dimensional environments that are conventionally used in cell motility assays. Cedric Gaggioli (London Research Institute) discussed methods for analyzing cell motility in 3D environments *in vitro* and referred to published methods in Hooper et al. (2006). Gels of Collagen I and Matrigel (1:1) can be used which combine fibrous and gel-like properties. Collagen I, 2–8mg/ml, and 2.5–8mg/ml Matrigel will give a 3D matrix rather than a coating. Fluorescently labelled collagen can be used for imaging the collagen fibres. There are several different configurations for invasion

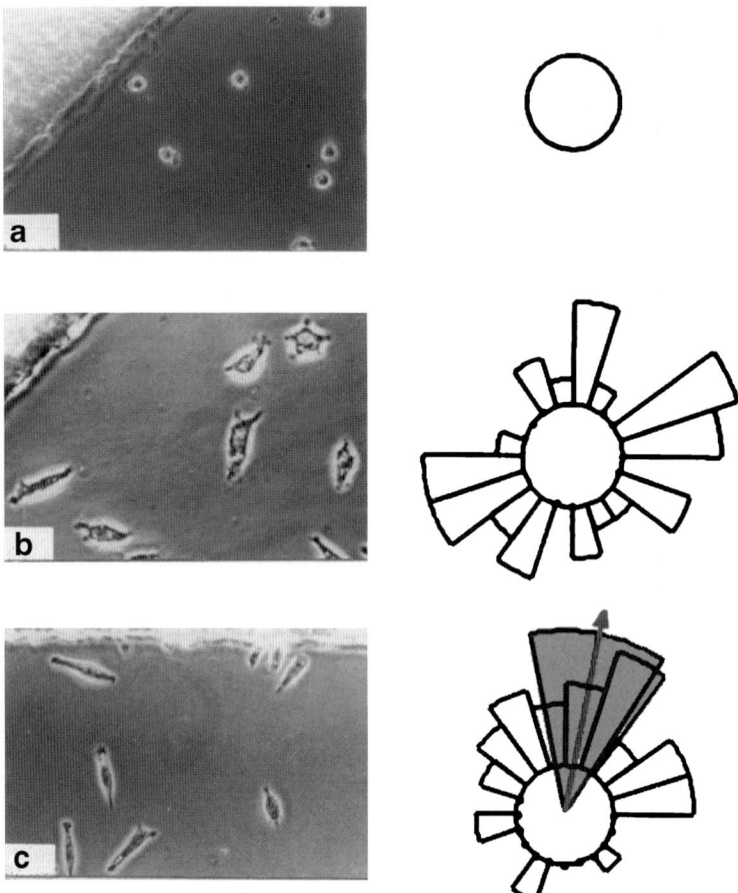

Fig. 1 Chemotaxis assays using the Dunn Chamber. Murine macrophages respond to the potent chemoattractant, CSF-1. If CSF-1 is withdrawn from the growth medium for 24 h, cells round up and cease migration (**a**). When restimulated with medium containing 10 ng/ml CSF-1, the cells rapidly flatten out, repolarise within 60 min and commence rapid migration over the substratum (**b**). If a gradient of CSF-1 is generated by adding CSF-1-containing medium only to the outer well of the Dunn chamber, cell migration takes on a directional component (**c**). Horizon plots quantify not only the number of cells that migrate beyond a selected distance from their origin, but also provide a statistical test of unidirectional migration. Whilst migration can be seen in the horizon plot given in **b**, only in **c** does the statistical test show that there is significant unidirectional migration up-gradient to the source of CSF-1

assays: in microwell plates with a base of coverslip glass that is suitable for imaging (MatTek Corporation) it is possible to measure (1) movement of cells up through submerged gels with cells seeded below the gel (Fig. 2c); or (2) movement down through submerged cells with cells seeded on top of the gel (Fig. 2d). In these wells, 50,000 cells are seeded in 50μl. In classical transwell assays, a chemoattractant can be used in the lower chamber (Fig. 2e). Alternatively, in inverted transwell assays, cells are seeded on the underside of the membrane, gels are formed inside the insert and a chemoattractant is placed above the gel such that the cells move up through the 8-μm pores and through the gel towards the chemoattractant (Fig. 2f). The gels can be fixed using 4% paraformaldehyde and 0.25% glutaraldehyde for 1h or overnight at 4°C. Permeabilised cells can be stained for F-actin. To examine 3D gels using laser scanning microscopy, an objective with a long working distance of >0.25mm is needed with water correction, not oil. Migration through the gel can be quantified by counting cells within individual z sections, and then expressing invasion as the percentage of cells that have invaded further than a threshold distance. The morphology of cells invading in a 3D matrix is very different to that of cells moving in 2D (Rhee et al. 2007).

Cell movement-contractility in collagen gels

It is now recognized that the 3D organisation of the extracellular matrix is as important as its biochemical composition in modulating cell behaviour. Fibroblast-populated collagen matrices have been widely used as an *in vitro* model for tissue contraction during wound healing. When seeded within one such matrix, usually composed of collagen I, fibroblasts typically contract the matrix within days, and the macroscopic contraction is easily monitored through measuring the gel surface area. Maryse Bailly (UCL) detailed how microscopic cell and matrix behaviour can be monitored qualitatively and quantitatively during the contraction process using 4D imaging with confocal or standard light and fluorescence microscopy. The cell behaviour in 3D can be recorded live by using either phase/DIC imaging or using cells that have

been labelled through transfection with a fluorescent marker such as EGFP, the latter allowing for greater automatism of the tracking procedure. Cell migration can be followed using the 4D Volocity software. DQ collagen or gelatine can be used to reveal where cells have degraded matrix. These are collagen or gelatine labelled with fluorophores at very high stoichiometry resulting in auto-quenching of fluorescence. When degraded, the collagen/gelatine fluoresces showing a "cell footprint". The diameter of the hole that the cell makes in the gel can be measured either by staining biotinylated collagen or by using DQ collagen (Fig. 3). Maryse's group have developed their own parameter, the dynamic index, to quantitatively analyse the cells' dynamic behaviour in the gels (Dahlmann-Noor et al. 2007). The remodelling of the matrix and local contraction can be analysed in parallel with the cell behaviour using live imaging

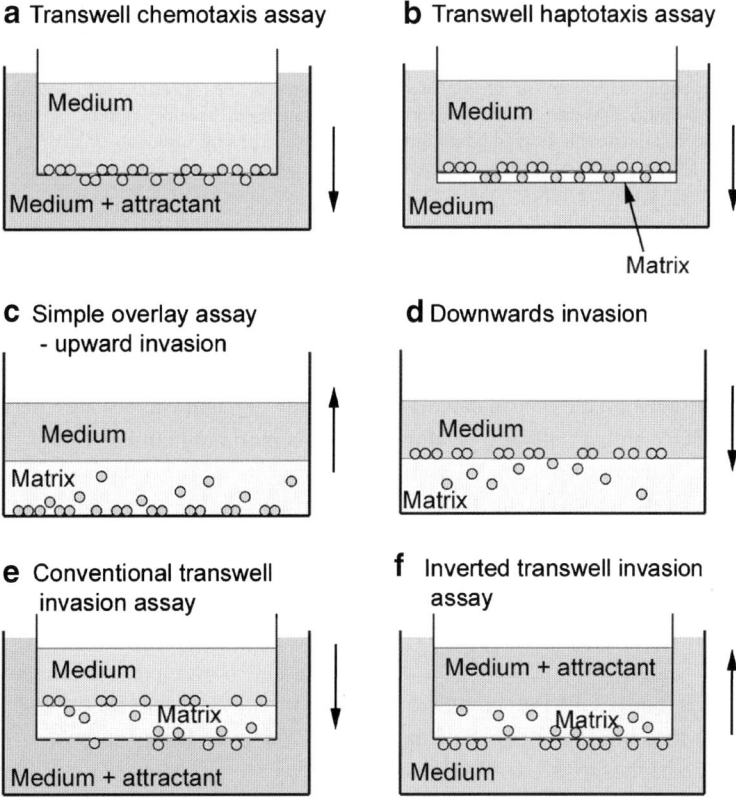

Fig. 2 Motility and invasion assays. **a** Transwell chemotaxis assay – cells move towards a chemoattractant in the base of the well and to the other side of the filter; **b** Transwell haptotaxis assay - cells move towards an extracellular matrix coating the base of the insert; **c** Simple overlay assay - cells move up into the matrix from the bottom of a dish; **d** Simple downwards invasion assay - cells plated on top of matrix invade down into it; **e** Conventional transwell invasion assay - cells plated on top of a transwell invade down to the underside of the filter; **f** Inverted transwell invasion assay – cells plated on the underside of a transwell migrate up through the filter and into the matrix inside the insert. *Arrows* indicate direction of movement (modified from Hooper et al 2006)

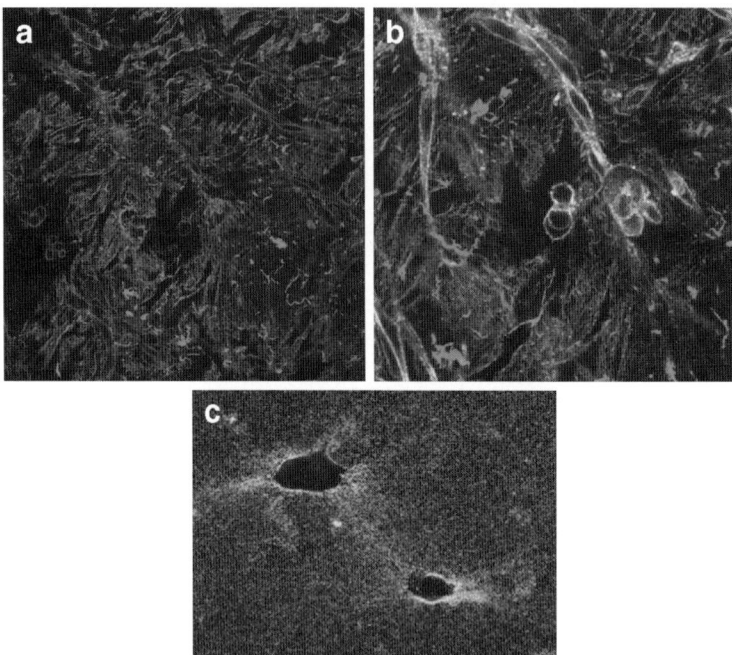

Fig. 3 Cell migration in a collagen matrix and matrix degradation. Fibroblasts (*blue* in **a**; *green* in **b**) within a 3D collagen matrix (*red*). The collagen shown is biotinylated collagen, identified using anti-biotin Cy3-conjugated antibodies. The cells (*blue or green*) are stained with labeled phalloidin (Alexa 488). Elongated cells are moving, round ones are dividing and degrading the matrix leaving black holes. **c** The use of the DQ gelatin to visualise degradation. The cells (*blue*) are visualised by DIC, while the collagen degradation is seen as a green label around the cells. Both collagen and its degradation fragments, i.e., gelatin, are degraded by the matrix metalloproteinases in this system, so either DQ collagen or DQ gelatin can be used to visualise the degradation (images courtesy of Maryse Bailly, University College London Institute of Ophthalmology)

of the matrix through confocal reflection microscopy. Movement of the actual matrix can be tracked manually by following individual fibres or automatically tracking beads embedded in the matrix. The local forces exerted by the cells on the matrix can also be evaluated using the DQA online software (Deformation Quantification and Analysis, Frederick Lanni, Carnegie Mellon University), which quantifies the local strains engendered by matrix remodelling.

Semaphorin-induced collapse assays

Collapse and retraction is normal in the growth of neurons. Collapse assays measure the collapse of the neuronal growth cone. Semaphorins are a family of growth cone guidance molecules. When associated with their receptors, plexins and neuropilins, they act either as chemorepellents and/or chemoattractants for an extensive range of neuronal populations. The prototypic semaphorin, Sema3A, has a potent inhibitory effect on sensory axons emanating from dorsal

root ganglia. Laura Turner (UCL) illustrated how this has formed the basis of the most famous assay for semaphorin activity, the dorsal root ganglia collapse assay. In recent years, an alternative, heterologous, highly tractable assay has been used to investigate semaphorin signalling. In this system, the binding of recombinant semaphorins to COS cells expressing plexins and neuropilins induces a morphological collapse that may correlate with growth cone collapse (Turner and Hall 2006). In her talk, Laura described how COS cells, fibroblasts of kidney origin, can be used as a non-neuronal model of a neuronal phenotype and how recombinant semaphorins, with an Fc tag to allow dimerisation, produce a similar response in COS cells as in neurons.

Imaging cell movement in embryos

Moving on from cell culture models, much can be learned from live cell imaging of simple embryos. Embryos heal wounds very rapidly and efficiently and without leaving a scar. Paul Martin (University of Bristol) is studying how they do this to learn about the natural morphogenetic movements of embryogenesis and to consider ways in which adult tissues could be made to repair more efficiently. Using live confocal imaging of transgenic *Drosophila* embryos expressing gfp-actin in epithelial tissues, his group is investigating the key actin machineries that drive the paradigm morphogenetic process of dorsal closure which appears to bear striking analogy with several mammalian morphogenetic episodes and with re-epithelialisation of skin wounds. Paul showed us dramatic movies of dorsal closure and illustrated how the actin cable pulls the dorsal cells together (Woolner et al. 2005). Transmission electron microscopy images showed interdigitating filopodia which facilitate formation of adherens junctions. Then, using embryos expressing mutant forms of the various small GTPases, Paul has tested the function of each of these actin-based elements – the actin cable and dynamic filopodia and lamellipodia – in both dorsal closure and the repair of laser-generated wound holes.

Experiments in embryonic chicks and mice and in the neonatal PU.1 null mouse, which has no macrophages, suggest that an inflammatory response is not essential for repair and may indeed be the cause of fibrosis in post-embryonic animals. Consequently, a microarray approach has been used with this mouse to identify a portfolio of candidate inflammation/fibrosis genes. Paul has also established models of inflammation in the *Drosophila* embryo and in the translucent zebrafish larval tail to dissect the genetics of inflammation, in particular, the signaling and cytoskeletal elements required to guide migration of macrophages towards wound sites; again, it appears that these wound-triggered migrations bear striking similarities to several developmental cell migrations. The tracking of fluorescent macrophages towards wounded tissues of a developing embryo is truly amazing (Redd et al. 2006).

The meeting provided insights into the breadth of the motility field, and useful tips for those of us interested to learn the practicalities and possibilities open to us for imaging and measuring dynamic cell behaviour. Importantly, the speakers were enthusiastic and happy to be contacted by anyone wishing to develop motility assays in their own laboratories. The reader is referred to Blow (2007) for further discussion of cell migration measurement.

References

Dahlmann-Noor AH, Martin-Martin B, Eastwood M, Khaw PT, Bailly M. Dynamic protrusive cell behaviour generates force and drives early matrix contraction by fibroblasts. Exp Cell Res. 2007;313:4158–69.

Denker SP, Barber DL. Cell migration requires both ion translocation and cytoskeletal anchoring by the Na-H exchanger NHE1. J Cell Biol 2002;159:1087–96.

Hodivala-Dilke KM, DiPersio CM, Kreidberg JA, Hynes RO. Novel roles for alpha3beta1 integrin as a regulator of cytoskeletal assembly and as a trans-dominant inhibitor of integrin receptor function in mouse keratinocytes. J Cell Biol 1998;142:1357–69.

Hodivala-Dilke KM, Reynolds AR, Reynolds LE. Integrins in angiogenesis: multitalented molecules in a balancing act. Cell Tissue Res 2003;314:131–44.

Hooper S, Marshall JF, Sahai E. Tumor cell migration in three dimensions. Methods Enzymol 2006;406:625–43.

Ivetic A, Florey O, Deka J, Haskard DO, Ager A, Ridley AJ. Mutagenesis of the ezrin–radixin–moesin binding domain of L-selectin tail affects shedding, microvillar positioning, and leukocyte tethering. J Biol Chem 2004;279:33263–72.

Jones GE, Ridley AJ, Zicha D. Rho GTPases and cell migration: measurement of macrophage chemotaxis. Methods Enzymol 2000;325:449–62.

Kellie S, Craggs G, Bird IN, Jones GE. The tyrosine phosphatase DEP-1 induces cytoskeletal rearrangements, aberrant cell-substratum interactions and a reduction in cell proliferation. J Cell Sci 2004;117:609–18.

Millán J, Williams L, Ridley AJ. An in vitro model to study the role of endothelial rho GTPases during leukocyte trans-endothelial migration. Methods Enzymol 2006;406:643–55.

Ramsay AG, Keppler MD, Jazayeri M, Thomas GJ, Parsons M, Violette S, et al. HS1-associated protein X-1 regulates carcinoma cell migration and invasion via clathrin-mediated endocytosis of integrin alphavbeta6. Cancer Res 2007; 67:5275–84.

Redd MJ, Kelly G, Dunn G, Way M, Martin P. Imaging macrophage chemotaxis in vivo: studies of microtubule function in zebrafish wound inflammation. Cell Motil Cytoskeleton 2006;63:415–22.

Rhee S, Jiang H, Ho CH, Grinnell F. Microtubule function in fibroblast spreading is modulated according to the tension state of cell–matrix interactions. Proc Natl Acad Sci U S A 2007;104:5425–30.

Turner LJ, Hall A. Plexin-induced collapse assay in COS cells. Methods Enzymol 2006;406:665–76.

Wells CM, Ahmed T, Masters JR, Jones GE. Rho family GTPases are activated during HGF-stimulated prostate cancer-cell scattering. Cell Motil Cytoskeleton 2005;62:180–94.

Woolner S, Jacinto A, Martin P. The small GTPase Rac plays multiple roles in epithelial sheet fusion–dynamic studies of *Drosophila* dorsal closure. Dev Biol 2005;282:163–73.

Further reading

Blow N. Cell migration: our protruding knowledge. Nature Methods 2007;4:589–94.

Protective action of fenugreek (*Trigonella foenum graecum*) seed polyphenols against alcohol-induced protein and lipid damage in rat liver

S. Kaviarasan · R. Sundarapandiyan ·
C. V. Anuradha

Originally published in the journal Cell Biology and Toxicology, Volume 24, Nos 4–5, 111–120.
DOI: 10.1007/s10565-007-9050-x © Springer Science + Business Media B.V. 2007

Abstract The study investigates the effect of fenugreek seed polyphenol extract (FPEt) on ethanol-induced damage in rat liver. Chronic ethanol administration (6 g kg^{-1} $day^{-1} \times 60$ days) caused liver damage that was manifested by excessive formation of thiobarbituric-acid-reactive substances, lipid hydroperoxides, and conjugated dienes, the end products of lipid peroxidation, and significant elevation of protein carbonyl groups and diminution of sulfhydryl groups, a marker of protein oxidation. Decreased activities of enzymic and non-enzymic antioxidant levels and decreased levels of thiol groups (both non-protein and protein) were observed in ethanol-treated rats. Further, ethanol significantly increased the accumulation of 4-hydroxynonenal protein adducts, nitrated and oxidized proteins in liver which was evidenced by immunohistochemistry. Administration of FPEt to ethanol-fed rats (200 mg kg^{-1} day^{-1}) significantly reduced the levels of lipid peroxidation products and protein carbonyl content, increased the activities of antioxidant enzymes, and restored the levels of thiol groups. The effects of FPEt were comparable with those of a positive control, silymarin. These findings show that FPEt ameliorates the pathological liver changes induced by chronic ethanol feeding.

Keywords Ethanol · Lipid peroxidation ·
Protein oxidation · Fenugreek seed polyphenols

Abbreviations

CAT	catalase
DNP	dinitrophenol
FPEt	fenugreek seed polyphenol extract
GPx	glutathione peroxidase
GR	glutathione reductase
GSH	reduced glutathione
GST	glutathione-*S*-transferase
H_2O_2	hydrogen peroxide
HNE	hydroxynonenal
NAD	nicotinamide adenine dinucleotide
NADH	nicotinamide adenine dinucleotide reduced
3-NT	3-nitrotyrosine
$NO^{\bullet}$	nitric oxide
$ONOO^{-}$	peroxynitrite
RNS	reactive nitrogen species
SM	silymarin
SOD	superoxide dismutase
TBARS	thiobarbituric acid reactive substances

S. Kaviarasan · C. V. Anuradha (✉)
Department of Biochemistry, Faculty of science,
Annamalai University,
Annamalai Nagar 608 002, India
e-mail: cvaradha@hotmail.com

R. Sundarapandiyan
Department of Pathology, Dr. ALM PG Institute of Basic
Medical Sciences, University of Madras,
Chennai, India

Introduction

The ability of ethanol to increase the production of reactive oxygen species and cause oxidative damage to lipids, proteins, and DNA has been demonstrated in a variety of systems, cells, and species including humans (Cederbaum 2001). Alterations in redox state (decrease in the NAD^+/NADH redox ratio), microsomal generation of hydroxyl radicals, production of the reactive metabolite acetaldehyde, and one-electron oxidation of ethanol to 1-hydroxy ethyl radical are documented to be the mechanisms of ethanol-induced oxidative stress and cell injury (Tsukamoto and Lu 2001).

Administration of antioxidants such as glutathione (GSH), *S*-adenosyl methionine, and vitamin E ameliorate the severity of ethanol-induced liver damage (Mato et al. 1999; Pares et al. 1998). Apart from pharmacological intervention, another potential measure could be to increase the dietary intake of flavonoids, compounds that are exceptionally efficient antioxidants and radical scavengers (Harborne and Williams 2000). Fenugreek (*Trigonella foenum graecum*) seeds are commonly used as spice in Indian homes. Fenugreek has a long history of traditional use as a medicinal herb for diabetes, and its antidiabetic potential has been experimentally evidenced (Sharma 1986). The seeds are reported to be rich in polyphenolic flavonoids (100 mg/g; Gupta and Nair 1999).We showed that the polyphenolic extract of fenugreek seeds has antioxidant activity in vitro (Kaviarasan et al. 2004) and prevents ethanol-induced apoptosis in Chang liver cells (Kaviarasan et al. 2006).To further explore the hepatoprotective action, we studied the effect of fenugreek seed polyphenol extract (FPEt) on ethanol-induced lipid and protein damage in the liver of alcohol-treated rats by measuring lipid peroxidation indices, antioxidant levels, protein carbonyl content (spectrophotometry and immunohistochemistry), and 4-hydroxynonenal (HNE)-protein adducts (immunohistochemistry) by localizing nitrated proteins (immunohistochemistry) and compared it with a standard hepatoprotective drug silymarin.

Materials and methods

Animals and chemicals

Healthy male albino Wistar rats (150–170 g) purchased from Central Animal House, Department of Experimental Medicine, Rajah Muthiah Medical College, Annamalai University were housed in polypropylene rat cages in a room with controlled temperature ($24\pm2°C$) and light (lights on 0600 to 1800). They were fed with standard pellet diet (Agro Corporation Private Limited, Bangalore, India) and water ad libitum. The pellet comprised 21% protein, 5% lipids, 4% crude fiber, 8% ash, 1% calcium, 0.6% phosphorous, 3.4% glucose, 2% vitamin, and 55% nitrogen-free extract (carbohydrates). It provided metabolizable energy of 3,600 kcal/kg. The experimental and animal handling procedures were approved by the Institutional Animal Ethics Committee. Silymarin was purchased from Hunan Kinglong Bio-Resource Co., Ltd. (China). Fine chemicals were obtained from Sigma (St. Louis, MO, USA). Rabbit anti-3-nitro-L-tyrosine (3-NT) polyclonal antibodies (Catalogue no. 06-284) were from Upstate (Lake Placid, NY, USA). Mouse 4-HNE monoclonal antibodies (Catalogue no. 24325) were from Oxis International Inc. (Portland, OR, USA). Goat anti-dinitrophenol (DNP) polyclonal antibodies (Catalogue no. J06) were from Biomeda Corporation (Foster City, CA, USA). Horse radish peroxidase (HRP) detection system was from Biogenex Laboratories, India. All other chemicals and solvents were of analytical grade.

Preparation of fenugreek seed extract

Fenugreek seeds (100 g) were finely powdered, mixed with 80% methanol, and kept at room temperature for 5 days. After 5 days, it was filtered and the solvent was evaporated. The residue was dissolved in water, and the aqueous layer was washed with petroleum ether several times until a clear upper layer of petroleum ether was obtained. The lower layer was then treated with ethyl acetate containing glacial acetic acid (10 ml/l). Extraction of polyphenols was carried out for 36 h at room temperature, and the combined ethyl acetate layer was concentrated (Xia et al. 1998). The residue was lyophilized and stored at −70°C. This yielded about 6–8 g per 100 g of seed powder. An aqueous extract (FPEt) was prepared and used for the studies. The polyphenolic content of the extract was assayed by the method of Singleton and Rossi (1965).

Study design

The animals were randomly divided into six groups of six rats in each. Alcoholic rats (toxicity control) received ethanol (6 g/kg) as an aqueous solution for 60 days by gastric intubation. Normal control rats received glucose solution equivalent to the calorific value of ethanol (5 ml of 40% glucose solution/100 g). After the induction of toxicity (i.e., initial 30 days), treatment groups received FPEt (200 mg kg^{-1} day^{-1}, i.e., 3 ml/day) and silymarin (SM; 100 mg kg^{-1} day^{-1}, i.e., 3 ml/day) for the next 30 days along with ethanol. This experimental design is depicted in Table 1. The total experimental duration was 60 days. Rats in all the groups were killed by decapitation 24 h after the last treatment. Blood was collected with heparin as anticoagulant. Plasma was separated by centrifugation at 2,000 rpm. The red blood cells were washed with ice-cold phosphate buffered saline, and hemolysate was prepared in ice-cold water. The liver tissue was sliced into pieces and homogenized in cold 50 mM phosphate buffer (pH 7.4) to give 10% homogenate (*w/v*). The homogenate was centrifuged at 1,000 rpm for 10 min at 0°C in a refrigerated centrifuge. The supernatant was separated and used for various estimations.

Biochemical estimations

The level of thiobarbituric acid reactive substances (TBARS) in plasma and liver was estimated by the method of Niehaus and Samuelsson (1968). Lipid hydroperoxides (LHP) was assayed by the method of Jiang et al. (1999). Conjugated dienes (CD) was estimated by the method of Rao and Recknagel (1968). The estimation of protein carbonyl was done by the method of Levine et al. (1990). The activity of superoxide dismutase (SOD) was assayed in hemolysate and liver by the method of Kakkar et al. (1984), and that of catalase and glutathione peroxidase (GPx) by the methods of Sinha (1972) and Rotruck et al. (1973), respectively. Glutathione reductase was esti-

mated by the method of Horn and Burns (1978). Reduced glutathione (Ellman 1959), ascorbic acid (Omaye et al. 1991), and α-tocopherol (Baker et al. 1980) were quantitated in plasma and liver. Total thiols, non-protein and protein thiols in liver were estimated according to the method of Sedlack and Lindsay (1968). Protein content was determined by the method of Lowry et al. (1951).

Immunohistochemical localization of 3-NT, DNP, and 4-HNE in liver

For immunohistochemistry, 4-μm sections were deparaffinized with xylene and dehydrated with graded concentration of isopropyl alcohol. Sections were incubated with peroxide blocking reagent for 10 min, rinsed with phosphate buffer, and again incubated with power block solution for 10 min. Nonspecific adsorption was minimized by leaving the sections in 3% bovine serum albumin in phosphate-buffered saline for 30 min. Sections were incubated overnight with a 1:700 dilution of anti-3-NT antibody or with a 1:500 dilution of anti-DNP antibody or with a 1:100 dilution of anti-4-HNE antibody. The sections were then rinsed well with phosphate buffer and incubated with super enhancer reagent for 30 min. After rinsing with phosphate buffer, incubation was done with poly HRP-reagent for 30 min. After washing thoroughly with phosphate buffer, the sections were incubated with diaminobenzidine substrate solution for 5 min. Sections were counterstained with hematoxylin and observed under light microscopy. All the sections from the various groups were incubated under the same conditions with the similar antibody concentration, and in the same running, to make the immunostaining comparable among the different experimental groups.

Table 1 Experimental design

Group	Treatment and duration	
	1–30 days	31–60 days
I	Isocaloric glucose (40% stock) twice a day (09.00 A.M. and 5.00 P.M.)	
II	Ethanol (3 g/kg twice a day, i.e., 6 g kg^{-1} day^{-1})	
III	Ethanol (6 g kg^{-1} day^{-1})	Ethanol + FPEt (100 mg/kg twice a day), i.e., 200 mg kg^{-1} day^{-1}
IV	Ethanol (6 g kg^{-1} day^{-1})	Ethanol + SM (50 mg/kg twice a day), i.e., 100 mg kg^{-1} day^{-1}
V	Glucos (40% stock)	Glucose (40% stock) + FPEt (100 mg/kg twice a day), i.e., 200 mg kg^{-1} day^{-1}
VI	Glucose (40% stock)	Glucose (40% stock) + SM (50 mg/kg twice a day), i.e., 100 mg kg^{-1} day^{-1}

Table 2 Initial and final body weights of control and experimental animals

Parameters	Group I	Group II	Group III	Group IV	Group V	Group VI
Body weight (g)						
Initial	175.83±9.70	173.33±5.16	175.0±4.47	175.0±7.74	175.0±7.07	170.0±8.37
Final	241.66±12.90[c]	208.33±9.31[a,c]	225.83±10.21[a,b]	226.67±11.69[a,b]	244.17±13.57 [c]	242.50±12.94[c]
Weight gain	70.83±7.36	35.83±3.76	45.0±4.47	50.83±4.92	71.67±6.06	69.17±4.92

Values are means ± SD of six animals. Group I—Control; Group II—Ethanol; Group III—Ethanol + FPEt;

Group IV—Ethanol + silymarin; Group V—Control + FPEt; Group VI—Control + silymarin

[a] Significant as compared to group I ($p<0.05$, DMRT)

[b] Significant as compared to group II ($p<0.05$, DMRT)

[c] Significant as compared to group III and IV ($p<0.05$, DMRT)

Statistical analysis

Statistical evaluation was done using one-way analysis of variance followed by Duncan's multiple range test (DMRT). Values are expressed as means ± SD of six rats in each group. A probability of $p<0.05$ was considered as significant.

Results

The total phenolic content was estimated to be 21.4± 1.2 mg gallic acid equivalents/100 mg of FPEt from triplicate measurements.

Table 2 shows the initial and final body weights and body weight gain in control and experimental animals.

The initial body weight in all the groups was within 150–170 g. Significant weight loss was observed in animals fed with ethanol as compared to control. Ethanol-fed animals co-treated with FPEt or silymarin did not lose weight during the experimental period.

Table 3 represents the levels of lipid peroxidation products such as TBARS, LHP, CD in plasma and liver of control and ethanol-fed rats and the level of protein carbonyl in liver of both the groups. Ethanol-treated rats showed increase in lipid peroxidation indices and protein oxidation. Treatment with FPEt or silymarin prevented the enhanced formation of oxidation products.

The activities of enzymic antioxidants such as SOD, catalase (CAT), GPx, and glutathione reductase (GR) in liver and hemolysate of control and ethanol-treated

Table 3 Effect of FPEt on plasma and liver lipid peroxidation products of control and experimental animals

Parameters	Group I	Group II	Group III	Group IV	Group V	Group VI
Plasma						
TBARS (mmol/dl)	1.09±0.04[c]	3.53±0.33[a,c]	1.86±0.16[a,b]	1.70±0.15[a,b]	0.96±0.03[c]	0.97±0.07[c]
LHP (nmol/dl)	0.87±0.04[c]	2.70±0.10 [a, c]	1.61±0.12[a,b]	1.59±0.13[a,b]	0.86±0.05[c]	0.87±0.09[c]
CD ($A_{233/215}$)	0.56±0.05[c]	1.64±0.07[a,c]	1.14±0.09[a,b]	1.10±0.54[a,b]	0.55±0.08[c]	0.58±0.05[c]
Liver						
TBARS (nmol/mg protein)	1.12±0.05[c]	2.56±0.16[a,c]	1.84±0.14[a,b]	1.91±0.17[a,b]	1.26±0.14[c]	1.23±0.11[c]
LHP (nmol/mg protein)	88.56±5.05[c]	160.71±15.96[a,c]	128.03±8.85[a,b]	122.02±8.42[a,b]	89.49±6.54[c]	92.02±4.69[c]
CD ($A_{233/215}$)	0.77±0.03[c]	1.70±0.03[a,c]	1.25±0.08[a,b]	1.20±0.06[a,b]	0.79±0.04[c]	0.78±0.06[c]
Protein carbonyl (nmol/mg protein)	0.72±0.04[c]	2.55±0.12[a,c]	1.60±0.04[a,b]	1.53±0.09[a,b]	0.71±0.05[c]	0.73±0.06[c]

Values are means ± SD of six animals. Group I—Control; Group II—Ethanol; Group III—Ethanol + FPEt;

Group IV—Ethanol + silymarin; Group V—Control + FPEt; Group VI—Control + silymarin

[a] Significant as compared to group I ($p<0.05$, DMRT)

[b] Significant as compared to Group II ($p<0.05$, DMRT)

[c] Significant as compared to Group III and IV ($p<0.05$, DMRT)

Table 4 Effect of FPEt on activities of enzymatic antioxidants in liver and hemolysate of control and experimental animals

Parameters	Group I	Group II	Group III	Group IV	Group V	Group VI
Liver						
SOD (A)	9.92±0.70[c]	5.39±0.46[a,c]	7.18±0.25[a,b]	7.59±0.37[a,b]	9.84±0.69[c]	9.99±0.69[c]
CAT (B)	74.51±6.18[c]	44.29±4.03[a,c]	58.25±5.53[a,b]	61.41±2.89[a,b]	73.44±5.01[c]	71.10±2.56[c]
GPx (C)	11.17±1.10[c]	4.68±0.36[a,c]	7.73±0.38[a,b]	8.03±0.31[a,b]	11.04±0.97[c]	11.26±0.91[c]
GR (D)	21.30±1.20[c]	11.00±1.08[a,c]	16.25±0.79[a,b]	17.16±1.58[a,b]	21.15±1.22[c]	21.13±1.23[c]
Hemolysate						
SOD (A)	8.34±0.29[c]	4.08±0.19[a,c]	6.46±0.23[a,b]	6.77±0.24[a,b]	8.35±0.39[c]	8.32±0.22[c]
CAT (B)	42.60±3.96[c]	23.95±2.19[a,c]	31.12±1.58[a,b]	33.55±2.04[a,b]	42.26±4.07[c]	43.05±4.27[c]
GPx (C)	13.60±0.47[c]	6.71±0.62[a,c]	9.09±0.84[a,b]	9.77±0.71[a,b]	13.38±0.31[c]	13.24±0.73[c]
GR (D)	4.56±0.44[c]	2.27±0.23[a,c]	3.20±0.24[a,b]	3.57±0.24[a,b]	4.47±0.45[c]	4.65±0.44[c]

Values are means ± SD of six animals. Group I—Control; Group II—Ethanol; Group III—Ethanol + FPEt;

Group IV—Ethanol + silymarin; Group V—Control + FPEt; Group VI—Control + silymarin

A—Units/mg protein for liver; Units/mg Hb for lysates, B—μmol min^{-1} mg^{-1} protein for liver; μmol min^{-1} mg^{-1} Hb for lysates, C—μg of GSH min^{-1} mg^{-1} protein for liver; μg of GSH min^{-1} mg^{-1} Hb for lysates, D—μmol of NADPH oxidized h^{-1} mg^{-1} protein for liver; μmol of NADPH oxidized h^{-1} mg^{-1} Hb for lysate

[a] Significant as compared to group I ($p<0.05$, DMRT)

[b] Significant as compared to group II ($p<0.05$, DMRT)

[c] Significant as compared to group III and IV ($p<0.05$, DMRT)

rats are shown in Table 4. Antioxidant enzymes registered a significant decrease in ethanol-treated group as compared to that of control. Upon treatment with FPEt or silymarin, the activities were near-normal.

The levels of non-enzymic antioxidants such as GSH, ascorbic acid, and α-tocopherol in plasma and liver of control and ethanol-fed rats are given in Table 5. Increased ethanol intake significantly lowered the levels of reduced glutathione (38%), ascorbic acid (70%), and α-tocopherol (66%) in plasma and liver. Co-administration of FPEt or silymarin prevented the decrease, and the levels of these antioxidants were brought back to near-normal values.

Table 6 depicts the levels of total, protein, and non-protein thiols in liver of control and ethanol-fed rats. The levels were significantly decreased ($p<0.001$) in

Table 5 Effect of FPEt on levels of non-enzymatic antioxidants of liver and plasma of control and experimental animals

Parameters	Group I	Group II	Group III	Group IV	Group V	Group VI
Liver						
GSH (A)	162.9±13.7[c]	100.2±8.1[a,c]	130.5±9.7[a,b]	134.0±12.2[a,b]	167.5±13.0[c]	157.2±12.0[c]
Vit-E (B)	6.04±0.61[c]	2.03±0.15[a,c]	4.75±0.32[a,b]	4.95±0.36[a,b]	5.89±0.54[c]	6.24±0.51[c]
Vit-C (B)	0.80±0.03[c]	0.24±0.02[a,c]	0.50±0.05[a,b]	0.54±0.05[a,b]	0.81±0.06[c]	0.84±0.02[c]
Plasma						
GSH (A)	97.16±8.23[c]	52.88±2.77[a,c]	76.60±5.35[a,b]	78.56±3.99[a,b]	95.17±4.50[c]	96.17±4.90[c]
Vit-E (B)	47.13±2.60[c]	29.69±1.68[a,c]	38.91±2.25[a,b]	40.07±2.46[a,b]	48.55±2.85[c]	47.57±2.76[c]
Vit-C (B)	2.53±0.24[c]	1.02±0.10[a,c]	1.82±0.12[a,b]	1.92±0.12[a,b]	2.43±0.23[c]	2.58±0.21[c]

Values are means ± SD of six animals. Group I—Control; Group II—Ethanol; Group III—Ethanol + FPEt;

Group IV—Ethanol + silymarin; Group V—Control + FPEt; Group VI—Control + silymarin

A—μmol/mg tissue for liver; μmol/dl for plasma, B—μg/mg protein for liver; mmol/dl for plasma

[a] Significant as compared to group I ($p<0.05$, DMRT)

[b] Significant as compared to group II ($p<0.05$, DMRT)

[c] Significant as compared to group III and IV ($p<0.05$, DMRT)

Table 6 Effect of FPEt on thiol groups (μmol/mg protein) of control and experimental animals

Parameters	Group I	Group II	Group III	Group IV	Group V	Group VI
T-SH	15.43 ± 1.21^c	$5.76 \pm 0.57^{a,c}$	$10.67 \pm 0.51^{a,b}$	$11.27 \pm 0.36^{a,b}$	15.27 ± 1.30^c	15.49 ± 1.15^c
P-SH	9.44 ± 0.42^c	$2.78 \pm 0.21^{a,c}$	$5.98 \pm 0.34^{a,b}$	$6.24 \pm 0.46^{a,b}$	9.35 ± 0.46^c	9.46 ± 0.48^c
NP-SH	6.00 ± 0.39^c	$2.59 \pm 0.13^{a,c}$	$4.09 \pm 0.32^{a,b}$	$4.18 \pm 0.22^{a,b}$	5.92 ± 0.43^c	6.02 ± 0.54^c

Values are means ± SD of six animals. Group I—Control; Group II—Ethanol; Group III—Ethanol + FPEt;

Group IV—Ethanol + silymarin; Group V—Control + FPEt; Group VI—Control + silymarin

[a] Significant as compared to group I ($p<0.05$, DMRT)

[b] Significant as compared to group II ($p<0.05$, DMRT)

[c] Sgnificant as compared to goup III and IV ($p<0.05$, DMRT)

animals given ethanol. Administration of FPEt or silymarin normalized the thiol content in liver of ethanol-fed rats.

Figures 1, 2 and 3 are the photomicrographs showing the immunostaining for 4-HNE, DNP, and 3-NT antibodies in liver of control and experimental rats. The intensity of staining for all three antibodies was more pronounced in ethanol-treated rat liver than in other groups. It is worthy to note that there was a marked reduction in immunoreactivity in the liver of rats treated with FPEt or silymarin. There was no apparent difference in the immunostaining for these antibodies in control rats and in control rats treated with FPEt or silymarin.

Discussion

Accumulation of oxidatively modified proteins and lipid peroxidation products in the liver of ethanol-

Fig. 1 Immunohistochemical localization of HNE protein adducts in liver. The figure shows representative staining for 4-HNE (DAB) against counterstain (hematoxylin) in liver of rats administered saline treatment (**a**; control group), ethanol (**b**), ethanol + FPEt (**c**), or ethanol + silymarin (**d**). **e** and **f** Groups treated with FPEt or silymarin alone. The liver sections of control animals are mainly negative. Liver sections of ethanol-exposed rats show more intensive staining as compared to other groups of animals

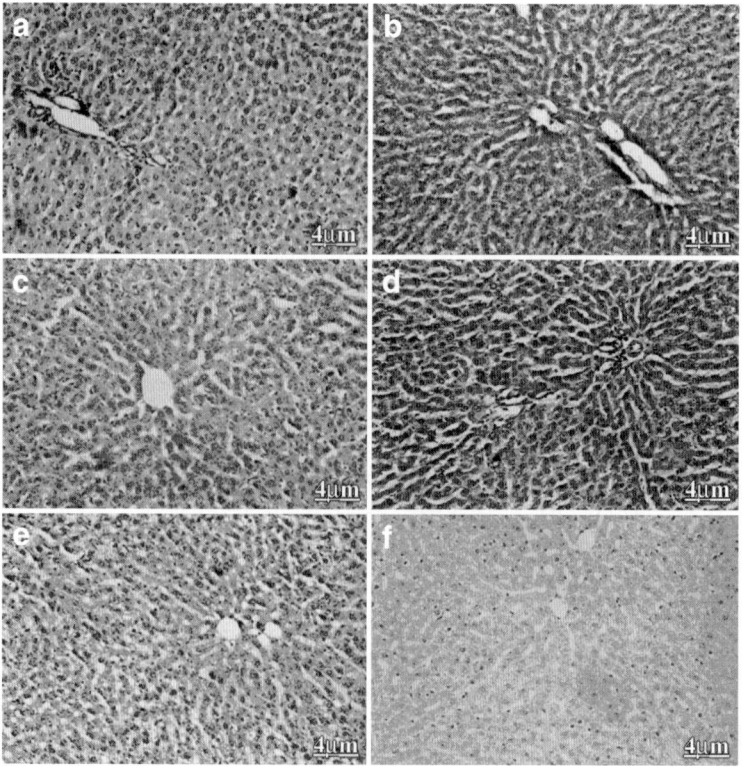

Fig. 2 Immunohistochemical localization of DNP in liver. The figure shows representative stainings for DNP (DAB) against counterstain (hematoxylin) in liver of rats administered saline (**a**; control group), ethanol (**b**), ethanol + FPEt (**c**), or ethanol + silymarin (**d**). **e** and **f** Control groups treated with FPEt or silymarin alone. The liver sections of control animals are mainly negative. Liver sections of ethanol-exposed rats show more intensive staining

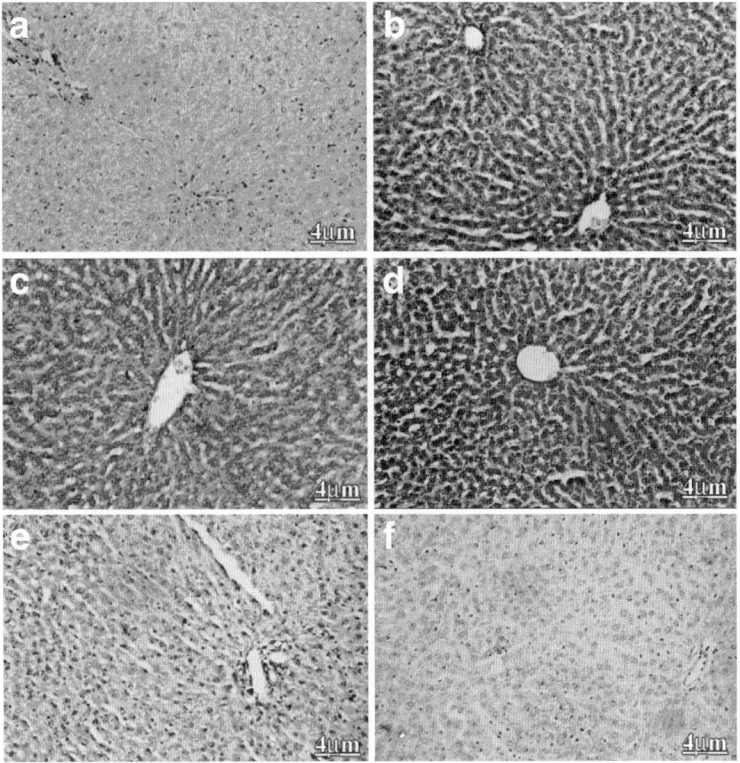

administered rats indicate excessive generation of free radicals. Indices of free radical damage such as the increase of malondialdehyde, 4-HNE protein adducts, and others associated with a depletion of antioxidants have been documented in alcoholic liver disease (Paradis et al. 1997; Ohhira et al. 1998; Rolla et al. 2000; Thirunavukkarasu et al. 2003). 4-HNE is an α, β-unsaturated aldehyde commonly used as a marker of lipid peroxidation, as it is produced in the peroxidative metabolism of arachidonic or linoleic acid (Toyokuni et al. 1994). HNE is a potent electrophile that rapidly modifies proteins on several amino acid residues especially lysine (Cohn et al. 1996) and is responsible for cellular protein modification and loss of function (Ando et al. 1997; Yoritaka et al. 1996).

Protein carbonyl content is the most general indicator and by far the most commonly used marker of protein oxidation (Beal 2002). Thiols, including glutathione, are protective antioxidants acting as free radical scavengers; therefore, the thioldisulfide balance can be an indication of oxidative damage in tissues. Significant increase in the protein carbonyl content, loss of protein thiols, and increased staining

for DNP antibody observed in ethanol-intoxicated rat liver suggest protein damage. Oxidative modifications alter the biological properties of proteins leading to their fragmentation, increased aggregation, and enzyme dysfunction (Levine 2002).

3-NT is a typical product between reactive nitrogen species (RNS) and tyrosine or its residues in proteins (Ischiropoulos et al. 1992). Formation of 3-NT has been used extensively as a marker of protein damage and a biomarker of inflammation (Greenacre and Ischiropoulos 2001). Interestingly, FPEt was also able to decrease 3-NT immunostaing in vivo, suggesting that FPEt might be able to scavenge in vivo RNS involved in protein nitration.

A deficiency of SOD activity would lead to an increased number of superoxide radicals, and that of GSH–Px would lead to increased levels of lipid peroxides. Low GSH and ascorbate levels may result from their increased utilization to scavenge free radicals and to protect other cellular constituents from oxidative damage. The mechanism of hepatoprotection by FPEt against ethanol toxicity could be mediated by enhancement of endogenous antioxidant defenses GSH, vitamins C and E, and restoring the

Fig. 3 Immunostaining for 3-nitrotyrosine in rat liver. The figure shows representative stainings for DNP (DAB) against counterstain (hematoxylin) in liver of rats administered saline (**b**). Strong staining for 3-NT was present in the liver of ethanol group as compared to control (**a**). Intensity of staining was decreased in the liver of FPEt or silymarin treated rats (**c** and **d**). Control groups treated with FPEt or silymarin showed negative staining (**e** and **f**)

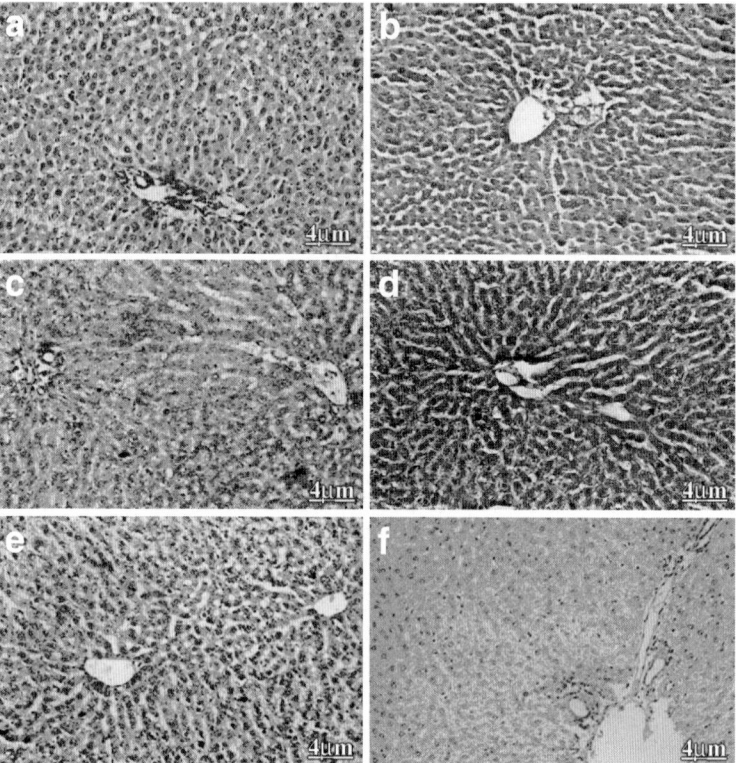

activities of these antioxidant enzymes possibly by reducing generation of free radicals.

Alcohol-fed rats showed decreased body weight due to reduction in adipose tissue astriceps which significantly reduced skin-fold thickness. FPEt treatment restored the body weight by restoring the thickening of adipose tissue.

FPEt supplementation was potentially effective in reducing lipid peroxidation, protein oxidation, and enhancing the thiol status, suggesting that antioxidant principles in FPEt are active against free radicals and prevent the process of protein and lipid oxidation. Earlier, we have shown that fenugreek seeds protect ethanol-induced changes in hepatic detoxification system, apoptosis, collagen, and lipid accumulation in rat liver (Kaviarasan and Anuradha 2007; Kaviarasan et al. 2007a).

A substantial body of evidence has revealed that supplementation of fenugreek seed prevents hyperlipidemia, atherosclerosis (Sharma et al. 1996), diabetes (Sharma 1986), cancer (Sur et al. 2001), and ulcer (Suja Pandian et al. 2002) in experimental animals. In a previous study, we found that FPEt was able to scavenge O_2^- and H_2O_2 (Kaviarasan et al. 2007b).

Different flavonoids namely vitexin, tricin, naringenin, quercetin, tricin-7-O-β-D-glucopyranoside (Shang et al. 1998a), N,N'-dicarbazyl, glycerol monopalmitate, stearic acid, beta-sitosteryl glucopyranoside, ethyl-alpha-D-glucopyranoside, D-3-O-methyl-chiroinositol, and sucrose (Shang et al. 1998b) have been identified. Dixit et al. (2005) reported the presence of gallic acid, o-coumaric acid, p-coumaric acid, rutin, and caffeic acid in aqueous extract of fenugreek seeds. We have identified the presence of quercetin and naringenin in FPEt, and it was found that these phytochemicals may effectively scavenge the free radicals and thereby limit the progression of liver disease.

Our data suggest that FPEt could restore antioxidant potential of hepatic cells and protect them from oxidative damage. Further exploration on the molecular mechanisms underlying FPEt action is essential.

Acknowledgments Financial support to Mr. S. Kaviarasan, one of the authors, in the form of Senior Research Fellowship (SRF) by the Indian Council of Medical Research (ICMR), New Delhi is gratefully acknowledged. The authors wish to thank Prof. Dr. Luke I. Szweda, University of Oklahoma Health Sciences Center, Prof. Dr. Ira Mellman, Yale University School of Medicine, and Prof. Dr. Dick Lightfoot, Childrens Hospital of Philadelphia for providing 4-HNE, DNP, and 3-NT antibodies.

References

Ando Y, Nyhlin N, Suhr O, Holmgren G, Uchida K, El Sahly M, et al. Oxidative stress is found in amyloid deposits in systemic amyloidosis. Biochem Biophys Res Commun 1997;232:497–502.

Baker H, Frank O, De Angelis B, Feingold S. Plasma tocopherol in man at various times after ingesting free or acetylated tocopherol. Nutr Rep Int 1980;21:531–6.

Beal MF. Oxidatively modified proteins in aging and disease. Free Radic Biol Med 2002;32:797–803.

Cederbaum AI. Introduction—serial review: alcohol, oxidative stress and cell injury. Free Radic Biol Med 2001;31:1524–6.

Cohn JA, Tsai L, Friguet B, Szweda LI. Chemical characterization of a protein-4-hydroxy-2-nonenal cross-link: immunochemical detection in mitochondria exposed to oxidative stress. Arch Biochem Biophys 1996;328:158–64.

Dixit P, Ghaskadbi S, Mohan H, Devasagayam TP. Antioxidant properties of germinated fenugreek seeds. Phytother Res 2005;19:977–83.

Ellman GL. Tissue sulphydryl groups. Arch Biochem Biophys 1959;82:70–7.

Greenacre SA, Ischiropoulos H. Tyrosine nitration: localization, quantification, consequences for protein function and signal transduction. Free Radic Res 2001;34:541–81.

Gupta R, Nair S. Antioxidant flavonoids in common Indian diet. South Asian J Prev Cardiol 1999;3:83–94.

Harborne JB, Williams CA. Advances in flavonoid research since 1992. Phytochemistry 2000;55:481–504.

Horn HD, Burns FH. Assay of glutathione reductase activity. In: Bergmeyer HV, editor. Methods of enzymatic analysis. New York: Academic Press; 1978. p. 142.

Ischiropoulos H, Zhu L, Chen J, Tsai M, Martin JC, Smith CD, et al. Peroxynitrite-mediated tyrosine nitration catalyzed by superoxide dismutase. Arch Biochem Biophys 1992;298:431–7.

Jiang ZY, Hunt JV, Wolf SP. Detection of lipid hydroperoxides using the FOX method. Anal Biochem 1999;202:384–9.

Kakkar P, Das B, Viswanathan PN. A modified spectrophotometric assay of superoxide dismutase. Ind J Biochem Biophys 1984;21:130–2.

Kaviarasan S, Anuradha CV. Fenugreek (*Trigonella foenum graecum*) seed polyphenols protect liver from alcohol toxicity: a role on hepatic detoxification system and apoptosis. Die Pharm 2007;62:299–304.

Kaviarasan S, Vijayalakshmi K, Anuradha CV. Polyphenol-rich extract of fenugreek seeds protect erythrocytes from oxidative damage. Plant Food Hum Nutr 2004;59:143–7.

Kaviarasan S, Ramamurty N, Gunasekaran P, Varalakshmi E, Anuradha CV. Fenugreek seed extract prevents ethanol-induced toxicity and apoptosis in Chang liver cells. Alcohol 2006;41:267–73.

Kaviarasan S, Naik GH, Gangabhagirathi R, Anuradha CV, Priyadarsini KI. In vitro studies on antiradical and antioxidant activities of fenugreek (*Trigonella foenum graecum*) seeds. Food Chem 2007a;103:31–37.

Kaviarasan S, Viswanathan P, Anuradha CV. Fenugreek seed (*Trigonella foenum graecum*) polyphenols inhibit ethanol-induced collagen and lipid accumulation in rat liver. Cell Biol Toxicol 2007b;23:373–83.

Levine RL. Carbonyl modified proteins in cellular regulation, aging and disease. Free Radic Biol Med 2002;32:790–6.

Levine RL, Garland D, Oliver CN, et al. Determination of carbonyl content of oxidatively modified proteins. Methods in enzymology, vol. 186. Florida: Academic; 1990. p. 464–78.

Lowry OH, Rosebrough NJ, Farr AL, Randall RJ. Protein measurement with the Folin's-Phenol reagent. J Biol Chem 1951;193:265–75.

Mato JM, Camara J, Fernandez de Paz J, Caballeria L, Coll S, Caballero A, et al. S-adenosylmethionine in alcoholic liver cirrhosis: a randomized placebo-controlled, double blind, multicentre clinical trial. J Hepatol 1999;30:1081–9.

Niehaus WG, Samuelsson B. Formation of malondialdehyde from phospholipids arachidonate during microsomal lipid peroxidation. Eur J Biochem 1968;6:126–30.

Ohhira M, Ohtake T, Matsumoto A, Saito H, Ikuta K, Fujimoto Y, et al. Immunohistochemical detection of 4-hydroxy-2-nonenal-modified-protein adducts in human alcoholic liver diseases. Alcohol Clin Exp Res 1998;22:145–9.

Omaye ST, Tarnbull JD, Sauberlich HE. Selected methods for the determination of ascorbic acid in animal cells, tissues and fluids. Method Enzymol 1991;62:1–11.

Paradis V, Kollinger M, Fabre M, Holstege A, Poynard T, Bedossa P. In situ detection of lipid peroxidation by products in chronic liver disease. Hepatology 1997;26:135–42.

Pares A, Planas R, Torres M, Caballeria J, Viver JM, Acero D, et al. Effects of silymarin in alcoholic patients with cirrhosis of the liver: results of a controlled, double-blind, randomized and multicenter trial. J Hepatol 1998;28:615–21.

Rao KS, Recknagel RO. Early onset of lipoperoxidation in rat liver after carbon tetrachloride administration. Exp Mol Pathol 1968;9:271–8.

Rolla R, Vay D, Mottaran E, Parodi M, Traverso N, Arico S, et al. Detection of circulating antibodies against malondialdehyde-acetaldehyde adducts in patients with alcohol-induced liver disease. Hepatology 2000;31:878–84.

Rotruck JT, Pope AL, Ganther HE, Swanson AB, Hafeman DG, Hoekstra WG. Selenium: biochemical role as a component of glutathione peroxidase. Science 1973;179:588–90.

Sedlack I, Lindsay RH. Estimation of total protein sulfhydryl groups in tissues with Ellman's reagent. Anal Biochem 1968;25:192–205.

Shang M, Cai S, Han J, Li J, Zhao Y, Zheng J, et al. Studies on flavonoids from fenugreek (*Trigonella foenum graecum* L). Zhongguo Zhong Yao Za Zhi. 1998a;23:614–6.

Shang M, Cai S, Wang X. Analysis of amino acids in *Trigonella foenum graecum* seeds. Zhong Yao Cai 1998b;21:188–90.

Sharma RD. Effect of fenugreek seeds and leaves on blood glucose and serum insulin responses in human subjects. Nutr Res 1986;6:1353–64.

Sharma RD, Sarkar A, Hazra DK, Misra B. Hypolipidaemic effect of fenugreek seeds: a chronic study in non-insulin dependent diabetic patients. Phytother Res 1996;10:332–4.

Singleton SL, Rossi JA. Colorimetry of total phenolics with phosphomolybdic—phosphotungstic acid reagents. Am J Enol Vitic 1965;16:144–58.

Sinha AK. Colorimetric assay of catalase. Anal Biochem 1972;47:389–94.

Suja Pandian R, Anuradha CV, Viswanathan P. Gastroprotective effect of fenugreek seeds (*Trigonella foenum graecum*) on experimental gastric ulcer in rats. J Ethnopharmacol 2002; 81:393–7.

Sur P, Das M, Gomes A, Vedasiromoni JR, Sahu NP, Banerjee S, et al. *Trigonella foenum graecum* (Fenugreek) seed extract as an antineoplastic agent. Phytother Res 2001;15:257–9.

Thirunavukkarasu V, Anuradha CV, Viswanathan P. Protective effect of fenugreek (*Trigonella foenum graecum*) seeds in experimental ethanol toxicity. Phytother Res 2003;17:737–43.

Toyokuni S, Uchida K, Okamoto K, Hattori-Nakakuki Y, Hiai H, Stadtman ER. Formation of 4-hydroxy-2-nonenal-modified proteins in the renal proximal tubules of rats treated with a renal carcinogen, ferric nitrilotriacetate. Proc Natl Acad Sci USA 1994;91:2616–20.

Tsukamoto H, Lu SC. Current concepts in the pathogenesis of alcoholic liver injury. FASEB J 2001;15:1335–49.

Xia J, Allenbrand B, Sun GY. Dietary supplementation of grape polyphenols and chronic ethanol administration on LDL oxidation and platelet function in rats. Life Sci 1998;63:383–90.

Yoritaka A, Hattori N, Uchida K, Tanaka M, Stadtman ER, Mizuno Y. Immunohistochemical detection of 4-hydroxynonenal protein adducts in Parkinson disease. Proc Natl Acad Sci USA 1996;93:2696–2701.

Genistein induces G₂/M cell cycle arrest via stable activation of ERK1/2 pathway in MDA-MB-231 breast cancer cells

Zhong Li · Jing Li · Baoqing Mo · Chunyan Hu · Huaqing Liu · Hong Qi · Xinru Wang · Jida Xu

Originally published in the journal Cell Biology and Toxicology, Volume 24, Nos 4–5, 121–129.
DOI: 10.1007/s10565-008-9054-1 © Springer Science + Business Media B.V. 2008

Abstract Genistein is an isoflavonoid present in soybeans that exhibits anti-carcinogenic effect. Several studies have shown that genistein can trigger G2/M cell cycle arrest and inhibit cell growth in human breast cancer cells. In the present study, we assessed the role of MEK-ERK cascade in regulation of genistein-mediated G2/M cell cycle arrest in the hormone-independent cell line MDA-MB-231. Flow cytometric analysis showed that treatment of MDA-MB-231 cells with genistein induced a concentration-dependent accumulation of cells in the G2/M phase of the cell cycle, with a parallel depletion of the percentage of cells in G0/G1. Genistein-mediated G2/M arrest was associated with a decrease in the protein levels of Cdk1, cyclinB1, and Cdc25C as determined by Western blot analysis. Genistein induced a slow and stable activation of phosphorylated ERK1/2 in a concentration- and time-dependent manner in MDA-MB-231 cells. MEK1/2-specific inhibitor PD98059 blocked genistein-induced activation of ERK1/2 and markedly attenuated genistein-induced G2/M arrest. Furthermore, genistein induced the expression of Ras and Raf-1 protein. Genistein also up-regulated steady-state levels of both c-Jun and c-Fos. PD98059 did not depress genistein-induced up-regulation of Ras and Raf-1 protein. However, it markedly blocked genistein-induced up-regulation of c-Jun and c-Fos. These results suggest that the Ras/MAPK/AP-1 signal pathway may be involved in genistein-induced G2/M cell cycle arrest in MDA-MB-231 breast cancer cells.

Keywords Genistein · Cell cycle arrest · ERK1/2 pathway · Breast cancer

Introduction

Genistein, the major isoflavonoid contained in soybeans, is believed to exert pleiotropic effects including potential estrogenic or growth promoting and/or anti-carcinogenic effects (Peterson and Barnes 1991; Fotsis et al. 1995; Zhou et al. 1998). Epidemiological studies, as well as work performed with animal models, suggest that it is responsible for chemopreventive effects on breast, colon, and skin tumors (Messina et al. 1994; Shao et al. 1998).

More recent studies have indicated that genistein can inhibit proliferation of cancer cells in culture by causing cell cycle arrest and/or apoptosis. In breast cancer cells, the effects of genistein are dependent on

Z. Li (✉) · H. Liu · H. Qi · X. Wang
The Key Laboratory of Reproductive Medicine
of Jiangsu Province, Institute of Toxicology,
Nanjing Medical University,
NO. 140 Hanzhong Rd, Jiangsu,
Nanjing 210029, China
e-mail: uiuclz@126.com

J. Li · B. Mo · C. Hu · J. Xu
Department of Nutrition & Food Science,
Nanjing Medical University,
Jiangsu,
Nanjing 210029, China

the estrogen receptor (ER) status. Genistein only stimulates cell growth at low concentration (<10 μM) in ER-positive breast cancer cells (Fioravanti et al. 1998; Zava and Duwe 1997; Hsieh et al. 1998). It suppresses cell growth at all concentrations in ER-negative cell lines (Monti and Sinha 1994). Genistein has also been reported to induce G2/M cell cycle arrest in normal and malignant breast epithelial cells (Upadhyay et al. 2001). The anti-cancer effects of several drugs are mediated by cell cycle arrest and involve modulation of the action of cyclins and cyclin-dependent kinases that regulate cell cycle progression (Sherr 1996). Previous studies suggest G2/M cell cycle arrest after genistein treatment; alterations in cyclinB1 and cdc2 proteins may be involved in the effects of genistein and other phytoestrogens in breast cancer cells (Traganos et al. 1992; Choi et al. 1998).

Signaling mediated by mitogen-activated protein kinases (MAPKs) has been shown to play critical roles in the regulation of cell proliferation and in the response of cells to DNA damage (Schaeffer and Weber 1999). On the basis of their sequence similarities and the nature of their upstream activators, MAPKs are grouped into four subfamilies: ERK1/2, JNK/SAPK, p38, and ERK5. MAPKs are activated by a variety of stimuli. The final signal commonly includes transcription of target genes leading to cellular responses such as proliferation, apoptosis, or cycle progression.

The G2/M checkpoint is essential for the proper repair of DNA damaged by genistein. Although extracellular signal-regulated kinase (ERK) is thought to play a key role in the proliferative process, recent studies suggest that persistent activation of ERK might mediate cell-cycle arrest (Tang et al. 2002). The MAP kinase pathway has been implicated in G2/M cell cycle regulation. In *Xenopus* oocytes, MAP kinase activity has been shown to be necessary for progression through G2 (Abrieu et al. 1997). The MEK1 and MEK2 activator, c-*mos*, has also been shown to be necessary for progression through G2 (Gotoh and Nishida 1995), and ionizing radiation activates the MAP kinase cascade in a specific manner to maintain G2/M checkpoint fidelity (Abbott and Holt 1999). Because the MAP kinase pathway is required for G2/M progression in a number of systems and because genistein leads to G2/M arrest, it is possible that genistein activates the MAP kinase cascade to exert an effect on G2/M checkpoint control.

In the present study, we determined the effect of genistein treatment on ERK1/2, particularly as they participate in the genistein-induced G2/M cell cycle block. Our data demonstrate for the first time, to our knowledge, that the Ras/MAPK/AP-1 signal pathway was involved in genistein-induced G2/M cell cycle arrest in breast cancer cells.

Materials and methods

Reagents and immunochemicals

Genistein was obtained from Sigma (USA). Leibovitz's L-15 medium and trypsinase were from Gibco (USA). Newborn fetal calf serum was obtained from PAA Laboratories (Austria). The MEK1/2 inhibitor (PD98059) was from Merk (Germany). NE-PER nuclear extraction kit was from Pierce (USA).

The antibodies against Cyclin B1, ERK1, and ERK2 were from NeoMarkers (USA), antibodies against phospho-ERK1/2, cyclin-dependent kinase 1 (Cdk1), Cdc25C, Raf-1 were from Santa Cruz Biotechnology (USA), and antibodies against c-Jun, c-Fos, Pan-ras, and actin were from Boster Corporation (China). The rabbit polyclonal anti-antibodies horseradish peroxidase conjugates of anti-rabbit and anti-mouse immunoglobulin G were from Bio-Rad Laboratories (USA). Enhanced chemiluminescence detection reagents were obtained from Amersham (USA).

Cell culture

The human breast cancer cell line, MDA-MB-231, obtained from the American Type Culture Collection (Rockville, MD), were routinely maintained in Leibovitz's L-15 medium, pH 7.3, supplemented with 100 IU/ml penicillin, 100 mg/ml streptomycin, and 10% fetal calf serum (FCS) and were grown at 37°. Genistein was dissolved in ethanol and was added directly to the culture media at different concentrations. The concentration of ethanol (0.1%) in the final working solution did not interfere with cell growth. Wherever indicated, the MEK1/2 inhibitor (PD98059) was dissolved in dimethyl sulfoxide (DMSO) and added to the culture media at final concentration of 15 and 30 μM. Control cultures received the same concentration of ethanol and/or DMSO similar to those used for the experimental cultures.

Cell cycle analyses

The distribution of cells at different stages in the cell cycle was estimated by flow cytometric DNA analysis. Briefly, 5×10^5 cells were incubated at 37°C overnight in triplicate 10-cm plastic dishes in medium containing 10% FCS, incubated for 48 h with or without various concentrations of genistein and PD98059. Cells from the different conditions were trypsinized, washed in cold phosphate-buffered saline (PBS) pH 7.4, fixed in 70% ethanol/30% PBS, and stored at 4°C until processing. An aliquot (1 ml) of fixed cell suspension containing 1×10^6 cells was washed twice in cold PBS. The fixed cells were treated for 30 min at 4°C in the dark with fluoro-chrome DNA staining solution (1 ml) containing 40 μg of propidium iodide and 0.1 mg of RNase A; then, the stained cells were analyzed by flow cytometry. The percentage of cells in each cell cycle phase (G0/G1, S, or G2/M) was calculated by using Lysis II Software, a minimum of 1.5×10^4 cells per sample being evaluated in each case.

Western blotting

The MDA-MB-231 cells were plated on culture dishes and allowed to attach for 24 h, followed by the addition of 5, 10, 20 μM genistein and/or 15, 30 μM PD98059 and incubation for 48 h. Control cells were incubated in the medium with ethanol using the same time points. After incubation, the cells were washed twice with ice-cold PBS and then scraped off in 0.2 ml of buffer [20 mM (4-(2-hydroxyethyl)-1-piperazineethanesulfonic acid), pH 6.8, 5 mM ethylenediaminetetraacetic acid, 10 mM [(2,2′-oxyproplylene-dinitrilo]tetraacetic acid, 5 mM NaF, 0.1 μg/ml okadaic acid, 1 mM dithiothreitol, 0.4 M KCl, 0.4% Triton X-100, 10% glycerol, 5 μg/ml leupeptin, 50 μg/ml phenylmethyl-sulfonyl fluoride, 1 mM benzamidine, 5 mg/ml aprotinin, 1 mM Na orthovanadate] and incubated on ice for 30 min followed by centrifugation at 12,000 rpm for 20 min. The supernatant was stored at −70°C. Protein concentration was then measured using bicinchoninic acid protein assay (Pierce, Rockford, IL). After the determination, all proteins were diluted to equal concentration, boiled for 5 min, and then separated by 12% sodium dodecyl sulfate–polyacrylamide gel electrophoresis (SDS-PAGE).

Proteins were then transferred to nitrocellulose membranes, which were probed with the primary antibodies overnight at 4°C. Membranes were then incubated with horseradish peroxidase-conjugated secondary antibodies for 1 h at room temperature before enhanced chemiluminescence (Amersham Biosciences) and exposure to film. Actin was used to normalize for protein loading. All the experiments were performed at least twice with similar results.

Statistical analyses

Data are expressed as means±SD. Statistical differences were analyzed using one-way analysis of variance. A value of $P<0.05$ was considered to indicate a statistically significant difference.

Results

Genistein-treated MDA-MB-231 cells are arrested in G2/M phase of the cell cycle

To determine at which phase the cells arrest after treatment with genistein, MDA-MB-231 cells were treated with 0, 5, 10, or 20 μM concentrations of genistein. After 48 h of treatment, cell cycle phase was determined by flow cytometry. Genistein treatment induced a significant accumulation of cells in the G2/M phase of the cell cycle in a concentration-dependent manner, with a parallel depletion of the percentage of cells in G0/G1 (Fig. 1). Treatment of cells with 0, 5, 10, or 20 μM genistein for 48 h resulted in G2/M phase accumulation of cells corresponding to 14, 34, 42, and 55%, respectively. The increase of the percentage of cells in the G2/M phase of the cell cycle after treatment with 20 μM genistein was fourfold in the case of MDA-MB-231 cells compared to the control ($P<0.05$, $n=3$).

As the cyclin B/Cdc2 complex performs an important function in controlling the G2/M phase, and as treatment of MDA-MB-231 cells with genistein resulted in a strong increase in G2/M phase cell population, we next conducted a detailed analysis of the molecules involved in G2/M phase of the cell cycle. To elucidate the mechanism for G2/M arrest in genistein-treated cells, we determined its effect on expression of proteins that are pivotal for G2/M transition, including cyclin B1, Cdk1, and Cdc25C, after treatment with

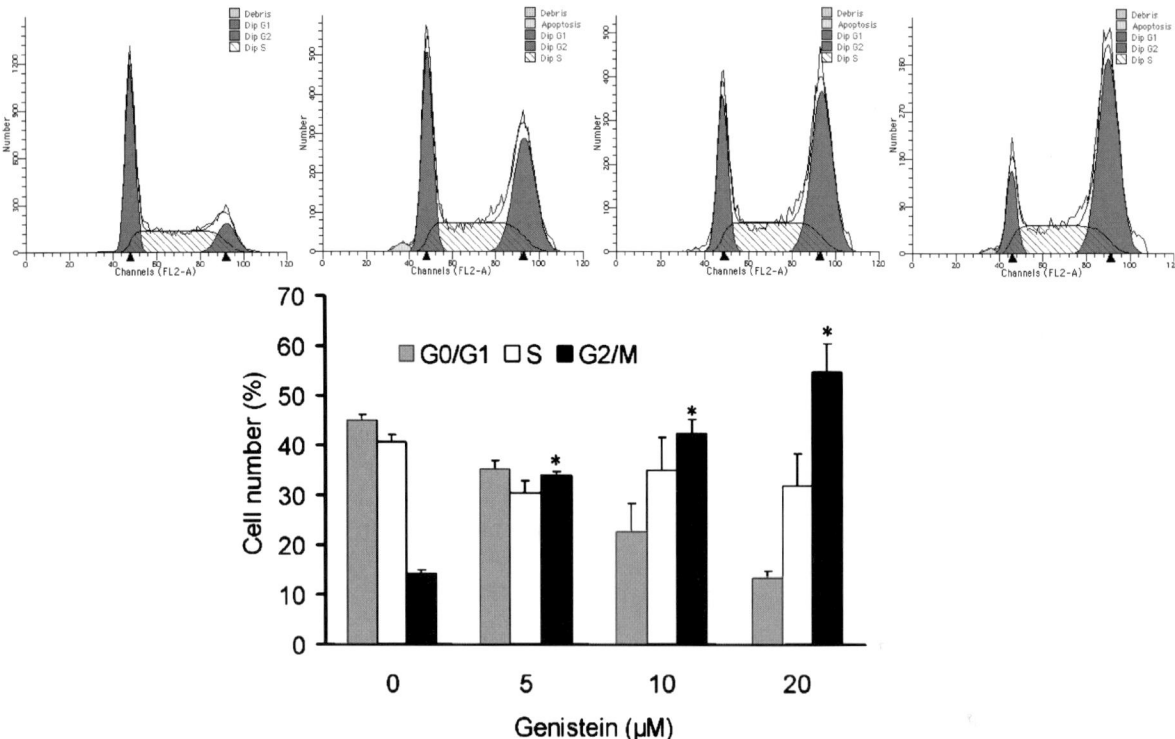

Fig. 1 Dose response of the cell cycle distribution in MDA-MB-231 cells treated with different concentrations of genistein. Cells were incubated with genistein at the concentration of 0, 5, 10, and 20 μM for 48 h, and the percentage of cells in each cell cycle phase (G1, S, and G2M) was determined by flow cytometry. *Asterisk* indicates significantly different from control, $P<0.05$ ($n=3$)

different concentrations of genistein for 48 h. Representative Western blots for the effect of genistein treatment on cyclin B1, Cdk1, and Cdc25C expression in MDA-MB-231 cells are depicted in Fig. 2. Immunoblotting revealed that genistein treatment resulted in a significant reduction in the protein levels of cyclin B1, Cdk1, and Cdc25C in a concentration-dependent manner. Taken together, these results suggested that genistein treatment might cause a reduction in the protein levels of cyclinB1, Cdk1, and Cdc25C. These cell cycle regulators may be responsible for genistein-induced G2/M phase cell cycle arrest.

Ras/ERK/AP-1 pathway is necessary
for genistein-induced G2/M cell cycle arrest
in breast cancer cells

To assess the effect of MEK1/2 inhibitor (PD98059) on genistein-induced G2/M cell cycle arrest, cells were treated with control or PD98059 (15, 30 μM) in the absence or presence of 20 μM genistein for 48 h. As shown in Fig. 3, PD98059 alone did not have a

significant effect on the cell cycle phase. When PD98059 was added to genistein-treated cells, it overrode genistein-induced cell G2/M arrest in a concentration-dependent manner. PD98059-induced G2/M depletion was associated with a corresponding increase in the percentage of cells in the G0/G1 phase of the cell cycle. Treatment of genistein-induced cells with 0, 15, and 30 μM PD98059 for 48 h resulted in G2/M phase depletion corresponding to 55, 45, and 29%, respectively. As PD98059 was a specific MEK1/2 inhibitor, these results suggested that MAPK signaling pathway was involved in genistein-induced G2/M cell cycle arrest.

To evaluate the effect of genistein in MDA-MB-231 cells in greater detail, we assessed the impact of genistein on the phosphorylation status of ERK1/2. As shown in Fig. 4a and b, untreated MDA-MB-231 cells expressed little or no phosphorylated ERK1/2; treatment with genistein increased ERK1/2 phosphorylation in a concentration- and time-dependent manner in MDA-MB-231 cells. Genistein induced a slow and stable activation of phosphorylated ERK1/2 starting at

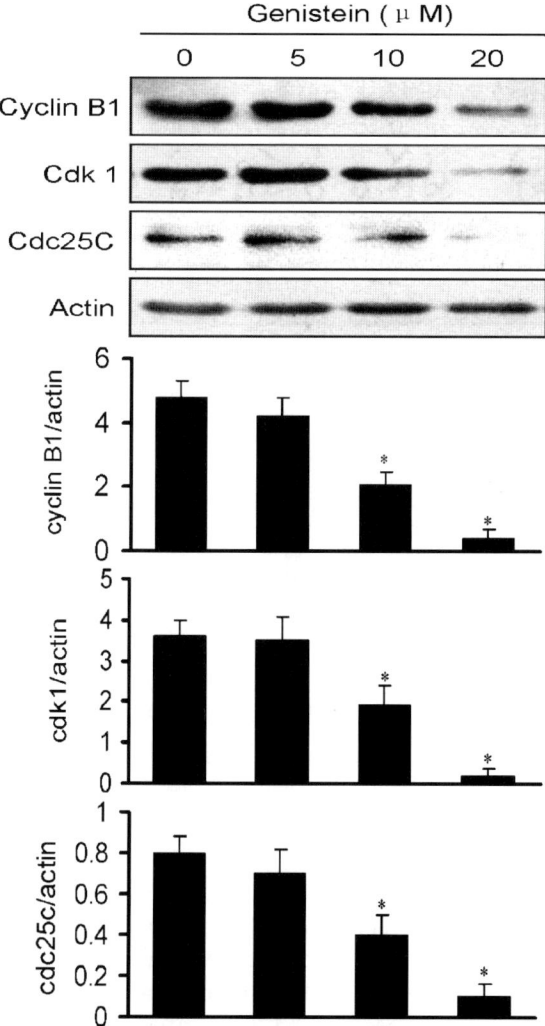

Genistein (μ M)

Fig. 2 The effects of genistein on cell cycle regulators. Cells were incubated with genistein at the concentration of 0, 5, 10, and 20 μM for 48 h. The representative Western blots for the expression of cyclin B1, Cdk1, and Cdc25C were presented. Actin protein was blotted as a control. Each experiment was repeated twice with similar results. Histograms represent densitometric measurement of specific bands using actin level as control. *Asterisk* indicates significantly different from control, $P<0.05$

24 h and was sustained for at least 48 h (Fig. 4a). In contrast, no change in total ERK1/2 (p42/p44) was observed during genistein treatment in MDA-MB-231 cells. Treatment of MDA-MB-231 cells with the MEK1/2 inhibitor PD98059 (15, 30 μM) largely decreased the phosphorylation of ERK1/2 induced by genistein in MDA-MB-231 cells (Fig. 4b). PD98059 had no effect on the expression of total ERK1/2, demonstrating the specificity of the inhibitor on

phosphorylation. Taken together, inhibition of ERK1/2 phosphorylation by PD98059 blocked genistein-induced G2/M cell cycle arrest. This study shows that stable activation of ERK1/2 is necessary for genistein-induced G2/M cell cycle arrest in MDA-MB-231 breast cancer cells.

Activation of ERK can be induced by a variety of extracellular stimuli. To further define the signaling molecules involved in genistein-induced ERK activation, we investigated whether the activation of ERK1/2 in MDA-MB-231 cells in response to genistein required activation of Ras and Raf-1. As shown in Fig. 2c, when MDA-MB-231 cells were treated with genistein for 48 h, the protein levels of Ras and Raf-1 were increased in concentration-dependent manner. When MDA-MB-231 cells were treated with PD98059 before genistein treatment, there was no significant inhibition of genistein-induced activation of Ras and Raf-1 (Fig. 4b). Together, these results indicate that genistein induces ERK1/2 activation in a Ras/Raf-1-dependent manner, and PD98059 blocks genistein-induced ERK1/2 activation, which is a downstream event of Ras/Raf-1 pathway.

The activator protein-1 (AP-1) transcriptional factor is composed of either homo- or heterodimers between members of Jun and Fos families. Expression of AP-1 subunits is regulated in response to various stimuli. To examine the effects of genistein exposure on the expression of AP-1 subunits, the nuclear protein levels of c-Jun and c-Fos were measured by Western blot analysis. As shown in Fig. 5, genistein significantly enhanced the nuclear protein level of both c-Jun and c-Fos in a dose-dependent manner within 48 h of treatment (Fig. 5). Genistein-induced expression of c-Jun and c-Fos were abrogated by addition of PD98059. Thus, these results indicate that the expression of c-Jun and c-Fos in MDA-MB-231 cells is mediated by ERK1/2 activation, and up-regulation of the AP-1 family might play an active role in the mediation of genistein-induced G2/M cell cycle arrest in MDA-MB-231 cells.

Discussion

Genistein is known to suppress tumor cell growth which is mediated by different types of cell cycle arrest in several tumor cell lines. Genistein arrests the cell cycle at the G2/M phases in hepatoma cells

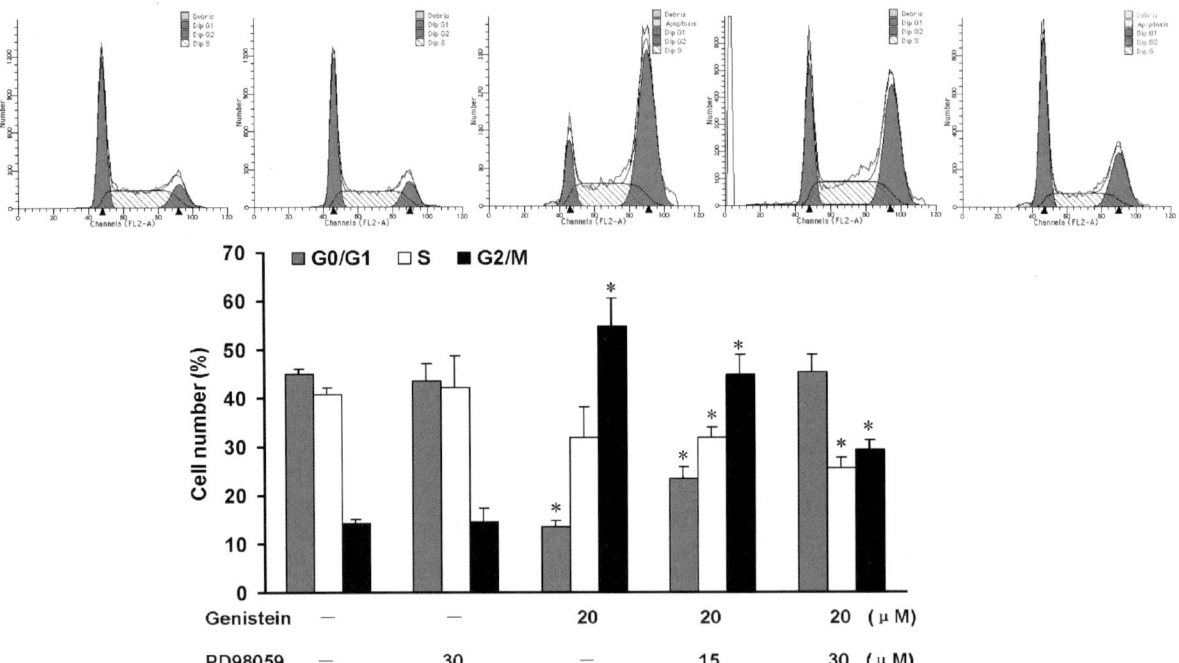

Fig. 3 PD98059 blocks genistein-induced G2/M cell cycle arrest in MDA-MB-231 cells. Cells were treated with genistein and incubated in the absence or presence of 15, 30 μM PD98059 for 48 h. The resulting cells were harvested, stained with PI, and analysed for DNA contents by flow cytometry. *Asterisk* indicates significantly different from control, $P<0.05$ ($n=3$)

(Chang et al. 2004), gastric cancer cells (Matsukawa et al. 1993), breast cancer cells (Nomoto et al. 2002), prostate cancer cells (Kobayashi et al. 2002), non-neoplastic human mammary epithelial cells (Frey et al. 2001), lung cancer cells (Lian et al. 1998), head and neck cancer cells (Alhasan et al. 2000), and intestinal cells (Chen and Donovan 2004). In terms of regulation of the cell cycle, cyclin-dependent kinases play a most critical role.

Eukaryotic cell cycle progression involves sequential activation of Cdks whose activation is dependent upon their association with cyclins. A complex formed by the association of Cdk1 and cyclin B1 plays a major role at entry into mitosis (Molinari 2000). In the present study, we observed that treatment of MDA-MB-231 cells with genistein results in arrest of cells in G2/M phase and that genistein-mediated G2/M arrest is associated with a decrease in the protein levels of Cdk1, cyclinB1, and Cdc25C. Thus, it is reasonable to postulate that genistein treatment may cause cell cycle arrest by reducing the activity of Cdk1/cyclin B kinase complex due to down-regulation of multiple G2/M regulating proteins.

The MAP kinase pathway is more often associated with cell survival (Xia et al. 1995; Cross et al. 2000). However, the importance of the MAP kinase pathway in all phases of cell cycle regulation is being increasingly recognized (Pumiglia and Decker 1997). Recently, the MAP kinase pathway has also been implicated in G2 cell cycle regulation. In *Xenopus* oocytes, MAP kinase activity has been shown to be necessary for progression through G2, possibly by inhibiting cyclin B/CDC2 kinase activity (Abrieu et al. 1997). In breast cancer cells, BRCA1-mediated G2/M cell cycle arrest requires ERK1/2 kinase activation (Yan et al. 2005). In this study, we investigated the specific effects of ERK1/2 signaling on the genistein-mediated G2/M arrest and found that the stable activation of ERK1/2 by genistein is necessary for genistein-mediated activation of G2/M arrest in MDA-MB-231 cells.

ERK activation in response to growth factors such as epidermal growth factor and platelet-derived growth factor classically proceeds via a Ras-mediated cascade that involves Raf-1, MEK, and MAPK/ERK activation (Sridhar et al. 2005). To determine whether

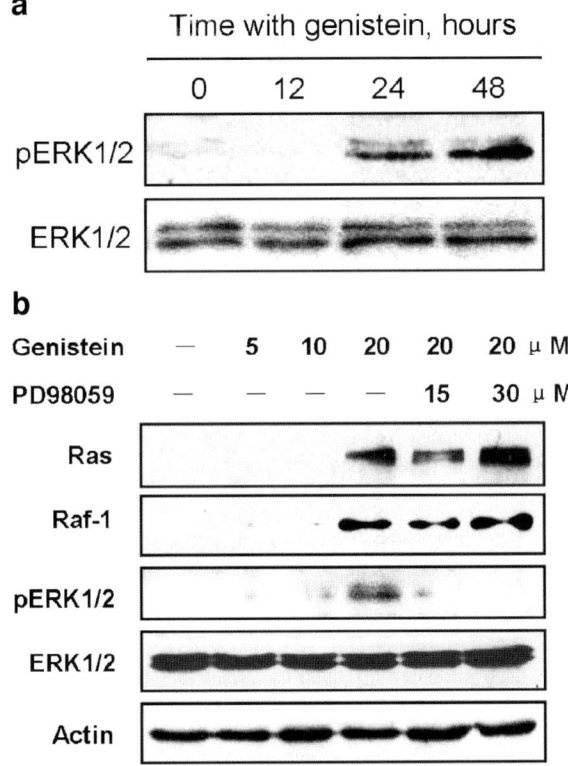

a

Time with genistein, hours

	0	12	24	48
pERK1/2				
ERK1/2				

b

Genistein	—	5	10	20	20	20 µM
PD98059	—	—	—	—	15	30 µM

Ras
Raf-1
pERK1/2
ERK1/2
Actin

Fig. 4 a Determination of phospho-ERK1/2 expression in lysate of MDA-MB-231 cells exposed to ethanol (control) or 20 µM of genistein for different time intervals. **b** PD98059 blocks genistein-induced activation of Ras/Raf-1/ERK1/2 pathways. MDA-MB-231 cells were treated with different concentrations of genistein in the absence or presence of 15, 30 µM PD98059 for 48 h. Western blot analyses of ras, raf-1, phospho-ERK1/2, and total ERK1/2 in MDA-MB-231 cells. Actin protein was blotted as a control. Each experiment was repeated twice with similar results

genistein seemed to involve AP-1. Genistein up-regulated steady-state levels of both c-Jun and c-Fos in MDA-MB-231 cells. Genistein-induced c-Jun and c-Fos expression was consistent with genistein-induced ERK1/2 activation, and both the expression of c-Jun and c-Fos, and phosphorylated ERK1/2 were inhibited by PD98059. Thus, genistein activates AP-1 through MAPK pathways, and correspondingly, deregulates AP-1-dependent cell cycle proteins. These findings strongly suggest an important role of the MAPK/AP-1 signal pathway in genistein-induced G2/M cell cycle arrest in MDA-MB-231 cells.

Need to note, in 2001, Dampier et al. (2001) evaluated the effects of genistein on cell growth, cell apoptosis, and cell cycle arrest in six breast cancer cell lines. The results suggest that induction of apoptosis, G2 cell cycle arrest and inhibition of c-fos expression, AP-1 transactivation, and ERK phosphorylation may contribute to the growth-inhibitory effect of genistein in some breast cell types. These results are quite different with ours. Dampier et al. stimulated cells with phorbol ester and then added genistein to block its action. ERK1/2 could be rapidly activated by growth factors, cytokines, and phorbol ester. Genistein and E2 also rapidly activate ERK1/2 in estrogen-receptor-positive cancer cells and stimulate cell growth (Borrás et al. 2006; Vivacqua et al. 2006). This activation is transient. In our studies, genistein induced cell growth inhibition in a dose-dependent manner (data not shown); genistein also

genistein activates ERK through Ras or by directly activating Raf and independently of Ras, we treated MDA-MB-231 cells with different concentrations of genistein for 48 h. Ras and Raf-1 were induced by genistein treatment, suggesting that the Ras/Raf/MEK pathway is involved in genistein-induced ERK1/2 activation.

The activation of the activating protein-1 (AP-1) family of transcription factors, including c-Fos and c-Jun family members, is one of the earliest nuclear events induced by growth factors that stimulate ERKs (Angel and Karin 1991). MAPK are responsible for the activation of Jun and Fos proteins. C-Jun and c-Fos can cooperate to regulate AP-1-dependent gene transcription. Thus, AP-1 is a major target of the MAPKs (Whitmarsh and Davis 1996). The action of

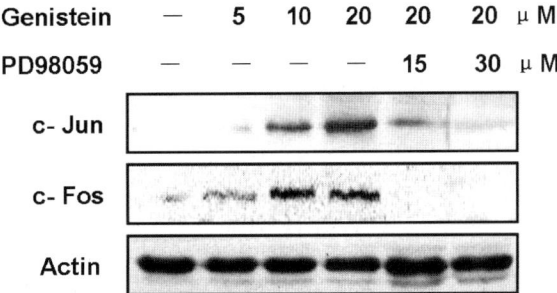

Genistein	—	5	10	20	20	20 µM
PD98059	—	—	—	—	15	30 µM

c-Jun
c-Fos
Actin

Fig. 5 PD98059 blocks genistein-induced c-Jun and c-Fos expression. MDA-MB-231 cells were treated with different concentrations of genistein in the absence or presence of 15,30 µM PD98059 for 48 h. Equal amounts of nuclear protein were fractionated on 12% SDS-PAGE gels and transferred to polyvinylidene difluoride membranes followed by immunoblotting with anti-c-Jun and anti-c-Fos polyclonal antibodies and analysis as described in "Materials and methods". Actin protein was blotted as a control. Each experiment was repeated twice with similar results

induced a slow and stable activation of ERK1/2 starting at 24 h and was sustained for at least 48 h in estrogen-receptor-negative breast cancer cell line MDA-MB-231. This activation profile is distinct from the rapid transient ERK1/2 activation. There are also reports suggesting that genistein induces apoptosis through a delayed and prolonged activation of p42/44 MAPK (Linford et al. 2001). Thus, different activation patterns of ERK1/2 may cause different cell responses.

The overall results of the present study suggest that the Ras/MAPK/AP-1 signal pathway is involved in genistein-induced G2/M cell cycle arrest in MDA-MB-231 cells. Our work provides new insights into the molecular mechanisms of genistein in breast cancer cells.

Acknowledgments We thank Drs. Ruiwen Zhang, Donald L. Hill, and Hui Wang for help in the preparation of the manuscript. This work was supported by grant 30271122 from National Natural Science Foundation of China, grant BK2002027 from Natural Science Foundation of Jiangsu Province (to Z. Li).

References

Abbott DW, Holt JT. Mitogen-activated protein kinase kinase 2 activation is essential for progression through the G2/M checkpoint arrest in cells exposed to ionizing radiation. J Biol Chem. 1999;274:2732–42.

Abrieu A, Fisher D, Simon MN, Doree M, Picard A. MAPK inactivation is required for the G2 to M-phase transition of the first mitotic cell cycle. EMBO J. 1997;16:6407–13.

Alhasan SA, Ensley JF, Sarkar FH. Genistein induced molecular changes in a squamous cell carcinoma of the head and neck cell line. Int J Oncol. 2000;16:333–8.

Angel P, Karin M. The role of Jun, Fos and the AP-1 complex in cell-proliferation and transformation. Biochim Biophys Acta. 1991;1072:129–57.

Borrás C, Gambini J, Gómez-Cabrera MC, et al. Genistein, a soy isoflavone, up-regulates expression of antioxidant genes: involvement of estrogen receptors, ERK1/2, and NFkappaB. FASEB J. 2006;20:2136–8.

Chang KL, Kung ML, Chow NH, Su SJ. Genistein arrests hepatoma cells at G2/M phase: involvement of ATM activation and upregulation of p21$^{waf1/cip1}$ and Wee1. Biochem Pharmacol. 2004;67:717–26.

Chen AC, Donovan SM. Genistein at a concentration present in soy infant formula inhibits Caco-2BBe cell proliferation by causing G2/M cell cycle arrest. J Nutr. 2004;134:1303–8.

Choi YH, Zhang L, Lee WH, Park KY. Genistein-induced G2/M arrest is associated with the inhibition of cyclin B1 and the induction of p21 in human breast carcinoma cells. Int J Oncol. 1998;13:391–6.

Cross TG, Scheel-Toellner D, Henriquez NV, et al. Serine/threonine protein kinases and apoptosis. Exp Cell Res. 2000;256:34–41.

Dampier K, Hudson EA, Howells LM, et al. Differences between human breast cell lines in susceptibility towards growth inhibition by genistein. Br J Cancer. 2001;85:618–24.

Fioranvanti L, Cappelletti V, Miodini P, et al. Genistein in the control of breast cancer cell growth: insights into the mechanism of action in vitro. Cancer Lett. 1998;130:143–52.

Fotsis T, Pepper M, Adlercreutz H, et al. Genistein, a dietary ingested isoflavonoid, inhibits cell proliferation and in vitro angiogenesis. J Nutr. 1995;125:790S–797S.

Frey RS, Li J, Singletary KW. Effects of genistein on cell proliferation and cell cycle arrest in nonneoplastic human mammary epithelial cells: involvement of Cdc2, p21$^{waf/cip1}$, p27^{kip1}, and Cdc25C expression. Biochem Pharmacol 2001;61:979–89.

Gotoh Y, Nishida E. Activation mechanism and function of the MAP kinase cascade. Mol Reprod Dev. 1995;42:486–92.

Hsieh CY, Santell RC, Haslam SZ, Helferich WG. Estrogenic effects of genistein on the growth of estrogen receptor-positive human breast cancer (MCF-7) cells in vitro and in vivo. Cancer Res. 1998;58:3833–8.

Kobayashi T, Nakata T, Kuzumaki T. Effect of flavonoids on cell cycle progression in prostate cancer cells. Cancer Lett 2002;176:17–23.

Lian F, Bhuiyan M, Li YW, et al. Genistein-induced G2-M arrest, p21^{WAF1} upregulation, and apoptosis in a non-small-cell lung cancer cell line. Nutr Cancer. 1998;31:184–91.

Linford NJ, Yang Y, Cook DG, Dorsa DM. Neuronal apoptosis resulting from high doses of the isoflavone genistein: role for calcium and p42/44 mitogen-activated protein kinase. J Pharmacol Exp Ther. 2001;299:67–75.

Matsukawa Y, Marui N, Sakai T, et al. Genistein arrests cell cycle progression at G2-M. Cancer Res 1993;53:1328–31.

Messina MJ, Persky V, Setchell KD, Barnes S. Soy intake and cancer risk: a review of the in vitro and in vivo data. Nutr Cancer 1994;21:113–31.

Molinari M. Cell cycle checkpoints and their inactivation in human cancer. Cell Prolif 2000;33:261–74.

Monti E, Sinha BK. Antiproliferative effect of genistein and adriamycin against estrogen-dependent and independent human breast carcinoma cell lines. Anticancer Res 1994;14:1221–6.

Nomoto S, Arao Y, Horiguchi H, Ikeda K, Kayama F. Oestrogen causes G2/M arrest and apoptosis in breast cancer cells MDA-MB-231. Oncol Rep 2002;9:773–6.

Peterson G, Barnes S. Genistein inhibition of the growth of human breast cancer cells: independence from estrogen receptors and the multi-drug resistance gene. Biochem Biophys Res Commun 1991;179:661–7.

Pumiglia KM, Decker SJ. Cell cycle arrest mediated by the MEK/mitogen-activated protein kinase pathway. Proc Natl Acad Sci U S A 1997;94:448–52.

Schaeffer H, Weber M. Mitogen-activated protein kinases: specific messages from ubiquitous messengers. Mol Cell Biol 1999;19:2435–44.

Shao ZM, Wu J, Shen ZZ, Barsky SH. Genistein exerts multiple suppressive effects on human breast carcinoma cells. Cancer Res 1998;58:4851–7.

Sherr CJ. Cancer cell cycle. Science 1996;274:1672–7.

Sridhar SS, Hedley D, Siu LL. Raf kinase as a target for anticancer therapeutics. Mol Cancer Ther 2005;4:677–85.

Tang D, Wu D, Hirao A, et al. ERK activation mediates cell cycle arrest and apoptosis after DNA damage independently of p53. J Biol Chem 2002;277:12710–7.

Tragados F, Ardelt B, Halko N, Bruno S, Darzynkiewicz Z. Effects of genistein on the growth and cell cycle progression of normal human lymphocytes and human leukemic MOLT-4 and HL-60 cells. Cancer Res 1992;52:6200–8.

Upadhyay S, Neburi M, Chinni SR, et al. Differential sensitivity of normal and malignant breast epithelial cells to genistein is partly mediated by p21^{WAF1}. Clin Cancer Res 2001;7:1782–9.

Vivacqua A, Bonofiglio D, Albanito L, et al. 17beta-estradiol, genistein, and 4-hydroxytamoxifen induce the proliferation of thyroid cancer cells through the g protein-coupled receptor GPR30. Mol Pharmacol 2006;70:1414–23.

Whitmarsh AJ, Davis RJ. Transcription factor AP-1 regulation by mitogen-activated protein kinase signal transduction pathways. J Mol Med 1996;74:589–607.

Xia Z, Dickens M, Raingeaud J, Davis RJ, Greenberg ME. Opposing effects of ERK and JNK-p38 MAP kinases on apoptosis. Science 1995;270:1326–31.

Yan Y, Spieker RS, Kim M, Stoeger SM, Cowan KH. BRCA1-mediated G2/M cell cycle arrest requires ERK1/2 kinase activation. Oncogene 2005;24:3285–96.

Zava DT, Duwe G. Estrogenic and antiproliferative properties of genistein and other flavonoids in human breast cancer cells in vitro. Nutr Cancer 1997;27:31–40.

Zhou JR, Mukherjee P, Gugger ET, et al. Inhibition of murine bladder tumorigenesis by soy isoflavones via alterations in the cell cycle, apoptosis, and angiogenesis. Cancer Res 1998;58:5231–8.

In vivo 5-flourouracil-induced apoptosis on murine thymocytes: involvement of FAS, Bax and Caspase3

Jose A. Aquino Esperanza · Maria V. Aguirre ·
Gualberto R. Aispuru · Carolina N. Lettieri ·
Julian A. Juaristi · Mirta A. Alvarez ·
Nora Cristina Brandan

Originally published in the journal Cell Biology and Toxicology, Volume 24, Nos 4–5, 131–142.
DOI: 10.1007/s10565-008-9056-z © Springer Science + Business Media B.V. 2008

Abstract Apoptosis is a highly regulated and pro-grammed cell breakdown process characterized by numerous changes. It was reported as the major mechanism of anticancer drug-induced cells death. Unfortunately, many of these drugs are non-specific and cause severe side effects. The effects of 5-flourouracil (5-FU) on the apoptotic events in normal murine thymus were evaluated using an in vivo model. A single dose of 5-FU (150 mg/kg ip) was injected to CF-1 mice. A multiparametric analysis of thymic weight, cellularity, viability, architectural organization, apoptosis, DNA fragmentation, and the expression of several apoptotic proteins was evaluated in 10 days time-course study post-5-FU dosing. Total organ weights, thymocyte counts, and cell viabilities diminished drastically from the second day. The thymus architecture assessed through electron scanning microscopy revealed deep alterations and the lost of cell–cell contact between the first and the third days. DNA fragmentation and apoptotic indexes (May Grünwald Giemsa staining, double flourescent dyes, and TdT-mediated dUTP nick-end labeling assay) revealed that cell death was maximal on the second day (three times over control). Furthermore, the pro-apoptotic proteins FAS and Bax were strongly up-regulated during the first 2 days. The aforementioned morphological and biochemical changes were also accompanied within the same period by caspase 3 activation. This study revealed that in vivo apoptosis in normal thymus after 5-FU administration is related to FAS, Bax, and Caspase 3 co-expressions under the current experimental conditions, these findings, therefore, contribute to a new insight into the molecular mechanisms involved during 5-FU administration upon the thymus and the possible events committed in the lymphophenia associated with chemotherapy.

Keywords 5-FU · Murine thymus · Apoptosis · FAS · Bax · Caspase 3

J. A. Aquino Esperanza · M. V. Aguirre · G. R. Aispuru ·
C. N. Lettieri · J. A. Juaristi · M. A. Alvarez ·
N. C. Brandan (✉)
Faculty of Medicine, Biochemistry,
Northeast National University,
Moreno 1240,
Corrientes 3400, Argentina
e-mail: nbrandan@med.unne.edu.ar

Introduction

Apoptosis is a well-controlled, tightly regulated physiological mechanism that is used extensively during the development, tissue homeostasis, and maintenance of the immune system in adult organisms (Jacobson 1997). This process involves the activation of several molecular events, leading to cell death that is characterized by morphological changes, chromatin condensation, and apoptotic bodies that are associated with DNA fragmentation and caspases activation (Kerr 2002). Caspases, also known as cysteine aspartate-specific proteases, are a family of intracellular proteins that exist as dormant proenzymes in healthy cells and are activated through proteolysis. Once activated, they cleave cellular substrates, leading to morphological hallmarks of apoptosis (Zhang et al. 2000a, b; Savill and Fadok 2000; Ashkenazi and Dixit 1998; Thornberry and Lazebnik 1998).

It has been reported that apoptosis is the major mechanism of anticancer drug-induced cells death (Ricci and Zong 2006). 5-Fluorouracil (5-FU) is an antimetabolic chemotherapeutic agent with multiple mechanisms of action, including inhibition of the synthesis of thymidine nucleotides and incorporation into RNA (Parker and Cheng 1990; Pritchard et al. 1997). Although 5-FU is a widely used antineoplastic agent, the cytotoxicity of 5-FU is not limited to tumor tissue. Hematopoietic cells and normal epithelial cells of gastrointestinal tract are susceptible to 5-FU-induced cytotoxicity, which produces severe leucopenia and intestinal toxicity, leading to lethal translocation of intestinal microflora (Yeager et al. 1983; Ijiri and Potten 1987; Rocha et al. 1994). In addition, in vitro and in vivo studies showed that 5-FU-induced apoptosis upon the thymus is partially mediated via death receptor CD95 (Eichhorst et al. 2001). Moreover, there is widespread evidence that another potential apoptotic-promoting system may be involved in the thymus post-5-FU, such as those involving the homodimerization of death promoting molecule Bax and/or Bak that regulate mitochondria-mediated apoptosis by direct modulation of mitochondrial permeabilization (Miyashita et al. 1995; Gottlieb and Oren 1998). Experimental evidence has suggested that Bax is one of the crucial proteins in apoptosis regulation upon 5-FU treatment. In vitro studies using oral squamous carcinoma cells (Takemura et al. 2005) and colon carcinoma cells (Kobayashi et al. 2000) showed an increased expression of Bax after 5-FU treatment. Furthermore, mutant colorectal cancer cells that lack functional Bax gene exhibit partial resistance to 5-FU (Zhang et al. 2000a, b). In addition, 5-FU induced-apoptosis was accompanied by increased expression of Bax in colon cancer cells with wild-type p53 (Nita et al. 1998). This in vitro experimental data strongly suggests that Bax expression is linked to 5-FU-induced apoptosis.

It is also noteworthy that degradation of antiapoptotic proteins such as Bcl-2 and Bcl-xL induces dimerization of Bax, involving the release of cytochrome c from mitochondria, caspases cascade activation, and cell death (Fincucane et al. 1999; Alnemri 1997; Henkart 1996; Martin and Green 1995; Chinnaiyan and Dixit 1996).

Although the apoptotic mechanisms are well known, cellular response triggered by 5-FU varies depending on experimental conditions. For instance, in vitro studies using HT 29 colon carcinoma cells could not show significant DNA fragmentation during the first 24 h after 5-FU (Horowitz et al. 1997), whereas LoVo colorectal cancer cells showed minimal DNA fragmentation at 48 h (Werner et al. 2007). Nevertheless, in vivo studies showed DNA fragmentation in breast cancer tissue removed after 5-FU treatment (Asaga et al. 2001). Unfortunately, little is known about the possible in vivo side effects of 5-FU, specifically upon normal thymic tissue and its apoptotic mechanism.

Therefore, in the current study, the effect of 5-FU on murine thymus using an in vivo normal model through several experimental procedures was studied. Thus, thymic weight and structure, apoptotic indexes (TdT-mediated dUTP nick-end labeling, TUNEL; DNA fragmentation; light; and fluorescence microscopy), as well as FAS, Bax, and caspase 3 expressions (immunoblottings) were evaluated after a single dose of 5-FU over a period of 10 days.

Experimental data strongly suggests that 5-FU induces thymocytes apoptosis 6 h post-drug dosing, reaching the maximum injury on the second day. In spite of the reduction of glands weight and the deep alterations of the thymic structure, the apoptotic related proteins (FAS, Bax, and Caspase 3) were expressed in a coordinated way along the acute apoptotic phase and the further recovery.

Data from this study may contribute to the understanding of 5-FU immunotoxicity and the underlying mechanisms involved in this process.

Material and methods

Animals

Adult female CF-1 Swiss mice (age, 5–6 weeks; average weight, 23–25 g) were used all through the experimental protocol. They were housed in cages in an air-conditioned room with controlled temperature (24°C) for 5 days before the experiment and maintained in a 12-h light–dark cycles. They were allowed to access freely to pelleted food and water. Experiments were conducted according to the principles in the "Guide for the Care and Use of Laboratory Animals" (NIH, Bethesda, MD, 1996).

Experimental design

Mice were divided randomly into three groups. The first group ($n=96$) was subdivided into two subsets. Mice of the first subset ($n=48$) were treated with saline for controls, whereas mice of the second subset ($n=48$) were injected with 5-FU (F 6627–5G; Sigma, St. Louis, MO). 5-FU was dissolved in sterile saline solution (NaCl 0.9%), and it was injected i.p. at a single dose of 150 mg/kg. Animals from the first group were used to assess cellularity, viability, thymic weight, and apoptotic assays. Six mice were used for control, and six ones were used for 5-FU-treated mice at each time point of the study for the above-mentioned assays.

The second group of animals ($n=18$) was used for DNA laddering assay and scanning electronic microscopy. Two animals were used at each time point for these assays.

Finally, the third group ($n=27$) was used to obtain thymic extracts for Western blotting. Three animals were used for obtaining lysates at each time point of the experimental schedule. Experimental data from 5-FU-injected mice of the second and third groups of rodents were compared to the control animals (day 0).

Animals were euthanized by cervical dislocation under pentobarbital (100 mg/kg i.p.) anesthesia at 0, 6, and 12 h, and 1, 2, 3, 5, 7, and 10 days, respectively, then glands were immediately removed and used for the different assays.

Determination of thymus cellularity and viability

Thymus tissue was placed in ice-cold phosphate buffer saline (PBS, pH 7.4) and passed through a sieve. Cell suspensions were washed several times with minimum essential medium (MEM, Alpha Modification Sigma Co., USA) and were centrifuged at 500 rpm for 10 min to avoid remaining debris.

Thymic cell suspensions were flushed with 500 μl of MEM, and cellularity, as well as viability, was determined using a hemocytometer. Viability was assessed by the Trypan Blue (0.2%) exclusion assay. Cellularities are expressed as total nucleated cells $\times 10^6$/thymus, and thymus viabilities are expressed as a percentage of viable cells.

Both parameters were determined in thymic cell suspensions from three independent experiments at the indicated time points after injection of 5-FU.

Scanning electronic microscopy

This technique aims to preserve the tissue, particularly for a direct observation of the thymic architecture during post-5-FU recovery. Thymi were removed and placed in fresh cold fixative solution (5% formaldehyde, 6% acetic acid, 65% ethanol, and 24% water) to be observed under the scanning electronic microscope. The samples were dehydrated and dried to critical point (Dento Drier). Then, they were exposed to gold–palladium coating for 3 min. The sections were examined through the scanning electronic microscope (Jepl-JSM-5800 L.V.) and images (1,500–2,000×) were obtained in triplicate at the indicated time points of the protocol.

Methodological aspects of apoptosis detection

(a) May Gründwald–Giemsa (MGG) staining

May Gründwald–Giemsa staining (Merck, Germany) was use on methanol-fixed cytospin preparations following the morphological criteria to identify apoptosis. Typical apoptotic findings consist of chromatin condensation, cell shrinkage, and formation of apoptotic bodies (Kerr et al. 1994).

Apoptotic indexes were evaluated from three independent assays by dividing the number of recognizable apoptotic cells to 1,000 cells counted randomly (400×). Results are expressed as apoptotic percentage at the indicated time points of the protocol.

(b) Fluorescence microscopic analysis of thymocytes death

A slight modified method of double fluorescent staining was used to evaluate thymocyte cell death (Jones and Senft 1985). Briefly, cells were incubated in PBS containing a combination of 75 μg/ml fluorescein diacetate and 100 μg/ml propidium iodide (IP). Fluorescein diacetate is cell permeant and metabolized in the cytosol to fluorescein, which is retained by cells with normally impermeant plasma membranes. Viable and early apoptotic cells exclude

PI, a nuclear stain; hence, this method is not suitable to distinguish between them. Moreover, late-apoptotic as necrotic cells take up IP because of cell membrane disruption, although it is also difficult to determine whether they are apoptotic or necrotic.

The identification of late-apoptotic cells was based on nuclear morphology and fluorescent brightness.

Apoptotic cells were counted in randomly selected fields (×400). A total of 500 cells were counted to determine the percentage of apoptosis at the indicated time points of the experimental protocol.

(c)   Apoptosis: TUNEL assay

Apoptosis in thymocytes after 5-FU treatment was confirmed by TUNEL assay as described previously (Romero Benitez et al. 2004). Briefly, samples fixed in 4% paraformaldehyde were assayed using the ApoptoTag fluorescein direct in situ apoptosis kit (Intergen Co., New York, USA) according to manufacturer's instructions. The assay was also performed in control slides. Apoptotic nuclei were identified under a fluorescence microscope. Nuclei of apoptotic cells were stained positive for green fluorescence, whereas counterstaining showed red fluorescence with PI staining.

The percentages of apoptotic cells were calculated from random fields on each slide. One hundred cells were counted up in each field. A total of 500 cells were counted up for every sample taken. Results obtained from thymic images, taken in triplicate (×400) are expressed as a percentage of apoptotic cells.

(d)   Isolation of apoptotic DNA fragments

Thymocytes (4×10^7) were treated in 0.2 ml of lysis buffer (50 mM Tris, pH 7.5, 20 mM ethylenediamine-tetra-acetic acid, and 1% Nonidet P-40) for 40 s. Supernatants with apoptotic DNA were collected after centrifugation at 2,000 rpm for 5 min at room temperature. They were treated with 6 μl of 100 mg/ml RNAase A (Sigma Co.) and 13 μl of 10% sodium dodecyl sulfate (SDS) plus 6 μl of water and were incubated at 56°C for 2 h. Then, 50 μl of proteinase K (100 μg/ml, Sigma Co.) were added to each sample. They were digested for 4 h at 37°C. DNA was precipitated by adding 450 μl of absolute ethanol. After precipitation, DNA was resuspended in 50 μl of water, and 10 μl of the samples were electrophoresed in 1.5% agarose gels containing 0.5 μg/ml ethidium bromide. DNA bands were visualized using 312 nm UV radiation.

Western blotting

To study FAS, Bax, and Caspase 3 expressions by Western blotting, different protein extractions were used.

FAS and Bax were performed essentially as described previously (Juaristi et al. 2007). Briefly, at each time points after 5-FU injection, thymi were treated with radioimmunoprecipitation assay buffer (50 mM Tris, 150 mM NaCl, 2.5 mg/ml deoxycholic acid, 1 mM EDTA, 10 μg/ml Nonidet-40, pH 7.4, supplemented with protease inhibitors: 2.5 mM phenylmethylsulfonyl fluoride).

Several authors have reported that cytosol is a suitable source of pro-caspase 3 and the cleaved forms of caspase 3 (Samali et al. 1999; Yang et al. 2005; Lee et al. 2006), consequently; caspase 3 was evaluated in cytosolic thymic extracts. Thymic cell suspensions were rinsed twice with PBS and then lysed with ice-cold buffer (10 mM 4-2-hydroxyethyl-1-piperazineethanesulfonic acid, pH 7.4, 10 mM KCl, 1.5 mM $MgCl_2$, 0.5 mM dithiotreitol, 0.1% Igepal (Sigma Co. 630), 2.5 mM phenylmethane-sulfonyl-fluoride, and supplemented with protease inhibitors: 2.5 μg/ml leupeptin, 0.95 μg/ml aprotinin) for 30 min. Cells were briefly sonicated, centrifuged at $14.000 \times g$ for 20 min at 4°C, and the supernatant was used as cytosolic fraction.

Proteins from whole cell lysates and cytoplasmatic extracts were loaded onto 12% SDS–polyacrylamide gel electrophoresis (40 μg/well). Proteins were transferred to nitrocellulose membranes to perform Western blottings. As blocking solution, 5% of low-fat milk in Tris-buffered saline–Tween (TBS-T) buffer (50 mM Tris(hydroxymethyl)aminomethane, 175 mM NaCl, adjusted to pH 7.5, with HCl and supplemented with 0.1% Tween-20) was used.

FAS rabbit polyclonal (SC-7886), Bax rabbit polyclonal (SC-6236), and Caspase 3 goat polyclonal (SC-1225; Santa Cruz Biotechnology Inc., Santa Cruz, CA, USA.) were used as primary antibodies. They were diluted in blocking solution at 1/200, 1/400, and 1/100 for FAS, Bax, and Caspase 3, respectively.

Secondary antibodies: IgG goat anti-rabbit (CN 111-035-045) and IgG donkey anti-goat (CN 705-035-147), horseradish peroxidase (HRP) labeled (Jackson Immunoresearch Inc.), were diluted 1/1,000 and 1/500, respectively, in blocking solution. Incubations were performed for 1 h at room temperature.

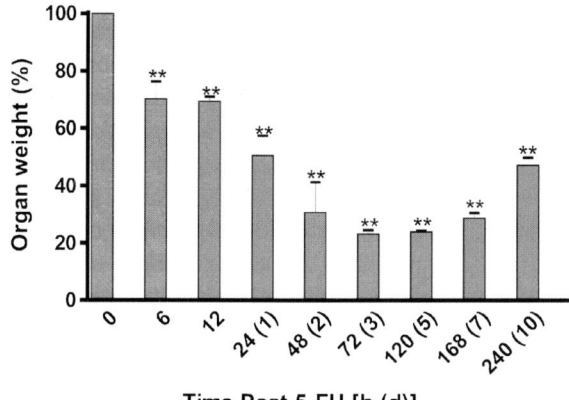

Time Post 5-FU [h (d)]

Fig. 1 5-FU induces time-dependent weight loss in murine thymus. The thymus was obtained at the indicated time points after 5-FU administration as described in "Materials and methods." Control weight was set as 100%. Organ weights diminished from 6 h after injection, reaching their lowest values between 48 and 120 h post-5-FU treatment (approximately 75% lower than control). Results were obtained from six mice/group (controls) and six mice/group (5-FU-treated animals) at each time points of the experimental study and expressed as mean ± SEM. **P<0.01 indicates significant differences between the control and the 5-FU-treated animals

Bound HRP was detected by Opti4CN kit (BioRad). Band intensities were quantified using Scion Image 3.0 Software.

Values that are expressed in arbitrary optical density units (UA) were obtained as previously described (Juaristi et al. 2007).

Image and statistical analysis

All results are expressed as mean ± standard error of mean (SEM). Thymocytes cellularities and viabilities from the 5-FU-treated and the control groups were statistically analyzed using a one-way analysis of variance (ANOVA) test corrected by Bonferroni. Data from all other experiences were compared by ANOVA followed by Dunnett's test. Analyses were performed using the software package Instat and Prism 4.0 (GraphPad Software Inc., San Diego, USA). A *P* value<0.05 was considered statistically significant. Correlation analyses between apoptosis-related proteins and apoptosis indexes were performed using Spearman rank correlations test.

Results

To assess whether 5-FU affects murine normal thymus, a time course study was designed (0–10 days) after a single dose of 5-FU (150 mg/kg) i.p., administration through several experimental procedures.

Thymic weight, cellularity, and viability post-5-FU dosing

Thymus of 5-FU-injected mice showed an acute weight reduction within the first 7 days (*p*<0.01).

Table 1 5-FU induces cell loss and viability reduction in murine thymus

Thymus cellularity and viability after 5-FU treatment

Time [h (d)]	Cellularity		Viability	
	Control (cells×10^6)	5-FU (cells×10^6)	Control (% of living cells)	5-FU (% of living cells)
6	97.2±8.12	76.02±4.13	97.75±1.18	88.03±1.23
12	101.52±12.32	85.95±11.05	95.58±0.98	84.03±1.53
24 (1)	87.6±6.36	60.16±3.83	96.49±1.10	79.56±2.46**
48 (2)	81.16±8.73	18.03±1.82**	97.12±2.03	73.70±0.57**
72 (3)	87.60±11.03	17.22±3.57**	97.41±1.78	72.25±3.44**
120 (5)	79.84±9.78	25.15±1.15**	98.13±1.97	66.23±7.44**
168 (7)	85. 70±7.46	32.22±3.33**	96.89±2. 17	74.83±0.62**
240 (10)	89.52± 12.03	28.90±6.60**	97.25±1.68	83.86±3.13

Thymocytes were isolated and counted. Subsequently, viability was determined by the Trypan Blue exclusion assay. Determinations were performed using hemocytometer as described in "Materials and methods." Results were expressed as mean×10^6 cells/thymus ± SEMs, and percentages of viable cells ± SEMs. Hypocellularity was noticeable 48 h after 5-FU treatment (five times below control values). Thymic cellularity increased gradually but failed to reach control values by the end of the experience. Thymic viability was reduced from 24 h after 5-FU dosing and returned to control values by the end of the study. Data are shown for six mice/group (controls) and six mice/group (5-FU-treated animals) at each time points of the study from three independent experiments. **P<0.01 indicates significant differences between control and 5-FU-treated animals.

Thymic mass loss started from the sixth hour after 5-FU dosing (80±0.2 mg), reaching low values between days 2 (35±0.10 mg) and 7 (34±0.4 mg) compared to control values (120±0.7 mg). Thymus weight failed to recover to normality through the experience (Fig. 1).

Reduction of this parameter was also reflected in thymocyte counts. Thymic cellularities decreased progressively during the experimental schedule, showing the minimal cell count from day 2 ($18.03 \pm 1.82 \times 10^6$ cells $p<0.01$) until the end of the study compared to control values ($80.33 \pm 12.01 \times 10^6$ cells). As regards thymus viabilities, they showed significant reduction between day 1 (79.6±2.5%) and 7 (74.8±0.6%), compared to control values (96.7±1.9%, $p<0.01$). Data is shown in Table 1.

Thymic morphologic changes

Interactions between stromal cells and thymocytes play a crucial role in T cell development (Anderson et al. 1996). To assess changes in the thymic architecture post-5-FU injury, scanning electronic microscopy (SEM) images were obtained from 5-FU-injected mice at each time points of the study (Fig. 2).

Architectural changes were observed from the 12th hour to the fifth day post-5-FU injection.

Important cell reductions, as well as the loss of cell–cell contact, were noticed between the first and the third day post-5-FU dosing. Thymus seemed to exhibit a moderate reorganization on day 7, and it was almost normal by day 10.

These results provide substantial evidence of 5-FU toxicity upon thymic tissue, suggesting that thymic hypocellularity is the additive result from the toxic effects of the drug and serious damage of the thymic microenvironment.

To determine whether apoptosis was involved in this process, additional experimental approaches were combined.

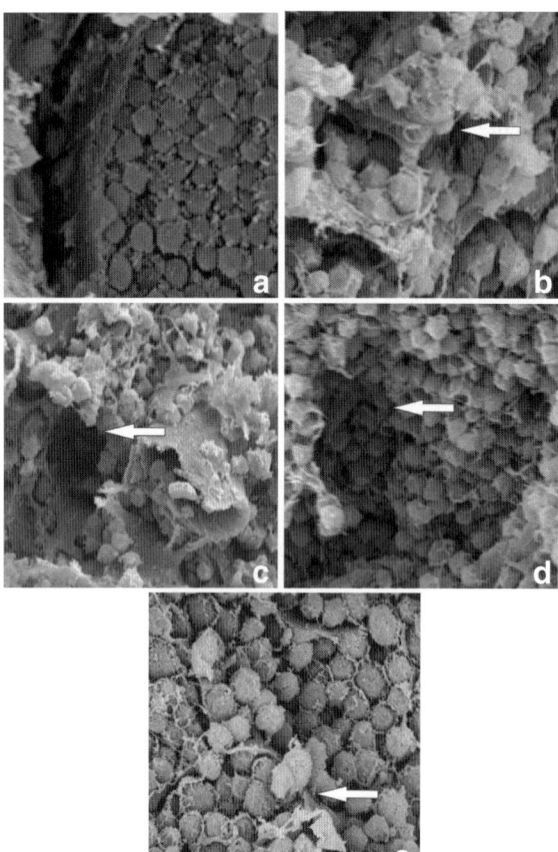

Fig. 2 Effects of 5-FU on thymic architecture. The figure depicts representative scanning electron microscopic images (×2,000) of thymic samples untreated (**a**) and 5-FU-treated mice at 12 h (**b**), 2 days (**c**), 7 days (**d**), and 10 days (**e**) post-5-FU. The main feature of 5-FU-induced damage is the acute alteration in the inner thymic architecture. *Arrowheads* indicate loss of cell–cell contact. Hypocellularity was noticed from the first 12 h (**b**) to the second day post-treatment (**c**). An apparent morphological recovery of the thymic architecture was seen from the seventh day onward (**d, e**). Two mice were used for each time point of the experimental schedule ($n=18$)

Fig. 3 5-FU-induced thymocyte apoptosis in vivo. Thymic ▶ cells were isolated from control and 5-FU-treated animals and fixed as described in "Materials and methods." Apoptotic biochemical and morphological changes were examined along the experience under light and fluorescence microscopes and TUNEL assay. Representative images were obtained from the control group and 5-FU-treated group 48 h post-injection. **a** May Grünwald–Giemsa (MG-G) staining of apoptotic cells exhibit shrinkages bodies, with nuclear condensation and fragmented nuclei. **b** Fluorescence assays with fluorescein diacetate (*DAF*) and propidium iodide (*IP*) show viable cells with homogeneous green fluorescence of their cytoplasm. In contrast, apoptotic cells show nuclei with irregular bright red fluorescence as a result of chromatin condensation and nuclear fragmentation. **c** TUNEL assay was used as a confirmatory technique to assess thymic apoptosis. Nuclei of apoptotic cells were stained positive for green fluorescence. **d** Percentages of apoptotic cells related to total cells (mean ± SEM) determined by TUNEL assays were represented. Five hundred cells were counted for each sample taken on the scheduled days. Results were obtained from six mice/group (controls) and six mice/group (5-FU-treated animals) at each time points of the experimental study and expressed as mean ± SEM. *$P<0.05$ and **$P<0.01$ indicate significant differences between apoptotic percentages of the untreated control group and the 5-FU-treated groups

Thymic apoptosis

Taking into account that apoptosis has been considered a major mechanism of chemotherapy-induced cell death (Ricci and Zong 2006), apoptosis values of the thymus were determined to elucidate whether this process is involved during 5-FU injury.

Apoptosis was assessed by May Grünwald–Giemsa staining (Fig. 3a), double fluorescent dyes (fluorescein diacetate and PI; Fig. 3b), and TUNEL assay (Fig. 3c), as described in "Materials and Methods." Percentages of apoptotic cells were obtained by TUNEL, a widely used confirmatory assay for programmed cell death (Fig. 3d).

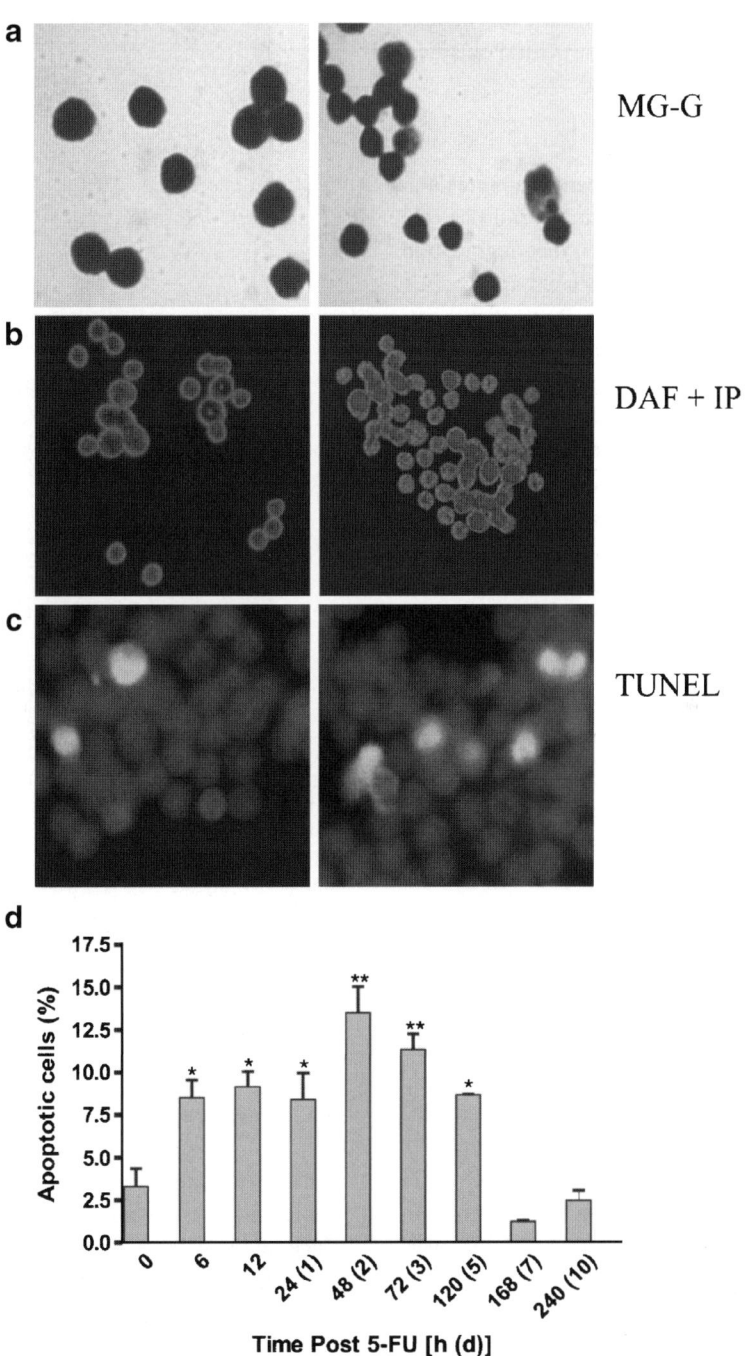

5-FU-injected mice showed an acute increase of apoptotic percentages from the sixth hour (8.5 ± 1.1, $p<0.05$) to the fifth day (8.7 ± 0.04, $p<0.05$), compared to the control group (3.3 ± 1.07). Maximal apoptotic values were observed on the second day (13.5 ± 1.5 $p<0.01$). Apoptotic percentages returned almost to basal values on day 7 (1.2 ± 0.06).

Experimental data shows temporal coincidence among maximal apoptotic values, minimal cellularities, low weight, and deep thymic structural changes.

Effect of 5-FU on DNA damage

Oligonucleosomal cleavage accompanies apoptosis in most of the systems. In this study, agarose gel electrophoresis was used to assess the degradation pattern of nuclear DNA in 5-FU induced apoptosis.

DNA damage was evident in the form of discernible fragmentation ladders in agarose gels (Fig. 4). Fragmented DNA was undetectable in the thymus control sample. Nonetheless, DNA obtained from 48 h post-5-FU-treated mice has revealed characteristic fragments composed of approximately 200 bp. On day 7, DNA degradation almost disappeared. The cleavage of DNA corroborates the previous morphological and biochemical analyses, indicating that in vivo 5-FU-induced apoptosis was maximal during the first 48 h.

FAS expression

It has been reported that the major proportion of thymic chemotherapeutic drug-induced-apoptosis in vitro is mediated by the CD95/CD95L system (Eichhorst et al. 2001). To determine if 5-FU-induced apoptosis is accompanied by FAS upregulation, immunoblottings were performed (Fig. 5).

FAS expression showed an abrupt increase from the sixth hour (8.8 ± 0.74) until the end of the study (8.3 ± 1.4), reaching approximately three times over control values from the 12th hour to the fifth day post-5-FU dosing (11.1 ± 0.2 and 17.6 ± 0.4, respectively, $p<0.01$). Interestingly, FAS upregulation was in agreement with the maximal apoptotic values. A direct and significant linear correlation was obtained between FAS overexpression and apoptotic indexes ($r=0.8490$, $p=0.007$). These data allow us to postulate that FAS is linked to 5-FU-mediated apoptosis in the thymus.

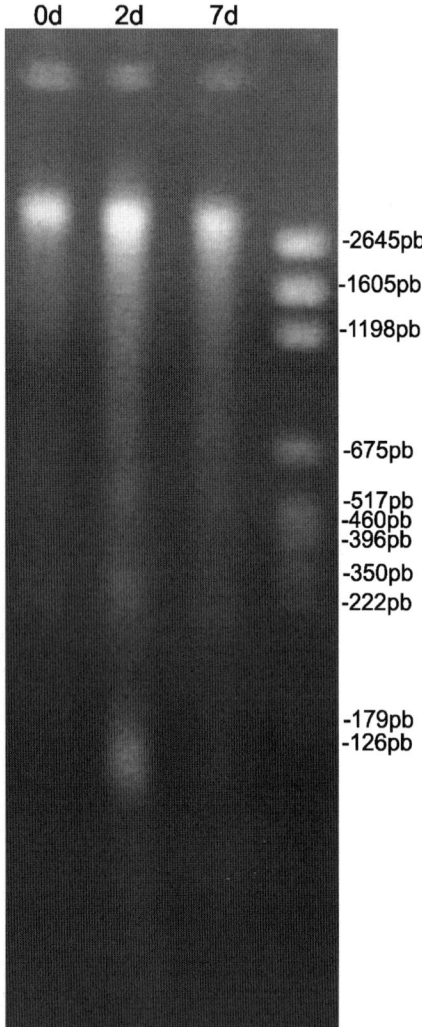

Fig. 4 Induction of DNA fragmentation in the thymus of mice after 5-FU administration. Samples from the control and the 5-FU-treated mice were obtained at each day of the experimental protocol ($n = 2$ mice/group). DNA molecules were extracted from 4×10^7 thymic cells and were electrophoretically separated on 1.5% agarose gels containing ethidium bromide. Internucleosomal DNA cleavage was visualized by UV transillumination. The figure shows the results of one representative experiment from three independent determinations at 0, 2, and 7 days post-5-FU

Bax expression

It has been shown in vivo that, blocking the CD95 system in the thymus, the apoptotic process takes place to a lesser extent (Eichhorst et al. 2001). It suggests that another potential mechanism might be involved in cell death, such as the Bax apoptotic pathway. To analyze this assumption, Bax immuno-

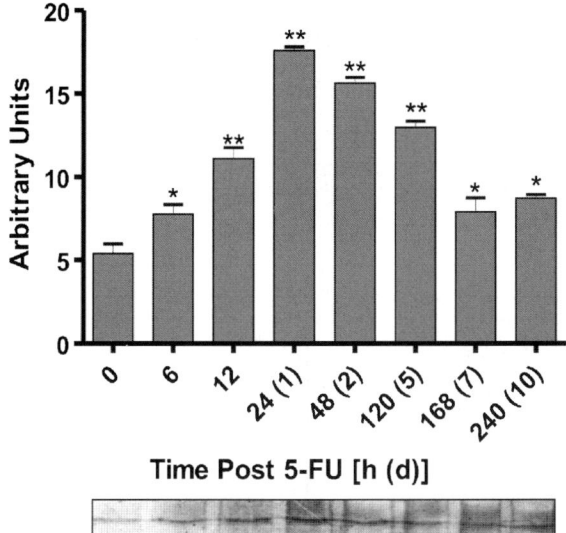

Fig. 5 Upregulation of FAS induced by 5-FU. Thymi were harvested from 5-FU-treated mice at the scheduled times; cell suspensions were obtained and lysed. Western Blotting analyses were performed as described in "Material and methods." A representative blot of three independent experiments is shown. FAS expression was noticeable along the study, showing an upregulation in the acute period of 5-FU injury until the fifth day. Thereafter, it returned to the control levels from day 7 onward. Results represent mean ± SEM of three mice per group; **P<0.01 indicates significant differences between protein expressions from the control group (day 0) and 5-FU-treated group

blottings were performed at each scheduled time (Fig. 6). Bax was overexpressed from the sixth hour (34.36±3.8, *p*<0.01) to the fifth day (31.07±1.85, *p*<0.01) post-5-FU, showing a total increase of two times over control values (39.28±1.03). This fact was almost coincident with the significant increase of the apoptotic values, the cleavage of DNA and FAS upregulation. More interestingly, Bax and FAS overexpressions showed a direct and significant correlation (*r*=0.8197, *p*=0.0127).

These results gave a novel approach to the 5-FU-induced-apoptosis mechanism involved in vivo model, which is consistent with previous in vitro studies.

Caspase 3 expression

To confirm whether pro-caspase 3 was activated during 5-FU treatment, the cleavages of this precursor were detected by immunoblottings. The activation of pro-caspase 3 was indicated by the disappearance of the 32 kd pro-enzyme form (Zhang et al. 2000a, b).

Indeed, control values of the inactive caspase 3 (11.6± 0.5) showed a remarkable decrease from the 24th hours (5.2±0.4, *p*<0.01) to the fifth day (2.8±0.1, *p*<0.01) post-5-FU. Moreover, the cleaved active forms of Caspase 3 (20 and 17 Kd) were overexpressed from the first day (11.14±1.6, *p<0.05*) to the fifth day (19.34±0.47, *p<0.01*) after 5-FU treatment (Fig. 7).

In addition, this pattern is coincident with the increase of the apoptotic values and DNA fragmentation. Furthermore, this fact is also concomitant with FAS and Bax overexpressions, which might reflect the interaction between these proteins during the apoptotic process.

Discussion

The regulation of cell survival and death is critical for the development and function of the mammalian immune system. The importance of apoptosis for the

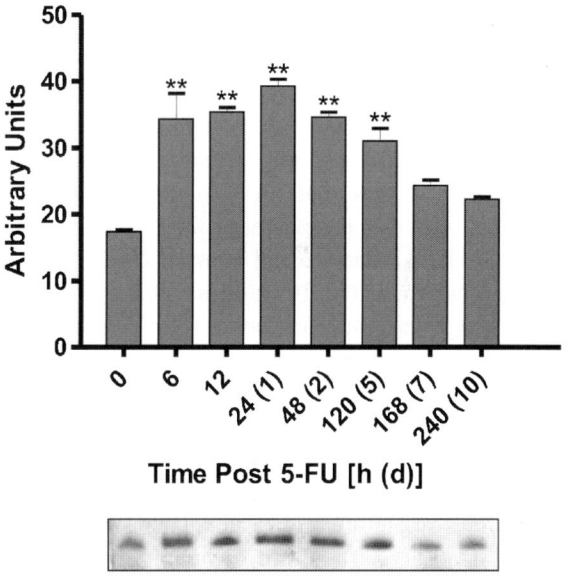

Fig. 6 Overexpression of Bax induced by 5-FU. Thymi were harvested from 5-FU-treated mice at the indicated time points; the cell suspensions obtained were lysed and subject to Western blotting analyses as described in "Material and methods." A representative blot of three independent experiments is shown. Bax expression was noticeable throughout the study, showing an overexpression in the acute period of 5-FU injury. Thereafter, it returned to control levels from day 5 onward. Results represent mean ± SEM of three mice per group; *P< 0.05 and **P<0.01 indicate significant differences between protein expressions from the control group (day 0) and 5-FU-treated group

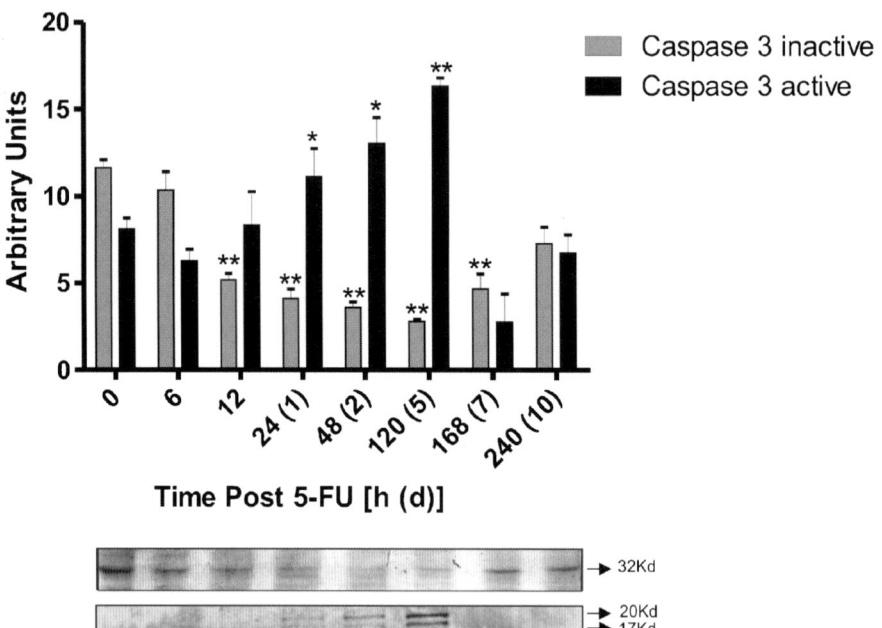

Fig. 7 Cleavage of the inactive pro-caspase 3 induced by 5-FU. Thymi were harvested from 5-FU-treated mice at the scheduled times; cell suspensions were obtained and lysed. Western blotting analyses were performed as described in "Material and methods." A representative blot of three independent experiments is shown. Cleavages of the inactive pro-caspase 3 were noticed from 12 h until the seventh day, indicating the presence of the active caspase 3 enzymes. Results represent mean ± SEM of three mice per group; **$P < 0.01$ indicates significant differences between protein expressions from the control group (day 0) and 5-FU-treated group

cell number maintenance, the deletion of useless or autoreactive cells, and the removal of expanded lymphocyte clones that are generated during an immune response have already been reported by several authors (Marsden and Strassen 2003; Newton et al. 1998; Smith et al. 1996; Ogasawara et al. 1995).

Although very little is known about apoptosis in thymus upon a chemotherapeutic insult. Severe side effects are caused by the fact that most of cytotoxic drugs are not able to distinguish between normal and tumoral cells (Guest and Uetrecht 2000).

It has been reported that 5-FU causes a reduction of the thymus weight during the first hours of treatment (Eichhorst et al. 2001). However, little is known about the thymus' behaviour in a longer period.

Experimental data from this in vivo model upon basic parameters of the thymus, taken together with other experimental approaches for evaluating apoptosis, have provided us with a novel scope of the response against 5-FU injury.

In this study, 5-FU induces loss of thymic weight, viability, and cellularity. Even more, thymic alterations of the structural organization, as well as the apoptotic percentages, were seriously altered, along the first 5 days post-5-FU. The aforementioned morphological thymic microenvironmental changes are linked to the enhancement of apoptosis. Thus, it is assumed that 5-FU might trigger the overexpression of key regulatory and executor molecules involved in apoptosis.

Nevertheless, the way in which this drug induces apoptosis is controversial (Fisher 1994). A possible mechanism may be the induction of apoptosis via death receptor, such as FAS (Fulda et al. 2000; Kasibhatla et al. 1998; Herr et al. 1997; Friesen et al. 1996; Krammer 1999).

This report shows that 5-FU induces an upregulation of FAS from the sixth hour onwards. Moreover, the chronological coincidence of this fact with maximal apoptosis and DNA fragmentation seemed to be strongly associated. These results are in agreement with other groups that have studied the mechanism involved during in vivo chemotherapy-induced apoptosis (Eichhorst et al. 2001). However, it has been reported that, when the CD95 system is blocked, apoptosis values are diminished, although not totally abrogated. Therefore, other potential mechanism might be involved in cell death. A possible protein committed in this alternative apoptotic event seemed to be the pro-apoptotic protein Bax (Takemura et al. 2005; Gottlieb and Oren 1998; Friedlander et al. 1996; Miyashita et al. 1995).

This study reveals that 5-FU induces an overexpression of Bax and FAS, both proteins share a similar pattern. Like FAS, Bax upregulation was coincident to maximal apoptotic indexes and the presence of intranucleosomal DNA degradation. These data provide a new insight regarding the expression of Bax during chemotherapy-induced apoptosis, which is consistent with the previously in vitro reported studies (Kobayashi et al. 2000; Zhang et al. 2000a, b; Fincucane et al. 1999; Nita et al. 1998; Martin and Green 1995).

The execution of the apoptotic program appears to be uniformly mediated through consecutive activation of the members of the caspase family (Marsden and Strassen 2003). Previous studies have suggested that caspase 3 is implicated in thymocyte cell death during T-cell development (Jiang et al. 1999; Zhang et al. 2000a, b). Nevertheless, data of caspase 3 activity during thymocyte-induced apoptosis in vivo post-chemotherapy are unavailable.

The current in vivo study provides a first approach about the role of caspase 3 during 5-FU treatment. Experimental data show an increase expression of cleaved caspase 3 from 24 h to 5 days post-5-FU. Interestingly, the occurrence of the active form of caspase 3 was in concordance with maximal apoptotic values, cleavage of DNA, and overexpressions of FAS and Bax.

In summary, in vivo effects of 5-FU showed that the morphological structure of the thymus was deeply altered, leading to hypocellularity, weight loss, and architectural changes. Therefore, this report revealed that 5-FU-induced apoptosis is related to the upregulation of the pro-apoptotic proteins FAS and Bax, and it is also linked to the overexpression of the active form of caspase 3.

Even more, this in vivo study offers a new insight about the pro-apoptotic proteins involved during 5-FU treatment upon the thymus and the possible mechanism involved in the lymphopenia associated with this chemotherapeutic agent.

Acknowledgment This work was supported by grants from SEGCyT-UNNE and CONICET, Argentina. We Thank Dr. M. Teresa De Jesus Saavedra and Dr. M. Barbara De Biasio for their expert help with DNA fragmentation. We also thank Professor Milagros Delfino for the English revision.

References

Alnemri ES. Mammalian cell death proteases: a family of highly conserved aspartate specific cysteine proteases. J Cell Biochem. 1997;64:33–42.

Anderson NC, Moore JJT, Jenkinson O, Jenkinson E. Cellular interactions in thymocyte development. Annu Rev Immunol. 1996;14:73–99.

Asaga T, Inaba M, Nagano A, Yanoma S. Induction of apoptosis in breast cancer cells by preoperative oral administration of 5-fluorouracil. Gan To Kagaku Ryoho. 2001;70:46–51.

Ashkenazi A, Dixit VM. Death receptors: signaling and modulation. Science. 1998;281:1305–8.

Chinnaiyan AM, Dixit VW. The cell-death machine. Curr Biol. 1996;6:555–62.

Eichhorst S, Muerkoster S, Weigand M, Kramer P. The chemotherapeutic drug 5-fluorouracil induces apoptosis in mouse thymocytes in vivo via activation of the CD95 (APO-1/Fas) system. Cancer Res. 2001;61:243–8.

Fincucane MD, Bossy-Wetzel E, Waterhouse NJ, Cotter TG, Green DR. Bax-induced caspase activation and apoptosis via cytochrome c release from mitochondria in inhibitable by Bcl-xL. J Biol Chem. 1999;74:2225–33.

Fisher DE. Apoptosis in cancer therapy: crossing the threshold. Cell. 1994;9:91–6.

Friedlander P, Haupt Y, Prives C, Oren MA. Mutant p53 that discriminates between p53-responsive genes cannot induce apoptosis. Mol Cell Biol. 1996;16:4961–71.

Friesen C, Herr I, Krammer PH, Debatin KM. Involvement of the CD95 (APO-1/Fas) receptor/ligand system in drug-induced apoptosis in leukemia cells. Nat Med. 1996;2:574–7.

Fulda S, Strauss G, Meyer E, Debatin KM. Functional CD95 ligand and CD95 death inducing signaling complex in activation-induced cell death and doxorubicin-induced apoptosis in leukemic T cells. Blood. 2000;95:301–8.

Gottlieb TM, Oren M. p53 and apoptosis. Semin Cancer Biol. 1998;8:359–68.

Guest L, Uetrecht J. Drugs toxic to the bone marrow the target stroma cells. Immunopharmacol. 2000;46:103–12.

Henkart PA. ICE family proteases: mediators of all apoptotic cell death? Immunity. 1996;4:195–201.

Herr I, Withelm D, Bohler T, Angel P, Debatin KM. Activation of CD95 (APO-1/Fas) signaling by ceramide mediates cancer therapy-induced apoptosis. EMBO J. 1997;16:6200–8.

Horowitz RW, Heerdt BG, Hu X, Schwartz EL, Walder S. Combination therapy with 5-Fluorouracil and INF-alfa2 induces a nonrandom increase in DNA fragments of less than 3 megabases in HT29 colon carcinoma cells. Clin Cancer Res. 1997;3:1317–22.

Ijiri K, Potten CS. Further studies on the response of intestinal cells of different hierarchical status to eighteen different cytotoxic agents. B J Cancer. 1987;55:113–23.

Jacobson MD. Programmed cell death: a missing key is found. Trends Cell Biol. 1997;7:467–9.

Jiang D, Zheng L, Lenardo MJ. Caspases in T-cell receptor-induced thymocyte apoptosis. Cell Death Differ. 1999;6:402–11.

Jones KH, Senft JA. An improved method to determine cell viability by simultaneous staining with fluorescein diacetate-propidium iodide. J Histochem Cytochem. 1985;33:77–9.

Juaristi AJ, Aguirre MV, Todaro JS, Alvarez MA, Brandan NC. EPO receptor, Bax and Bcl-xL expressions in murine erythropoiesis after cyclophospamide treatment. Toxicology. 2007;231:188–99.

Kasibhatla S, Brunner T, Genestier L, Echeverri F, Mahboubi A, Green DR. DNA damaging agents induce expression of Fas ligand and subsequent apoptosis in T lymphocytes via activation of NF-κB and AP-1. Mol Cell. 1998;1:543–51.

Kerr JF. History of the events leading to the formulation of the apoptosis concept. Toxicology. 2002;27:181–2.

Kerr JF, Winterford CM, Harmon BV. Apoptosis. Its significance in cancer and cancer therapy. Cancer. 1994;35:796–807.

Kobayashi T, Sawa H, Morikawa J, Zhang W, Shiku H. Bax induction activates apoptotic cascade via mitochondrial cytochrome c release and bax overesspression enhances apoptosis induced by chemotherapeutic agents in DLD-1 colon cancer cells. Jpn J Cancer Res. 2000;91:1264–8.

Krammer PH. CD95 (APO-1/Fas)-mediated apoptosis: live and let die. Adv Immunol. 1999;71:163–210.

Lee H, Kim YJ, Kim HW, Lee DH, Sung M-K, Park T. Induction of apoptosis by *cordycep militaris* through activation of caspase-3 in leukemia HL-60 cells. Biol Pharm Bull. 2006;29:670–4.

Marsden VS, Strassen A. Control of apoptosis in the immune system: Bcl-2, BH3-only proteins and more. Annu Rev Immunol. 2003;21:71–105.

Martin SJ, Green DR. Protease activation during apoptosis: death by a thousand cuts. Cell. 1995;82:349–52.

Miyashita T, Krajewski S, Krajewska M, Wang HG, Lin HK, Liebermann DA, Hoffman B, Reed JC. Tumor suppressor p53 is a regulator of bcl-2 and bax gene expression in vitro and in vivo. Oncogene. 1995;9:293–9.

Newton K, Harris AW, Bath ML, Smith KGC, Strasser A. A dominant interfering mutant of FADD/Mort1 enhances deletion of autorreactive thymocytes and inhibitions of proliferation of mature T lymphocytes. EMBO J. 1998;17:706–18.

Nita ME, Nagawa H, Tominaga O, Tsuno N, Fuji S, Sasaki S, Fu CG, Takenoue T, Tsuruo T, Muto T. 5-Fluorouracil induces apoptosis in human colon cancer cell lines with modulation of Bcl-2 family proteins. Br J Cancer. 1998;78:986–92.

Ogasawara J, Suda T, Nagata S. Selective apoptosis of CD4 + CD8 + thymocytes by the anti-Fas antibody. J Exp Med. 1995;181:485–91.

Parker WB, Cheng YC. Metabolism and mechanism of action of 5-fluorouracil. Pharmacol Ther. 1990;48:381–95.

Pritchard DM, Watson AJM, Potten CS, Jackman AL, Hickmann JA. Inhibition by uridine but not thymidine of p53-dependent intestinal apoptosis initiated by 5-fluorouracil: evidence for the involvement of RNA perturbation. Proc Nat Acad Sci U S A. 1997;94:1795–9.

Ricci S, Zong W. Chemotherapeutic approaches for targeting cell death pathways. Oncologist. 2006;11:342–57.

Rocha B, Vassalli P, Guy-Grand D. Thymic and extrathymic origins of gut intraepithelial lymphocyte population in mice. J Exp Med. 1994;180:681–6.

Romero Benitez MM, Aguirre MV, Juaristi JA, Alvarez MA, Trifaro JM, Brandan NC. In vitro erythroid recovery following paclitaxel injury: Correlation between GATA-1, c-MYB, NF-E2, Epo receptor expressions and apoptosis. Toxicol Appl Pharmacol. 2004;194:230–8.

Samali A, Cai J, Zhivotovsky B, Jones DP, Orrenius S. Presence of a pre-apoptotic complex of pro-caspase-3, Hsp60 and Hsp10 in the mitochondrial fraction of Jurkat cells. EMBO J. 1999;18:2040–8.

Savill J, Fadok V. Corpse clearance defines the meaning of cell death. Nature. 2000;12,407:784–8.

Smith KGC, Strassen A, Vaux DL. CrmA expression in T lymphocytes of transgenic mice inhibits CD95 (Fas/APO-1)-transducing apoptosis, but does not cause lymphadenophaty on autoimmune disease. EMBO J. 1996;15:5167–76.

Takemura K, Noguchi M, Ogi K, Tokino T, Kubota H, Miyazaki A, Kohama G, Hiratsuka H. Enhanced Bax in oral SCC in relation to antitumor effects of chemotherapy. J Oral Pathol Med. 2005;34:93–9.

Thornberry NA, Lazebnik Y. Caspases: enemies within. Science. 1998;281:1312–6.

Werner JM, Eger K, Jurgen Steinfelder H. Comparison of the rapid pro-apoptotic effect of trans-beta-nitrostyrenes with delayed apoptosis induced by the standard agent 5-fluorouracil in colon cancer cells. Apoptosis. 2007;12:235–46.

Yang MY, Serrine S, Monks L, Monks TJ. 2,3,5-Tris(Glutation-S-yl)hydroquinone (TGHQ)-mediate apoptosis of human promyelocytic leukemia cells is preceded by mitochondrial cytochrome *c* release in the absence of a decrease in the mitochondrial membrane potential. Tox Sci. 2005;86:92–100.

Yeager AM, Levin J, Levin FC. The effects of 5-fluorouracil on hematopoiesis: studies of murine megakaryocyte-CFC, granulocyte-macrophage-CFC, and peripheral blood cell levels. Exp Hematol. 1983;11:944–52.

Zhang J, Mikecz K, Finnega A, Glant TT. Spontaneous thymocyte apoptosis is regulated by a mitochondrion-mediated signaling pathway. J Immunol. 2000a;165:2970–4.

Zhang L, Yu J, Park BH, Kinzler KW, Volgestein B. Role of Bax in the apoptotic response to anticancer agents. Science. 2000b;290:989–92.

Abstracts

Originally published in the journal Cell Biology and Toxicology, Volume 24, Nos 4–5, 143–190.
DOI: 10.1007/s10565-008-9079-5 © Springer Science + Business Media B.V. 2008

An invited paper presented in the symposium "Copper in neurologic and neurodegenerative diseases".

Overview of the Role of Copper in Neurodegenerative Diseases and Potential Treatment with Tetrathiomolybdate

George J. Brewer[1,2]
Departments of Human Genetics[1] and Internal Medicine[2]
University of Michigan Medical School, Ann Arbor
MI, 48109, USA

Goals of this symposium

The main purposes of this symposium were to focus on recent data on the role of copper in Alzheimer's disease (AD) and characterize the potential of tetrathiomolybdate (TM), which might be a treatment for AD. However, copper may be playing an important role in other diseases of neurodegeneration, and these diseases and the role of copper are mentioned briefly in the next section.

Roles of copper in diseases of neurodegeneration other than AD

In Huntington's disease, Fox et al. (2007) have shown a higher level of copper in the striatum and cortex of brains of transgenic mice with the human Huntington's disease inserted, than in controls. In a mouse model of prion disease, Sigurdsson et al. (2003) showed that the copper chelator, D-penicillamine, significantly inhibited the onset of clinical disease. In a mouse model of amyotrophic lateral sclerosis (ALS), Hottinger et al. (1997) showed that treatment with D-penicillamine significantly prolonged the onset of clinical disease. Kiaei et al. (2004) made mice doubly mutant with ALS and with a mutant gene of ATP7 causing deficiency of copper. The doubly deficient mice had a slower onset of ALS symptoms than the mice with the ALS mutation alone. Rasia et al. (2005) showed that copper promotes aggregation of α-synuclein into Lewy bodies, the aggregation found in the neurons of Parkinson's patients. These are only a few of the studies in the literature which weave copper into the possible onset or progression of many of the diseases of neurodegeneration.

Recent data on the role of copper in ad and cognitive decline discussed at this symposium

Sparks and colleagues (Sparks and Schreurs 2003; Sparks et al. 2006) have produced some very exciting data, showing that adding trace amounts of copper (0.12 ppm) to the drinking water of rabbits in a rabbit model of AD greatly increases the amyloid plaque burden in the rabbits' brains, and decreases their performance on cognitive tasks. If relevant to humans, this means the EPA allowance of 1.3 ppm copper in human drinking water is enhancing the development and/or severity of AD.

Squitti et al. (2005; 2006) in Italy presented exciting work showing that free copper, that is the non-ceruloplasmin copper of the blood, is, on average, significantly elevated in AD patients. Since this free copper is potentially toxic copper, as known in Wilson's disease, these findings directly implicate possible copper toxicity in the pathogenesis and/or the progression of AD.

Morris et al. (2006) in Chicago have shown a dramatic effect of high copper intake, mostly from copper supplements, on damaging cognition in the presence of a high fat diet. Although, AD was not shown to be produced in this study, the implication of a high copper intake on reducing cognition is an obvious connection.

Finally, James Camakaris (White et al. 1999; Bellingham et al. 2004) provided insights on the role of copper in human neurodegenerative diseases by using a variety of preclinical model systems. All in all, it is becoming clear that copper is intimately involved with AD, and that lowering copper levels by use of an anticopper drug may be a useful therapy in AD. In the next section, we review the development and use of TM as an anticopper drug, and then suggest a trial of TM in AD.

The anticopper drug tetrathiomolybdate (TM)

We first developed tetrathiomolybdate (TM) for the initial treatment of neurologically presenting Wilson's disease (Brewer et al. 2003a; 2006a). We have found that penicillamine and trientine, when used initially, cause neurologic worsening in these patients 50% (Brewer et al. 1987) and 26% (Brewer et al. 2006a) of the time, respectively, probably by mobilizing hepatic copper and temporarily elevating brain copper further. The other anticopper drug on the market, zinc is too slow acting for these acutely ill patients, taking about 9 months to control copper toxicity, during which time the disease may progress due to its own natural history. TM controls copper toxicity in an average of about 2 weeks, and 96% of the time stabilizes neurologic function, allowing recovery in the ensuing 12–24 months. Beyond this, in a series of animal model studies, we have shown that by lowering copper levels to an intermediate level with TM, using ceruloplasmin (Cp) levels to gauge the degree of free copper availability, we can produce antifibrotic,

antiinflammatory, and antiautoimmune disease effects (Brewer 2003).

In the fibrosis area, using the bleomycin mouse model of pulmonary fibrosis, we have completely prevented the development of fibrosis (Brewer et al. 2003b), while inhibiting the fibrosis cytokine, transforming growth factor beta (TGF$_\beta$) and the inflammatory cytokine, tumor necrosis factor alpha (TNFα), in the lung (Brewer et al. 2004). In separate experiments we showed that fibrosis inhibition still occurred if TM was started after full TNFα expression, showing that the effect wasn't due just to inhibition of inflammation. Fibrosis was also inhibited in the carbon tetrachloride mouse model of cirrhosis, again with inhibition of TGF$_\beta$ (Askari et al. 2004).

In the inflammation area, TM has been shown to strongly inhibit acetaminophen hepatitis (Ma et al. 2004), and doxorubicin heart damage in mice (Hou et al. 2005). Inhibition of the inflammatory cytokines TNFα and interleukin-1-beta (IL-1$_\beta$) was shown in these studies. In the antiautoimmune disease area, TM has been shown to inhibit concanavalin A hepatitis (Askari et al. 2004), bovine collagen 2 arthritis (McCubbin et al. 2006), and prolong the development of diabetes in the non-obese diabetic (NOD) mouse model of type I diabetes (Brewer et al. 2006b).

This preclinical work has led to a small uncontrolled clinical trial of TM in idiopathic pulmonary fibrosis, with encouraging results, and to a double blind clinical trial in primary biliary cirrhosis, which is currently underway. Given the data suggesting a role for copper in the development and/or pathogenesis of AD, partially reviewed earlier, we believe a clinical trial of TM in AD is indicated. This is further supported by a preclinical trial by Quinn et al. of TM in a rodent model. The amyloid plaque burden was reduced 40% in these studies (Wadsworth et al. 2007). Accordingly, a clinical trial of TM in AD has been planned, in collaboration with Dr. Squitti and her Italian colleagues, sponsored by Pipex Therapeutics Inc, developers of TM (trade name Coprexa®).

Acknowledgements

This work was supported in part by Pipex Therapeutics, Inc, Ann Arbor, MI, USA. The University of Michigan has recently licensed the antifibrotic and antiinflammatory uses of TM to Pipex Therapeutics,

Inc, Ann Arbor, MI, USA. Dr. Brewer has equity in and is a paid consultant to Pipex Therapeutics, Inc.

References

Askari FK, Dick RB, Mao M, Brewer GJ. Tetrathiomolybdate therapy protects against concanavalin A and carbon tetrachloride hepatic damage in mice. Exp Bio Med. 2004;229:857–63.

Bellingham SA, Ciccotosto GD, Needham BE, Fodero LR, White AR, Masters CL, Cappai R, Camakaris J. Gene knockout of amyloid precursor protein and amyloid precursor-like protein-2 increases cellular copper levels in primary mouse cortical neurons and embryonic fibroblasts. J Neurochem. 2004;91:423–8.

Brewer GJ. Copper lowering therapy with tetrathiomolybdate produces antiangiogenic, anticancer, antifibrotic and antiinflammatory effects. Semin Integr Med. 2003;1:181–90.

Brewer GJ, Askari F, Lorincz MT, Carlson M, Schilsky M, Kluin KJ, Hedera P, Moretti P, Fink JK, Tankanow R, Dick RB, Sitterly J. Treatment of Wilson disease with ammonium tetrathiomolybdate: IV. Comparison of tetrathiomolybdate and trientine in a double-blind study of treatment of the neurologic presentation of Wilson disease. Arch Neurol. 2006a;63:521–7.

Brewer GJ, Dick R, Ullenbruch MR, Jin H, Phan SH. Inhibition of key cytokines by tetrathiomolybdate in the bleomycin model of pulmonary fibrosis. J Inorg Biochem. 2004;98:2160–7.

Brewer GJ, Dick R, Zeng C, Hou G. The use of tetrathiomolybdate in treating fibrotic, inflammatory, and autoimmune diseases, including the non-obese diabetic mouse model. J Inorg Biochem. 2006b; 100:927–30.

Brewer GJ, Hedera P, Kluin KJ, Carlson M, Askari F, Dick RB, Sitterly J, Fink JK. Treatment of Wilson disease with ammonium tetrathiomolybdate: III. Initial therapy in a total of 55 neurologically affected patients and follow-up with zinc therapy. Arch Neurol. 2003a;60:379–85.

Brewer GJ, Terry CA, Aisen AM, Hill GM. Worsening of neurologic syndrome in patients with Wilson's disease with initial penicillamine therapy. Arch Neurol. 1987; 44: 490–3.

Brewer GJ, Ullenbruch MR, Dick RB, Olivarez L, Phan SH. Tetrathiomolybdate therapy protects against bleomycin-induced pulmonary fibrosis in mice. J Lab Clin Med. 2003b;141:210–6.

Fox JH, Kama JA, Lieberman G, Chopra R, Dorsey K, Chopra V, Volitakis I, Cherny RA, Bush AI, Hersch S. Mechanisms of copper ion mediated Huntington's disease progression. PLoS ONE. 2007;2:e334.

Hottinger AF, Fine EG, Gurney ME, Zurn AD, Aebischer P. The copper chelator D-penicillamine delays onset of disease and extends survival in a transgenic mouse model of familial amyotrophic lateral sclerosis. Eur J Neurosci. 1997;9:1548–51.

Hou G, Dick R, Abrams GD, Brewer GJ. Tetrathiomolybdate protects against cardiac damage by doxorubicin in mice. J Lab Clin Med. 2005;146:299–303.

Kiaei M, Bush AI, Morrison BM, Morrison JH, Cherny RA, Volitakis I, Beal MF, Gordon JW. Genetically decreased spinal cord copper concentration prolongs life in a transgenic mouse model of amyotrophic lateral sclerosis. J Neurosci. 2004; 24:7945–50.

Ma S, Hou G, Dick RD, Brewer GJ. Tetrathiomolybdate protects against liver injury from acetaminophen in mice. J Appl Res Clin Exp Ther. 2004;4:419–26.

McCubbin MD, Hou G, Abrams GD, Dick R, Zhang Z, Brewer GJ. Tetrathiomolybdate is effective in a mouse model of arthritis. J Rheumatol. 2006; 33:2501–6.

Morris MC, Evans DA, Tangney CC, Bienias JL, Schneider JA, Wilson RS, Scherr PA. Dietary copper and high saturated and trans fat intakes associated with cognitive decline. Arch Neurol. 2006;63:1085–8.

Rasia RM, Bertoncini CW, Marsh D, Hoyer W, Cherny D, Zweckstetter M, Griesinger C, Jovin TM, Fernandez CO. Structural characterization of copper (II) binding to alpha-synuclein: Insights into the bioinorganic chemistry of Parkinson's disease. Proc Natl Acad Sci USA. 2005;102:4294–9.

Sigurdsson EM, Brown DR, Alim MA, Scholtzova H, Carp R, Meeker HC, Prelli F, Frangione B, Wisniewski T. Copper chelation delays the onset of prion disease. J Biol Chem. 2003;278:46199–202.

Sparks DL, Friedland R, Petanceska S, Schreurs BG, Shi J, Perry G, Smith MA, Sharma A, Derosa S, Ziolkowski C, Stankovic G. Trace copper levels in the drinking water, but not zinc or aluminum, influence CNS Alzheimer-like pathology. J Nutr Health Aging. 2006;10:247–54.

Sparks DL, Schreurs BG. Trace amounts of copper in water induce beta-amyloid plaques and learning deficits in a rabbit model of Alzheimer's disease. Proc Natl Acad Sci USA. 2003;100:11065–9.

Squitti R, Barbati G, Rossi L, Ventriglia M, Dal Forno G, Cesaretti S, Moffa F, Caridi I, Cassetta E, Pasqualetti P, Calabrese L, Lupoi D, Rossini PM. Excess of nonceruloplasmin serum copper in AD correlates with MMSE, CSF [beta]-amyloid, and h-tau. Neurology. 2006;67:76–82.

Squitti R, Pasqualetti P, Dal Forno G, Moffa F, Cassetta E, Lupoi D, Vernieri F, Rossi L, Baldassini M, Rossini PM. Excess of serum copper not related to ceruloplasmin in Alzheimer disease. Neurology. 2005;64:1040–6.

Wadsworth TL, Bishop JA, Domes CM, Ralle M, Brewer G, Quinn JF. Copper complexing with tetrathiomolybdate in a murine model of Alzheimer's Disease. In: Society for Neuroscience Annual Meeting, San Diego, CA. 2007.

White AR, Multhaup G, Maher F, Bellingham SA, Camakaris J, Zheng H, Bush AI, Beyreuther K, Masters CL, Cappai R. The Alzheimer's disease amyloid precursor protein modulates copper-induced toxicity and oxidative stress in primary neuronal cultures. J Neurosci. 1999;19:9170–9.

Copper and cognition in Alzheimer's disease and Parkinson's disease

D. Larry Sparks[1], Chuck Ziolkowski[1], Donald Connor[1], Tom Beach[1], Charles Adler[2], Marwan Sabbagh[1], et al.
[1]Sun Health Research Institute, Sun City, AZ, USA;
[2]Mayo Clinic, Scottsdale, AZ, USA

Correspondence:
DL Sparks SHRI, 10515 W. Santa Fe Drive Sun City, AZ 85351, USA

Trace metals including copper, zinc and iron have been implicated in the etiology of Alzheimer's disease (AD; Plantin et al. 1987; Deibel et al. 1996; Religa et al. 2006). Blood levels of copper and ceruloplasmin (circulating copper chaperone) have been shown to be elevated in AD compared to controls by many, but not all investigators (Snaedal et al. 1998). Squitti et al. have reported a significant increase in circulating copper in AD and a trend for increased ceruloplasmin (Squitti et al. 2005), and they have suggested that free copper has the greatest influence in AD (Babiloni et

al. 2007). These authors also reported a significant negative correlation in AD between increased copper/ceruloplasmin and decreased scores on the MMSE, AVLT-A7 and the clock draw (Squitti et al. 2005; 2006). Similarly, we have shown that there are significant increases in circulating copper and ceruloplasmin in AD compared to age-matched controls and that increases were related to decreased performance on the MMSE and Rey's AVLT-A7 (Sparks et al. 2005). Copper ion has also been implicated in promoting production or toxicity of Aβ in AD (Moir et al. 1999; Atwood et al. 2000). The binding of copper to Aβ (Atwood et al. 2000) produces aggregates that are more (soluble; Moir et al. 1999) and thus possibly more toxic.

We have shown, in the setting of elevated circulating cholesterol, that adding copper to the drinking water of rabbits promotes AD-like neuropathology and causes 80% memory deficits (Sparks and Schreurs 2003). High dietary copper intake (7 mg/day) in humans compared with normal intake significantly lowers absorption and increases excretion, but not enough to preclude significantly increased retention of copper (Rosenson et al. 2005). Epidemiologic data suggests that increased dietary copper significantly hastens the progression of AD in the setting of increased saturated and trans fat intake compared to the progression of AD among individuals on a low copper diet (Morris et al. 2006). Chelation of copper has been shown to reduce the levels of Aβ in the brains of transgenic mouse models of AD (Cherny et al. 2001) and the copper/zinc chelator clioquinol and the copper chelator D-penicillamine are in clinical trials to test for benefit in the treatment of AD (Finefrock et al. 2003). We report herein cortical zinc, iron, and copper levels, and CSF copper levels among individuals grouped according to their clinically established cognitive status and performance prior to death.

Methods

Anterior superior temporal cortex and CSF samples were obtained at autopsy from clinically well-characterized individuals assessed annually for cognitive function. Each individual was administered standardized clinical instruments including, but not limited to, the MMSE (Folstein et al. 1975), Rey's AVLT (Rey 1964), and the digit span (Wechsler 1997).

Individuals obtained a consensus neurologic diagnosis based on clinical judgment, and the interval between an individual's last clinical evaluation and demise was less than 12 months in all cases. Postmortem measures were correlated to cognitive performance and diagnosis at the previous yearly clinical evaluation.

Ninety individuals were grouped for comparison into control ($N=32$), mild cognitive impairment (MCI; $N=7$), AD ($N=32$), Parkinson's disease—cognitively normal (PD-CogNL; $N=12$) and Parkinson's disease—dementia (PDD; $N=5$) populations. We further sub-grouped controls based on cognitive performance (Sparks et al. 2005), and compared trace metal levels, clinical and neuropathologic variables for 16 individuals considered high-function controls (HFC; MMSE=30 and AVLT-A7>12) and 16 individuals considered low-function controls (LFC; MMSE=27–29 and AVLT-A7=5–11). Individuals with PD were investigated as an alternate neurologic disorder group, and PD individuals with a concomitant neuropathologic diagnosis of AD were excluded. Neuropathologic evaluation was performed on paraffin sections from the middle temporal gyrus stained for α-synuclein (LB509 antibody) to identify Lewy bodies (LB). Frozen sections from the same region were stained using the Gallyas and Thioflavine S methods for senile plaques (SP) and neurofibrillary tangles (NFT).

Sections were graded (0—none, to 3—frequent) for densities of SP and NFT (using the CERAD criteria, Mirra et al. 1991), and Lewy-bodies (LB) by a single investigator (TB). Mean densities of SP, NFT and LB in sections of cortex from middle temporal cortex (level of the amygdala) were utilized for group comparisons and correlation to trace metal levels in the anterior superior temporal gyrus and copper levels in postmortem CSF.

Triplicate one-gram samples of temporal cortex were excised, freeze-dried and re-weighed. Trace metal levels in brain were determined by atomic absorption spectrophotometric methods (AOAC 1990). A blank was run in parallel with each sample. Standard solutions were prepared daily from certified atomic standards (Fisher Scientific, NJ). Copper, zinc, and iron levels were quantified by reference to standard curves using an Aanalyst-200 Perkin-Elmer Spectrometer. Brain trace metals are presented as microgram per gram wet tissue weight. Copper levels in autopsy CSF were determined by a commercial laboratory (Galbraith Labs) and presented in parts per billion.

Differences between the populations for trace metals, clinical and neuropathologic indices were assessed by ANOVA followed by two-tailed Student's *t-tests; significance was set at $p < 0.05$.*

Results

Trace metal levels were compared for significant differences in postmortem samples from 90 individuals grouped according to their cognitive status (consensus diagnosis); 32 controls (sub-grouped as HFC and LFC), 32 AD, seven MCI, 12 PD-CogNL, and five PDD subjects. The group of individuals with MCI tended to be older than the control and AD groups, and the demented individuals with PD tended to be younger than the non-demented PD group (Table 1).

Mean copper levels in temporal cortex and CSF were significantly reduced in AD compared to normal controls (Table 1). Although reduced compared to the control group, the mean cortical and CSF copper levels in MCI were not significantly different from either AD or control levels of copper. Mean cortical copper levels were lower in LFC subjects compared to HFC subjects, but the difference was not significant (Table 1). The mean cortical copper level in MCI was significantly reduced compared to the HFC group ($p < 0.05$), but not the LFC or control populations. Copper levels in PD-CogNL patients were not different from controls without PD. Consistent with AD, cortical copper levels were significantly reduced in PDD patients compared to PD-CogNL, and there was a trend for reduced CSF copper levels.

Mean zinc levels in temporal cortex were not different between the control (sub-grouped), MCI, and AD populations, but levels were significantly lower in PDD than PD-CogNL (Table 1). Cortical iron levels were significantly elevated in AD compared to control, while levels in MCI were intermediate between the two populations; iron levels in PD-CogNL were not significantly different from any other group and variability attenuated significance of increased iron in PDD (Table 1).

The number of NFT in the temporal cortex was similar in the control, MCI, PD-CogNL, and PPD groups and significantly increased in AD compared to all other groups, likewise the severity of SP deposition was similar in control, MCI, PD-CogNL, and PDD patients and increased in AD compared to all other groups (Table 1). Increased density of LB in

Table 1 Mean age, cortical trace metal levels (microgram per gram wet weight) and CSF copper levels (parts per billion) and density scores for neurofibrillary tangles (NFT), senile plaques (SP) and Lewy bodies (LB) in temporal cortex, and scores on the MMSE, AVLT, AVLT-A7 and digit span instruments (±SEM) for the groups

Group	N	Age	Brain Cu	CSF Cu	Brain Zn	Brain Fe	NFT	SP	LB	MMSE	AVLT	AVLT-A7	Digit span
Control	32	85.2±1.0	3.79±0.19	19.6±1.3	20.7±0.6	36.7±1.2	0.33±0.17	1.39±0.26	0.0	29.1±0.19	40.5±1.4	7.4±0.6	17.1±0.6
HFC	16	85.3±1.1	4.04±0.20	21.3±2.7	20.2±0.9	36.7±1.8	0.43±0.18	1.18±0.34	0.0	Defined		Defined	17.0±0.7
LFC	16	85.1±1.0	3.55±0.20	17.9±2.4	21.1±0.9	36.8±1.6	0.22±0.15	1.48±0.41	0.0	Defined		Defined	17.2±0.8
MCI	7	91.1±2.3*	2.94±0.25	12.4±2.4	17.9±1.3	38.2±2.6	0.40±0.24	1.36±0.46	0.0	26.6±0.92	26.4±0.9*	3.5±1.0*	13.9±0.7*
AD	32	87.6±1.0	2.76±0.16*	15.4±1.6*	20.6±0.7	43.8±2.2 ****	1.73±0.23	2.52±0.16*	0.32±0.12	9.8±1.7*	9.7±2.7*	0.7±0.3*	12.7±0.9
PD-CogNL	12	85.3±1.4	3.65±0.20	17.4±4.3	17.0±0.8	41.3±1.2	0.25±0.15	1.36±0.30	0.54±0.22	27.3±1.2	35.3±3.7	7.2±1.4	15.9±2.2
PDD	5	78.6±2.2**	2.88±0.27***	10.0±1.1**	20.8±1.4***	46.8±9.1	0.0±0.0	1.25±0.48	1.28±0.29	13.9±3.1***	18.7±2.3***	1.0±0.7***	13.1±1.7

$*P<0.05$ compared to controls

$**P<0.10$ compared to the PD-CogNL group

$***P<0.05$ compared to the PD-CogNL group

$****P<0.01$ compared to control and <0.05 compared to LFC and HFC

temporal cortex of PDD patients was significantly increased compared to all other groups except the PD-CogNL population (Table 1).

Based on the employed clinical groupings, there was a significant decrease in the mean performance on the MMSE and Rey's AVLT between control and MCI, and a further significant decrease between MCI and AD. A significant decrease on the MMSE was identified in the PDD population compared to both the PD–ND and control populations (Table 1). Mean scores on the digit span were significantly reduced to comparable levels in MCI and AD compared to controls.

Discussion

We investigated a group of individuals rigorously evaluated clinically predicated on their willingness to donate their brain via rapid autopsy (<5 h PMI in each case) upon demise. We measured cortical trace metal levels and CSF copper concentration among these individuals and compared sub-populations grouped according to clinical performance and consensus clinical diagnosis of normal control, MCI, AD, PD–CogNL, or PDD without AD.

The data indicated that in contrast to circulating blood levels, brain, and CSF copper levels may gradually decrease with increasingly severe deterioration of cognitive performance in both AD and PD. A similar relationship was not found for brain levels of zinc or iron and gradual cognitive decline. Increased production of APP and Aβ have been associated with reduced CNS copper levels, while increased brain copper levels correlate with reduced brain Aβ levels (Maynard et al. 2005). In contrast, studies found that Aβ co-injected (at physiologic concentrations found in AD) with iron, copper, or zinc into rat cortex indicated that Aβ-Fe and Aβ-Zn were more toxic that Aβ alone, while Aβ-copper was non-toxic (Bishop and Robinson 2004). This could support the hypothesis suggesting that binding of copper by Aβ is a scavenger mechanism by which the peptide aggregates with copper, thus inactivating the metal ion and possibly Aβ (Robinson and Bishop 2002). In the case of AD, it would seem possible that as brain copper levels wane so goes the capacity to inactivate Aβ thus enhancing neurotoxicity.

Acknowledgments

This study was made possible via funding from the Arizona Biomedical Research Commission, the NIA—Arizona Alzheimer Research Center, and the Michael J. Fox Foundation.

References

AOAC (1990). Official Methods of Analysis. 15th ed. Arlington, VA., Association of Official Analytical Chemists.

Atwood CS, Scarpa RC, Huang X, Moir RD, Jones WD, Fairlie DP, Tan RE, Bush AI. Characterization of copper interactions with Alzheimer amyloid beta peptides: identification of an attomolar-affinity copper binding site on amyloid beta1–42. J Neurochem 2000;75(3): 219–1233.

Babiloni C, Squitti R, Del Percio C, Cassetta E, Ventrigila MC, Ferreri F, Frisoni G, Binetti G, Curzi M, Salinari S, Zappasodi F, Rossini PM. Free copper and resting temporal EEG rhythms correlate across cognitive impairment and Alzheimer's disease subjects. Clin Neurophysiol 2007;118(6):1244–60.

Bishop GM, Robinson SR. The amyloid paradox: amyloid-beta-metal complexes can be neurotoxic and neuroprotective. Brain Pathol 2004;14:448–52.

Cherny RA, Atwood CS, Xilinas ME, Gray DN, Jones WD, McLean CA, Barnham KJ, Volitakis I, Fraser FW, Kim Y, Huang X, Goldstein LE, Moir Rd, Lim JT, Beyreuther K, Zheng H, Tankzi RE, Maters CL, Bush AI. Treatment with a copper–zinc chelator markedly and rapidly inhibits beta-amyloid accumulation in AD transgenic mice. Neuron 2001;30(3): 665–76.

Deibel MA, Ehmann WD, Markesbery WR. Copper, iron and zinc imbalances in severely degenerated brain regions in AD: possible relation to oxidative stress. J Neurol Sci 1996;143:137–42.

Finefrock AE, Bush AI, Doraiswarny PM. Current status of metals as therapeutic targets in AD. J Amer Geriatr Soc 2003;51:1143–8.

Folstein MF, Folstein SE, McHugh PR. "Mini-Mental State": a practical method for grading the cognitive state of patients for the clinician. J Psychiatr Res 1975;12:189–98.

Maynard CJ, Bush AI, Masters CL, Cappai R, Li QX. Metals and amyloid-beta in Alzheimer's disease. Int J Exp Pathol 2005;86:147–59.

Mirra SS, Heyman A, McKeel D, Sumi SM, Crain BJ, Brownlee LM, Vogel FS, Hughes JP, van Belle G, Berg L. The consortium to establish a registry for Alzheimer's disease (CERAD). Part II. Standardization of the neuropathologic assessment for Alzheimer's disease. Neurology 1991;41:479–86.

Moir RD, Atwood CS, Romano DM, Laurans MH, Huang X, Bush AI, Smith JD, Tanzi RE. Differential effects of apolipoprotein E isoforms on metal-induced aggregation of Abeta using physiological concentrations. Biochemistry 1999;38:4595–603.

Morris MC, Evans DA, Tangney CC, Bienias JL, Schneider JA, Wilson RS, Scherr PA. Dietary copper and high saturated and trans fat intakes associated with cognitive decline. Arch Neurol 2006;63:1085–8.

Plantin LO, Lying-Tunell U, Kristensson K. Trace elements in the human central nervous system studied with neutron activation analysis. Biol Trace Element Res 1987;13:69–75.

Religa D, Strozyk D, Cherny RA, Volitakis I, Haroutunian V, Winblad B, Naslund J, Bush AI. Elevated cortical zinc in Alzheimer disease. Neurology 2006;67: 69–75.

Rey A. (1964). L'examen clinique en psychologie. Paris, Presses Universitaires de France.

Robinson SR, Bishop GM. Ab as a bioflocculant: implications for the amyloid hypothesis of Alzheimer's disease. Neurobiol Aging 2002;23: 1051–72.

Rosenson RS, Tangney CC, Levine DM, Parker TS, Gordon BR. Association between reduced low density lipoprotein oxidation and inhibition of monocyte chemoattractant protein-1 production in statin-treated subjects. J. Lab Clin Med 2005;Feb(145 (2)):83–7.

Snaedal J, Kristinsson J, Gunnarsdottir S, Olafsdottir A, Baldvinsson M, Johannesson T. Copper, ceruloplasmin and superoxide dismutase in patients with Alzheimer's disease. Dementia Geriatr Cog Dis 1998; 9:239–42.

Sparks DL, Petanceska S, Sabbagh M, Connor D, Soares H, Adler C, Lopez J, Ziolowski C, Lochhead J, Browne P. Cholesterol, copper and Ab in controls, MCI, AD and the AD Cholesterol-Lowering Treatment trial (ADCLT). Curr Alz Res 2005;2:527–39.

Sparks DL, Schreurs BG. Trace amounts of copper in water induce b-amyloid plaques and learning deficits in a rabbit model of Alzheimer's disease. PNAS (track II) 2003;100:1065–9.

Squitti R, Barbati G, Rossi L, Ventriglia M, Dal Forno G, Cesaretti S, Moffa F, Caridi I, Cassetta E, Pasqualetti P, Calabrese L, Lupoi D, Rossini PM. Excess of nonceruloplasmin serum copper in AD correlates with MMSE, CSF B-amyloid, and h-tau. AAN Enterprises, inc. 2006:76–82.

Squitti R, Pasqualetti P, Dal Forno G, Moffa F, Cassetta E, Lupoi D, Vernieri F, Rossi L, Baldassini M, Rossini PM. Excess of serum copper not related to ceruloplasmin in Alzheimer disease. Neurology 2005; 64:1040–6.

Wechsler D. Wechsler Adult Intelligence Scale. San Antonio, TX, The Psychological Corp, Harcourt Brace 1997: 217.

An invited paper presented in the symposium "Copper in neurologic and neurodegenerative diseases".

Copper Studies in Alzheimer's Disease Patients

Rosanna Squitti[1] and P. M. Rossini[1,2,3]

[1]Department of Neuroscience, AFaR—Ospedale Fatebenefratelli, Rome, Italy; [2]Clinica Neurologica, Università Campus Biomedico, Rome, Italy; [3]IRCCS San Raffele, Pisana, Rome, Cassino, Italy

Corresponding Author:
E-mail address: rosanna.squitti@afar.it

Metallochemistry in AD

Alzheimer's disease (AD) is an irreversible, progressive neurodegenerative disorder, characterized by gradual cognitive deficits, leading to dementia. These deficiencies are related to progressive loss of neurons, and presence of dystrophic neuritis and synapses. At the microscopic level, it is characterized by amyloid plaques and neurofibrillary tangles in the brain cortex. The plaques are made up of beta-amyloid ($A\beta$), a peptide of 39–43 amino acids.

Current research hypotheses on AD focus on oxidative stress and metal (such as iron, zinc and copper) levels imbalance as potential factors inducing the accumulation of $A\beta$ in the brain (Bush 2002; 2003).

The metallochemistry of AD has gradually developed in the mid 90s, with the observation that the $A\beta$'s precursor protein (APP) possesses selective zinc and copper binding sequences. It is now established that $A\beta$ is a high-affinity copper protein and APP is known to be a chaperone involved in copper trafficking (White et al. 1999; Bellingham et al. 2004). Copper, as also zinc and iron, has been demonstrated to induce amyloidal plaque deposition in vitro (Bush et al. 1994; Multhaup et al. 1996) that is completely reversed by chelation (Cherny et al. 2001) as observed in post mortem AD brain samples. Copper and iron, aside from metal dependent aggregation, confer redox activity to APP-$A\beta$ peptide, triggering Fenton's-like reactions of oxidative stress (White et al. 1999).

Clinical Studies in AD

Our group has contributed to collect evidence supporting the hypothesis (Bush 2002) of an implication of copper in the pathogenesis of AD on setting clinical trials. We previously measured copper, iron, total hydro- and lipoperoxides, transferrin and ceruloplasmin levels and the antioxidant capacity (Total Radical Trapping Antioxidant capacity or TRAP) in serum on patients affected by AD, vascular dementia (VAD) and normal subjects (Squitti et al. 2002, 2003). We also aimed to determine the correlation between these biological variables of metals and oxidative stress and functional or anatomical deficits in the AD brain. Primary results indicated that copper levels were higher in AD patients than in normal elderly controls (Squitti et al. 2002).

Elevated copper levels in particular, as well as low TRAP capacity, were correlated with typical neuropsychological deficits found in AD patients and a positive correlation between isolated medial temporal lobe atrophy was found, estimated by visual inspection of brain MRI, and serum TRAP and copper levels (Squitti et al. 2002). Serum copper levels were found directly correlated with cognitive deficits of AD but had no effect in serum of VAD patients. More recent studies investigated the possible effects in AD of copper-enzymes that were copper, zinc superoxide dismutase (Cu, Zn SOD) and ceruloplasmin.

AD patients had higher Cu, Zn SOD activity than controls (Rossi et al. 2002). Both copper:ceruloplasmin and copper:transferrin ratios showed disequilibrium, and were higher in AD patients than in VAD or in healthy subjects (Squitti et al. 2005). In our study, about 56% of serum copper variability in normalcy could be explained by ceruloplasmin variation. On this basis, we initially computed two copper measures: the first, copper "explained by ceruloplasmin", corresponded to the expected level of copper, given a ceruloplasmin level; the second, copper "not explained by ceruloplasmin", corresponded to the residual copper (Squitti et al. 2005). AD patients had higher copper unexplained by ceruloplasmin than controls and VAD subjects (Squitti et al. 2005). In a subsequent study (Squitti et al. 2006), we calculated that on average a unit micromole per liter of ceruloplasmin could account for 6.68 μmol/L copper explained by ceruloplasmin, consistent with the notion that ceruloplasmin contains six copper atoms per molecule.

Moreover, we compared the portion of copper bound to ceruloplasmin (CB), that can be easily calculated as a 0.3% of ceruloplasmin (Walshe 2003), with the estimated explained copper. The mean value of the CB obtained in the control population did not differ from the explained copper (Squitti et al. 2006). The unexplained copper could thus be referred to as non-ceruloplasmin-copper, also named 'free' copper (Walshe 2003). 'Free' copper is the serum biological marker of Wilson's disease, the paradigmatic disease of copper accumulation or intoxication (Walshe 2003). Moreover, we performed experiments of ultrafiltration to find a filterable copper in the AD serum, which revealed a 3.7 fold higher concentration of copper in patients than in controls (Squitti et al. 2006). Recently, these observations were confirmed by two other groups (Hoogenraad 2007; Althaus, personal communication). In particular, hard data from the Althaus' study indicated that the 'free' copper level in AD sera nearly doubled the one in normal sera (AD 2.27±0.16 μmol/L; normal 1.56± 0.29 μmol/L). Furthermore, even though results from previous AD studies regarding absolute serum copper (i.e., total of serum copper, both bound and not bound to ceruloplasmin) appear controversial (Snaedal et al. 1998; Gonzalez et al. 1999; Squitti et al. 2002; Ozcankaya and Delibas 2002; Kessler et al. 2006; Sedighi et al. 2006), the controversy does not dispute the ceruloplasmin–copper relationship, i.e., the evidence of 'free' copper in AD. In fact, some authors confirm our findings of a copper/ceruloplasmin dyshomeostasis in AD (Snaedal et al. 1998; Kessler et al. 2006; Sedighi et al. 2006), some of whom have published earlier. In particular, in their study, Snaedal et al. (1998) found similar levels of absolute serum copper in AD and controls, but significantly lower concentrations of ceruloplasmin. This means a higher concentration of 'free' copper in AD than in controls.

Kessler et al. (2006) reported data coherent with a 2.5-fold increase of 'free' copper in AD with respect to normal values (<1.6 μmol/L; Walshe 2003); Sedighi et al. (2006) a 40% increase of 'free' copper in AD than in controls, even though the authors found similar levels of copper and ceruloplasmin.

Normally, the majority of human serum copper is considered to be tightly bound to ceruloplasmin (Walshe 2003). The remaining copper, i.e., 'free' copper, would be distributed and exchanged among albumin, amino acids (e.g. histidine), and small-molecular-weight complexes (0.5–5%), which can easily cross the brain blood barrier (BBB). Since APP is a copper chaperone and copper-binding APP has been hypothesized to represent a mean for removing excess copper from brain tissue (White et al. 1999; Bellingham et al. 2004). The excess of serum copper we have defined in AD could be explained by an efflux from cortical cells, as also proposed by some authors (Bush 2003). Alternatively, our results could be ascribed to a failure of copper incorporation into APP in the liver. In fact, a hepatic origin of copper abnormalities have been suggested by some authors (Bush and Strozyk 2004) coherently with the APP−/− mouse model in which ablation of the APP molecule determines a copper increase by 80% in the liver and 40% in the brain (White et al. 1999). This idea is supported by recent results suggesting abnormal incorporation of copper into ceruloplasmin in AD patients (Squitti et al. 2006). In particular, the serum of patients with higher percentage of biologically inactive apo-form of ceruloplasmin had increased 'free' copper concentrations (Squitti et al. 2006). In fact, when impairment of copper incorporation into the protein occurs, generally because of a dysfunction of the copper-transporting ATPase 7b (like in Wilson's disease), ceruloplasmin apo-protein is excessively secreted by hepatocytes. Moreover, we explored the relationship between a typical panel of liver function markers and biological variables of copper metabolism in a sample of AD patients and control subjects. It was found that AD patients with no evidence of additional pathological conditions, including liver dysfunctions of any origin, had higher 'free' copper, longer PT and lower albumin levels than controls matched for age, sex and risk factors for cardiovascular diseases and medications intake (Squitti et al. 2007), concluding a potential hepatic effect on copper abnormalities in AD.

As some authors (Strozyk et al. 2007) recently reported evidence of an inverse correlation between copper and Aβ concentrations in the CSF, our results show that the 'free' copper pool is correlated with Aβ and copper levels in the CSF (Squitti et al. 2006). The finding of a decrease of active ceruloplasmin in the CSF of AD patients associated with an increase of their CSF copper not bound to this protein (Capo et al. 2008) also supports the idea of a copper imbalance as a factor disturbing the brain. The idea of a flux of an excess of a low-molecular-weight copper from the serum to the brain disturbing brain functioning is also supported by the finding that the typical abnormalities of the AD brain on the organization of electroencephalographic rhythmic activity well correlated with higher levels of serum 'free' copper (Babiloni et al. 2007) and that this relationship resulted even stronger in apolipoprotein E-ε4 carriers (in progress).

Conclusions

Alzheimer's disease is, nowadays, considered a multifactorial disease stemming from the interaction between genetic predisposition, environmental factors as well as anamnestic factors (i.e. educational level, severe head trauma, etc.). Our recent results seem to support, also from a clinical point of view, the model proposed of a significant role on copper pathogenesis in AD (Bush 2002). In particular, we propose that, along with other, yet non-mutually exclusive hypothesis of AD neurodegeneration, a mechanism involving a deregulation of the 'free' copper serum pool may be operating, acting a toxic effect by crossing the BBB and interacting with Aβ, possibly resulting in catalytic generation of peroxides (H_2O_2) and Aβ aggregation (Opazo et al. 2002).

Acknowledgments

This review was supported by Grants of the Italian Ministero della Salute, RF conv.58/2006.

References

Bellingham SA, Ciccotosto GD, Needham BE, Fodero LR, White AR, Masters CL, Cappai R, Camakaris J. Gene knockout of amyloid precursor protein and amyloid precursor-like protein-2 increases cellular copper levels in primary mouse cortical neurons and embryonic fibroblasts. J Neurochem. 2004;91:423–28.

Babiloni C, Squitti R, Del Percio C, Cassetta E, Ventriglia MC, Ferreri F, Tombini M, Frisoni G, Binetti G, Gurzi M, Salinari S, Zappasodi F, Rossini PM. Free copper and resting temporal EEG rhythms correlate across healthy, mild cognitive impairment, and Alzheimer's disease subjects. Clin Neurophysiol. 2007;118:1244–60.

Bush AI, Pettingell WH, Multhaup G, d Paradis M, Vonsattel JP, Gusella JF, Beyreuther K, Masters CL, Tanzi RE. Rapid induction of Alzheimer A beta amyloid formation by zinc. Science. 1994;265:1464–67.

Bush AI. Metal complexing agents as therapies for Alzheimer's disease. Neurobiol Aging. 2002;23:1031–38.

Bush AI. The metallobiology of Alzheimer's disease. Trends Neurosci. 2003; 26:207–14.

Bush AI, Strozyk D. Serum copper: a biomarker for Alzheimer disease? Arch Neurol. 2004;61:631–32.

Capo CR, Arciello M, Squitti R, Cassetta E, Rossini PM, Calabrese L, Rossi L. Features of ceruloplasmin in the cerebrospinal fluid of Alzheimer's disease patients. Biometals. 2008;21:367–72.

Cherny RA, Atwood CS, Xilinas ME, Gray DN, Jones WD, McLean CA, Barnham KJ, Volitakis I, Fraser FW, Kim Y, Huang X, Goldstein LE, Moir RD, Lim JT, Beyreuther K, Zheng H, Tanzi RE, Masters CL, Bush AI. Treatment with a copper–zinc chelator markedly and rapidly inhibits beta-amyloid accumulation in Alzheimer's disease transgenic mice. Neuron. 2001;30:665–76.

Gonzalez C, Martin T, Cacho J, Brenas MT, Arroyo T, Garcia-Berrocal B, Navajo JA, Gonzalez-Buitrago JM. Serum zinc, copper, insulin, and lipids in Alzheimer's disease epsilon 4 apolipoprotein E allele carriers. Eur J Clin Invest. 1999; 29:637–42.

Hoogenraad TU. Measuring hypercupremia in blood of patients with Alzheimer's disease is logical, but the utility of measuring free-copper has to be proven. In: Frijns CJM, Kappelle, LJ, Klijn, CJM, Wokke, JHJ. Neurologie. Utrechts Tijdschrift voor. 2007: 111–2.

Kessler H, Pajonk FG, Meisser P, Schneider-Axmann T, Hoffmann KH, Supprian T, Herrmann W, Obeid R, Multhaup G, Falkai P, Bayer TA. Cerebrospinal fluid diagnostic markers correlate with lower plasma copper and ceruloplasmin in patients with Alzheimer's disease. J Neural Transm. 2006;113:1763–9.

Multhaup G, Schlicksupp A, Hesse L, Beher D, Ruppert T, Masters CL, Beyreuther K. The amyloid precursor protein of Alzheimer's disease in the reduction of copper (II) to copper(I). Science. 1996;271:1406–9.

Opazo C, Huang X, Cherny RA, Moir RD, Roher AE, White AR, Cappai R, Masters CL, Tanzi RE, Inestrosa NC, Bush AI. Metalloenzyme-like activity of Alzheimer's disease beta-amyloid. Cu-dependent catalytic conversion of dopamine, cholesterol, and biological reducing agents to neurotoxic H_2O_2. J Biol Chem. 2002:277;40302–8.

Ozcankaya R, Delibas N. Malondialdehyde, super-oxide dismutase, melatonin, iron, copper and zinc blood concentrations in patients with Alzheimer Disease: cross-sectional study. Croat Med J. 2002;43:28–32.

Rossi L, Squitti R, Pasqualetti P, Marchese E, Cassetta E, Forastiere E, Rotilio G, Rossini PM, Finazzi-Agro A. Red blood cell copper, zinc super-oxide dismutase activity is higher in Alzheimer's disease and is decreased by D-penicillamine. Neurosci Lett. 2002;329:137–40.

Sedighi B, Shafa MA, Shariati M. A study of serum copper and ceruloplasmin in Alzheimer's disease in Kerman, Iran. Neurology Asia. 2006;11:107–9.

Snaedal J, Kristinsson J, Gunnarsdottir S, Olafsdottir Baldvinsson M, Johannesson T. Copper Ceruloplasmin and superoxide dismutase in patients with Alzheimer's disease, a case-control study. Dement Geriatr Cogn Disord. 1998;9:239–42.

Squitti R, Lupoi D, Pasqualetti P, Dal Forno G, Vernieri F, Chiovenda P, Rossi L, Cortesi M, Cassetta E, Rossini PM. Elevation of serum copper levels in Alzheimer's disease. Neurology. 2002;59:1153–61.

Squitti R, Pasqualetti P, Cassetta E, Dal Forno G, Cesaretti S, Pedace F, Finazzi-Agrò A, Rossini PM. Elevation of serum copper levels discriminates Alz-heimer's disease from vascular dementia. Neurology. 2003;60:2013–14.

Squitti R, Pasqualetti P, Dal Forno G, Moffa F, Cassetta E, Lupoi D, Vernieri F, Rossi L, Baldassini M, Rossini PM. Excess of serum copper not related to ceruloplasmin in Alzheimer disease. Neurology. 2005;64:1040–6.

Squitti R, Barbati G, Rossi L, Ventriglia M, Dal Forno G, Cesaretti S, Moffa F, Caridi I, Cassetta E, Pasqualetti P, Calabrese L, Lupoi D, Rossini PM. Excess of nonceruloplasmin serum copper in AD correlates with MMSE, CSF [beta]-amyloid, and h-tau. Neurology. 2006;67:76–82.

Squitti R, Ventriglia M, Barbati G, Cassetta E, Ferreri F, Dal Forno G, Ramires S, Zappasodi F, Rossini PM. 'Free' copper in serum of Alzheimer's disease patients correlates with markers of liver function. J Neural Transm. 2007;114:1589–94.

Strozyk D, Launer LJ, Adlard PA, Cherny RA, Tsatsanis A, Volitakis I, Blennow K, Petrovitch H, White LR, Bush AI. Zinc and copper modulate Alzheimer Abeta levels in human cerebrospinal fluid. Neurobiol Aging. 2007; doi: 10.1016/j.neurobiolaging. 2007.10.012, in press.

Walshe JM. Clinical Investigations Standing Com-mittee of the Association of Clinical Biochemists. Wilson's disease: the importance of measuring serum caeruloplasmin non-immunologically. Ann Clin Bio-chem. 2003;40 (Pt 2):115–21.

White AR, Reyes R, Mercer JF, Camakaris J, Zheng H, Bush AI, Multhaup G, Beyreuther K, Masters CL, Cappai R. Copper levels are increased in the cerebral cortex and liver of APP and APLP2 knockout mice. Brain Res. 1999;842:439–44.

An invited paper presented in the symposium "Cop-per in neurologic and neurodegenerative diseases".

Dietary Fat and Copper Effects on Cognition

Martha Clare Morris, Sc.D.
Department of Internal Medicine, Rush University Medical Center, Chicago, IL, USA

Corresponding Author:
Email address: Martha_C_Morris@rush.edu

Introduction

Dementia is a progressive and heterogeneous disorder that is common in old age. Because of increased life expectancy, this devastating and irreversible condition is becoming a major public health problem in the Western hemisphere. By the year 2050, we can expect that approximately 25% of the population will be 65 years and older, and more than one third will likely develop dementia (Hebert 2001). The complex inter-action of fatty acids, cholesterol, and biological metals is key to the neurodegenerative processes that underlie dementia. These dietary components are essential to the normal structure and functioning of neuronal cells. However, dyshomeostasis in their regulation and metabolism is linked to susceptibility to Alzheimer and vascular pathology. There is increasing evidence that dietary consumption of fats and biological metals are linked to brain levels and functioning, and, thus, have the potential to modulate the risk of becoming demented.

Brain Neuropathology

Alzheimer disease is the most common dementia, representing at least 80% of clinical cases (Evans 1989). It is characterized neuropathologically by extra-cellular deposition of β-amyloid (Aβ) in senile plaques, intra-neuronal formation of neuro-fibrillary tangles composed of hyper-phosphorylated tau protein, and loss of neurons and synapses in the neocortex, hippocampus, and other subcortical areas of the brain. Vascular dementia caused by cerebral infarcts is the second most common form of dementia in the US. In one study, only one third of persons with clinical expression of Alzheimer disease exhibited pure Alzheimer's disease pathology. Over 57% had mixed pathology, that is, Alzheimer pathology with infarction, Lewy bodies, or both. Further, whereas both Alzheimer neuropathology and cerebral infarcts were each independently and strongly associated with increased odds of dementia, their combined presence had a multiplicative effect. In late onset Alzheimer disease, the accumulation of amyloid plaque neuropathology is the result of a complex interplay between genetic and environmental factors affecting the generation, clearance, and aggregation of Aβ peptide. An intriguing theory is that Aβ-lipid membrane interactions are central to the cause of Aβ I-42 neurotoxicity in Alzheimer disease (Smith 2006). These interactions are fostered by copper and result in changes in membrane fluidity leading to depolarization and disorder (Eckert 2005), leading to ion-channel formation and disrupted calcium homeostasis (Kagan 2002), lipid peroxidation, cholesterol oxidation and the production of reactive oxygen species (Butterfield 2004; Puglielli 2005). This cascade of events results in cell death and amyloid plaque formation.

Cholesterol, Neuropathology, and Alzheimer Disease Risk

The brain has the highest cholesterol content of any organ in the human body. Physiologically, cholesterol is an integral membrane component required for normal cell functioning (signaling, adhesion and motility), and its metabolism is tightly regulated by the cell. Cholesterol regulates both the generation and clearance of Aβ from the brain (Refolo 2000). Elevated cholesterol increases Aβ in cellular and animal models of Alzheimer disease (Refolo 2000; Mori 2001; Sparks 1994), and drugs that inhibit cholesterol synthesis lower Aβ in these models (Fassbender 2001). One theory is that increased intracellular cholesterol increases the secretion and immunoreactivity of Aβ, leading to the accumulation of amyloid deposit load and size (Puglielli 2003). The extent of amyloid deposition may be influenced by the rate of amyloid clearance which, in turn, may be influenced by other factors, such as the level of biological metals. For example, poor clearance of amyloid in certain individuals may exacerbate amyloid deposition.

The primary genetic risk factor for late onset Alzheimer disease encodes apolipoprotein E (APOE) which plays a central role in cholesterol uptake and transport in the brain. Persons with two copies of the APOE-ε4 allele have elevated serum cholesterol levels and increased risk of developing Alzheimer disease and cardiovascular disease (Evans 2003). A number of epidemiologic studies have reported that high mid-life serum cholesterol level increased the risk of late-life dementia (Notkola 1998; Kivipelto 2002), and that use of cholesterol-lowering medications reduced the risk (Wolozin 2000; Jick 2000). A hypercholesterolemic diet has been shown to increase Alzheimer pathology in transgenic mice (Refolo 2000) and rabbits (Sparks 2003; Greenwood 1996) and impair cognitive function in animal models (Sparks 1994; Greenwood 1996). In humans, a diet that is high in saturated and trans fats and low in polyunsaturated and monounsaturated fats is a primary cause of hypercholesterolemia. Of five prospective epidemiologic studies that examined the effect of dietary fat intake on the development of Alzheimer's disease, four (Luchsinger 2002; Laitinen 2006; Morris 2003; Kalmijn 1997) observed associations with fat composition. In the Chicago Health and Aging Project, older persons whose diets were high in saturated and trans fats had a significantly faster rate of cognitive decline over 6 years than persons with low intakes of these fats (Morris 2004). Thus, these several lines of evidence provide support for the hypothesis that dietary consumption of fats and blood cholesterol are related to the development of brain neuropathology and dementia.

Biological Metals and Neuropathology

Copper, zinc, and iron are three biological metals known to be essential for normal brain functioning and development (Pollitt 2000; Danks 1988). However, disrupted homeostasis of brain levels of these metals are thought to play a central role in the formation and neurotoxicity of amyloid-β (Aβ; Huang 2004; Bartzokis 2004). β-amyloid (Aβ) is a copper/zinc-metalloprotein that aggregates and becomes redox-active in the presence of these metals (Atwood 1998; Bush 1994). This explains the pooling of high concentrations of copper, zinc, and iron in amyloid plaques, and the rescue of amyloid pathology by the genetic ablation of the neocortical zinc transporter, ZnT3 (Friedlich 2004; Lee 2004). Previous observations indicate that both Aβ (Atwood 1998; Atwood 2000) and the amino terminus of amyloid protein precursor (APP; Hesse 1994) possess high-affinity, selective Cu2+ binding sites. APP gene transcription is sensitive to copper (Bellingham 2004), and its translation is sensitive to iron. Recent reports suggest that a function for the Cu2+ binding site on Aβ is that the peptide can sequester Cu2+ and prevent the metal ion from generating damaging reactive oxygen species (Kontush 2001; Zouk 2002). Therefore, Aβ may be part of a metal clearance system, which becomes corrupted in Alzheimer disease (Bush 2003). The distribution of copper in the brain changes markedly with aging (Maynard 2002) so that it is less bioavailable. The abnormal decoration of Aβ with Cu2+ leads to two principal abnormal reactions: redox activity leading to H_2O_2 production (Huang 1999; Opazo 2002) and aggregation (Atwood 1998; 2000). Aβ-Cu+2 complexes lead to lipid peroxidation and reactive oxygen species, and cell death. The lipid peroxidation can be inhibited by the use of the metal-complexing agent clioquinol, which potently inhibits AD-like amyloid neuropathology in transgenic mice (Cherny 2001). A second-generation derivative of clioquinol is currently being tested in clinical trials. In health, the brain strictly regulates the movement of these metals across the blood–brain barrier (BBB), which is relatively impermeable to fluctuations in blood levels.

The Interaction Effects of Dietary Fat and Copper on Cognition

A recent animal study suggested that increased neuronal Aβ immunoreactivity and senile plaque-like structures in the brain induced by a hypercholesterolemic diet were exacerbated by consumption of trace amounts of copper in drinking water (Sparks 2003). These study findings were later replicated in several animal species: spontaneously hypercholesterolemic Watanabe rabbits, cholesterol-fed beagles and rabbits, and PS1/APP transgenic mice (Sparks 2006). There is only one published study of the interaction of dietary fat and copper on cognitive function in humans. The study was of 3,718 participants of the Chicago Health and Aging Project (CHAP), a geographically defined population-based study of persons 65 years and older (Morris 2006). Cognitive function among the CHAP participants was assessed three times over a 6-year period using four cognitive tests: the East Boston Test of Immediate Memory (Albert 1991), the East Boston Test of Delayed Memory (Albert 1991), the Mini-Mental Status Examination (Folstein 1975), and the Symbol Digit Modalities Test (Smith 1984). Scores from the tests were standardized and averaged to form a single global measure of cognitive function at each of the three measurement periods. Diet and multivitamin use was assessed a median of 1.2 years after the baseline cognitive assessment using a comprehensive food frequency questionnaire. For analysis, study participants were grouped according to whether or not they consumed a high saturated/trans fat diet. The grouping was determined based on saturated fat intake in the highest 20% of the study population and trans fat intake in the upper 60%. This high fat diet was consumed by 16.2% of the study population. These arbitrary cut-points were based on previous findings from the CHAP study showing statistically significant increased risk of incident Alzheimer's disease at these intake levels.

Mixed-effects models (Laird 1982) were used to examine whether cognitive decline was accelerated among persons whose diets were high in saturated/trans fat and who also consumed high amounts of copper. Remarkably, there was a strong statistical interaction between high intakes of saturated/trans fat and copper on the rate of cognitive decline (Morris 2006). Persons whose dietary intake of saturated and trans fats was high and whose copper intake (from food and multivitamins) was in the highest quintile had a 145% increase in the rate of cognitive decline compared with those in the lowest quintile of copper intake. The increase in rate was the equivalent of 19 years of older age. There was also a statistically significant increase in the rate of decline among persons who had a high fat diet and high copper intake from food sources only. The strongest association was observed among persons consuming vitamin supplements containing copper. In comparison to the decline rate in persons who did not consume a vitamin supplement containing copper, there was a linear increase in the rate of cognitive decline with increasing copper dose among the high-fat consumers. There was no evidence of association of high copper intake with cognitive decline among persons who did not consume a high fat diet.

The copper content of multivitamins is typically 2 mg/d, two times the RDA of 0.9 mg/d. The study did not have information on copper intake from tap water sources. The low concentration of copper in the drinking water of the Sparks et al. animal model was 1/10th the maximum contaminant level goal of 1.3 ppm of copper for drinking water set by the Environmental Protections Agency. These findings are intriguing because they suggest that Aβ metabolism is extraordinarily sensitive to small changes in copper concentrations that might be transduced across the blood brain barrier as a result of environmental exposure to copper. These findings hold enormous public health implications given the widespread exposure of the population to copper in drinking water, multivitamins, and food, and the high dietary intake of saturated and trans fats. Furthermore, the cognitive deterioration that was observed in the CHAP study could have been due to an acceleration of Alzheimer's disease pathology induced by Cu, as seen in animal studies.

References

Albert MS, Smith LA, Scherr PA, et al. Use of brief cognitive tests to identify individuals in the community with clinically-diagnosed Alzheimer's disease. Internatl J Neurosci 1991;57:167–78.

Atwood CS, Moir RD, Huang X, Scarpa RC, Bacarra NM, Romano DM, et al. Dramatic aggregation of Alzheimer abeta by Cu(II) is induced by conditions representing physiological acidosis. J Biol Chem 1998;273(21):12817–26.

Atwood CS, Scarpa RC, Huang X, Moir RD, Jones WD, Fairlie DP, et al. Characterization of copper interactions with alzheimer amyloid beta peptides: identification of an attomolar-affinity copper binding site on amyloid beta1–42. J Neurochem 2000;75(3): 1219–33.

Bartzokis G. Age-related myelin breakdown: a developmental model of cognitive decline and Alzheimer's disease. Neurobiol Aging 2004;25(1):5–18.

Bellingham SA, Lahiri DK, Maloney B, La Fontaine S, Multhaup G, Camakaris J. Copper depletion down-regulates expression of the Alzheimer's disease amyloid-beta precursor protein gene. J Biol Chem 2004;279:20378–86.

Bush AI, Pettingell WH, Multhaup G, Paradis M, Vonsattel JP, Gusella JF, et al. Rapid induction of Alzheimer A beta amyloid formation by zinc. Science 1994;265(5177):1464–7.

Bush AI. Copper, zinc, and the metallobiology of Alzheimer disease. Alzheimer Dis Assoc Disord 2003;17(3):147–50.

Butterfield DA, Boyd-Kimball D. Amyloid beta-peptide(1–42) contributes to the oxidative stress and neurodegeneration found in Alzheimer disease brain. Brain Pathol 2004;14(4):426–32.

Cherny RA, Atwood CS, Xilinas ME, Gray DN, Jones WD, McLean CA, et al. Treatment with a copper–zinc chelator markedly and rapidly inhibits beta-amyloid accumulation in Alzheimer's disease transgenic mice. Neuron 2001;30(3):665–76.

Danks DM. Copper deficiency in humans. Annu Rev Nutr 1988;8:235–57.

Eckert GP, Wood WG, Muller WE. Membrane disordering effects of beta-amyloid peptides. Subcell Biochem 2005;38:319–37.

Evans DA, Funkenstein HH, Albert MS, Scherr PA, Cook NR, Chown MJ, et al. Prevalence of Alzheimer's disease in a community population of older persons. Higher than previously reported. JAMA 1989;262 (18):2551–6.

Evans DA, Bennett DA, Wilson RS, Bienias JL, Morris MC, Scherr PA, et al. Incidence of Alzheimer's disease in a biracial urban community: relation to apolipoprotein E allele status. Arch Neurol 2003;60:185–9.

Engelhart MJ, Geerlings MI, Ruitenberg A, van Swieten JC, Hoffmann A, Witteman JC, et al. Diet and risk of dementia: Does fat matter? Neurology 2002;59:1915–21.

Fassbender K, Simons M, Bergmann C, Stroick M, Lutjohann D, Keller P, et al. Simvastatin strongly reduces levels of Alzheimer's disease beta-amyloid peptides Abeta 42 and Abeta 40 in vitro and in vivo. Proceedings of the National Academy of Sciences of the United States of America 2001;98(10):5856–61.

Folstein MF, Folstein SE, McHugh PR. "Mini-mental state". A practical method for grading the cognitive state of patients for the clinician. J Psych Res 1975;12(3):189–98.

Friedlich AL, Lee JY, van Groen T, Cherny RA, Volitakis I, Cole TB, et al. Neuronal zinc exchange with the blood vessel wall promotes cerebral amyloid angiopathy in an animal model of Alzheimer's disease. J Neurosci 2004;24(13):3453–9.

Greenwood CE, Winocur G. Cognitive impairment in rats fed high-fat diets: a specific effect of saturated fatty-acid intake. Behavioral Neuroscience 1996;110 (3):451–9.

Hebert LE, Beckett LA, Scherr PA, Evans DA. Annual incidence of Alzheimer disease in the United States projected to the years 2000 through 2050. Alzheimer Disease & Associated Disorders 2001;15 (4):169–73.

Hesse L, Beher D, Masters CL, Multhaup G. The beta A4 amyloid precursor protein binding to copper. FEBS Lett 1994;349(1):109–16.

Huang X, Cuajungco MP, Atwood CS, Hartshorn MA, Tyndall JD, Hanson GR, et al. Cu(II) potentiation of alzheimer abeta neurotoxicity. Correlation with cell-free hydrogen peroxide production and metal reduction. J Biol Chem 1999;274(52):37111–6.

Huang X, Moir RD, Tanzi RE, Bush AI, Rogers JT. Redox-active metals, oxidative stress, and Alzheimer's disease pathology. Ann N Y Acad Sci 2004; 1012:153–63.

Jick H, Zornberg GL, Jick SS, Seshadri S, Drachman DA. Statins and the risk of dementia. Lancet 2000;356 (9242):1627–31.

Kagan BL, Hirakura Y, Azimov R, Azimova R, Lin MC. The channel hypothesis of Alzheimer's disease: current status. Peptides 2002;23(7):1311–5.

Kalmijn S, Launer LJ, Ott A, Witteman JC, Hofman A, Breteler MM. Dietary fat intake and the risk of incident dementia in the Rotterdam Study. Annals of Neurology 1997;42(5):776–82.

Kivipelto M, Helkala EL, Laakso MP, Hanninen T, Hallikainen M, Alhainen K, et al. Apolipoprotein E epsilon4 allele, elevated midlife total cholesterol level, and high midlife systolic blood pressure are independent risk factors for late-life Alzheimer disease. Ann Intern Med 2002;137(3):149–55.

Kontush A, Mann U, Arlt S, Ujeyl A, Luhrs C, Muller-Thomsen T, et al. Influence of vitamin E and C supplementation on lipoprotein oxidation in patients with Alzheimer's disease. Free Radical Biology & Medicine 2001;31(3):345–54.

Laird N, Ware J. Random-effects models for longitudinal data. Biometrics 1982;38:963–974.

Laitinen MH, Ngandu T, Rovio S, Helkala EL, Uusitalo U, Viitanen M, et al. Fat intake at midlife and risk of dementia and Alzheimer's disease: a population-based study 6. Dement Geriatr Cogn Disord 2006;22(1):99–107.

Lee JY, Kim JH, Hong SH, Lee JY, Cherny RA, Bush AI, et al. Estrogen decreases zinc transporter 3 expression and synaptic vesicle zinc levels in mouse brain. J Biol Chem 2004;279(10):8602–7.

Luchsinger JA, Min-Xing T, Shea S, Mayeux R. Caloric intake and the risk of Alzheimer disease. Arch Neurol 2002;59:1258–63.

Maynard CJ, Cappai R, Volitakis I, Cherny RA, White AR, Beyreuther K, et al. Overexpression of Alzheimer's disease amyloid-beta opposes the age-dependent elevations of brain copper and iron. J Biol Chem 2002;277(47):44670–6.

Mori T, Paris D, Town T, Rojiani AM, Sparks DL, Delledonne A, et al. Cholesterol accumulates in senile plaques of Alzheimer disease patients and in transgenic APP(SW) mice. J Neuropathol Exp Neurol 2001;60(8):778–85.

Morris MC, Evans DA, Bienias JL, Tangney CC, Bennett DA, Aggarwal N, et al. Dietary fats and the risk of incident Alzheimer's disease. Arch Neurol 2003;60:194–200.

Morris MC, Evans DA, Bienias JL, Tangney CC, Wilson RS. Dietary fat intake and 6-year cognitive change in an older biracial community population. Neurology 2004;62:1573–9.

Morris MC, Evans DA, Tangney CC, Bienias JL, Schneider JA, Wilson RS, et al. Dietary copper and high saturated and trans fat intakes associated with cognitive decline. Arch Neurol 2006;63 (8):1085–8.

Notkola IL, Sulkava R, Pekkanen J, Erkinjuntti T, Ehnholm C, Kivinen P, et al. Serum total cholesterol, apolipoprotein E epsilon 4 allele, and Alzheimer's disease. Neuroepidemiology 1998;17(1):14–20.

Opazo C, Huang X, Cherny RA, Moir RD, Roher AE, White AR, et al. Metalloenzyme-like activity of Alzheimer's disease beta-amyloid. Cu-dependent catalytic conversion of dopamine, cholesterol, and biological reducing agents to neurotoxic H_2O_2. J Biol Chem 2002;277(43):40302–8.

Pollitt E. Developmental sequel from early nutritional deficiencies: conclusive and probability judgements. J Nutr 2000;130(2S Suppl):350S–3S.

Puglielli L, Tanzi R, Kovacs D. Alzheimer's disease: the cholesterol connection. Nature Neurosci 2003;6:345–51.

Puglielli L, Friedlich AL, Setchell KD, Nagano S, Opazo C, Cherny RA, et al. Alzheimer disease beta-amyloid activity mimics cholesterol oxidase. J Clin Invest 2005;115(9):2556–63.

Refolo LM, Malester B, LaFrancois J, Bryant-Thomas T, Wang R, Tint GS, et al. Hypercholesterolemia accelerates the Alzheimer's amyloid pathology in a transgenic mouse model. Neurobiol Dis 2000;7 (4):321–31.

Smith A. Symbol Digit Modalities Test Manual—Revised. Los Angeles, CA: Western Psychological. 1984.

Smith DP, Smith DG, Curtain CC, Boas JF, Pilbrow JR, Ciccotosto GD, et al. Copper-mediated amyloid-beta toxicity is associated with an intermolecular histidine bridge. J Biol Chem 2006; 281 (22):15145.

Sparks DL, Scheff SW, Hunsaker JC3, Liu H, Landers T, Gross DR. Induction of Alzheimer-like beta-amyloid immunoreactivity in the brains of rabbits with dietary cholesterol. Experimental Neurology 1994;126(1):88–94.

Sparks DL, Schreurs BG. Trace amounts of copper in water induce beta-amyloid plaques and learning deficits in a rabbit model of Alzheimer's disease. Proc Natl Acad Sci U S A 2003;100(19):11065–9.

Sparks DL, Friedland R, Petanceska S, Schreurs BG, Shi J, Perry G, et al. Trace copper levels in the drinking water, but not zinc or aluminum influence CNS Alzheimer-like pathology. J Nutr Health Aging 2006;10(4):247–54.

Wolozin B, Kellman W, Ruosseau P, Celesia GG, Siegel G. Decreased prevalence of Alzheimer disease associated with 3-hydroxy-3-methyglutaryl coenzyme A reductase inhibitors. Arch Neurol 2000;57(10):1439–43.

Zou K, Gong JS, Yanagisawa K, Michikawa M. A novel function of monomeric amyloid beta-protein serving as an antioxidant molecule against metal-induced oxidative damage. J Neurosci 2002;22 (12):4833–41.

An invited introduction presented in the symposium "Health effects of low dose exposure to toxic metals".

Health effects of low dose exposure to toxic metals: introduction and research recommendations

Gunnar Nordberg[1] and Staffan Skerfving[2]
[1]Umea University, Umea, Sweden; [2]Lund University, Lund, Sweden

Background

"Declaration of Brescia"

At the ICOH Congress in Milan, 2006, the President suggested that Scientific Committees develop policy documents with recommendations based on evaluations of existing scientific evidence. The Scientific Committee on the Toxicology of Metals (SCTM) and the Scientific Committee on Neurotoxicology prepared such a document at a symposium on Neurotoxic Metals, Brescia, Italy, June 2006 and published as the "Declaration of Brescia on Prevention of the Neurotoxicity of Metals" (Landrigan et al. Am J Ind Med 50, 709–11, 2007). In the document, items were specified as required to reduce existing adverse effects caused by toxic metals in human population groups and to prevent the occurrence of such effects in the future:

–Intensified attention must be paid to early warnings of neurotoxicity.

–All uses of lead, including recycling, should be reviewed.

–Tetraalkyl lead must be eliminated without delay from gasoline supplies of all nations.

–Current exposure standards for lead need urgently to be reduced.

–Exposures of pregnant women and women of reproductive age to methylmercury need to be reduced.

–Exposures of pregnant women and young children to manganese need to be reduced to prevent subclinical neurotoxicity.

–The addition of organic manganese compounds to gasoline should be halted immediately.

–Exposure standards for manganese need to be reconsidered.

–Economic impacts of the neurotoxicity caused by metals must be considered.

–The need is great for continuing research into the neurotoxicity of metals and such research should include studies on delayed consequences of developmental toxicity; prospective and retrospective cohort studies; neurotoxicity of other metals, e.g. arsenic, aluminium and interactions; genetic and other susceptibility factors; determinants of the rearing environment including exposure to metals; the impact of global warming on exposure to neurotoxic metals, e.g. mercury.

Recent studies employing sensitive biomarkers have indicated that adverse effects on human health occurs at very low exposures to toxic metals such as cadmium. Effects may occur even at "background" exposures. These effects may be due to a combination of factors (e.g. genetic) in addition to the actual metal exposure.

Aims

The present symposium displayed and discussed recent findings in this field, as a basis for recommendations about future research, employing modern technologies (proteomics, metabolomics and genomics) of investigation.

Presentations and research recommendations

During the symposium, presentations were given by Drs. Fowler (read by G. Nordberg), Barregard, Lucchini, Akesson and Jin. The following research needs related to neurotoxicity (in addition to those identified in the "Declaration of Brescia") were identified:

–Interactions between manganese, lead, copper and zinc for the development of Parkinson's disease should be further studied.

–Interactions should be studied of the neurotoxicity of metals and persistent organic pollutants such as polychlorinated biphenyls (PCB) and dioxins.

–Neurotoxic effects of elemental mercury vapor released from amalgam tooth fillings should be further studied.

The present symposium was not limited to adverse effects of metals on the nervous system, and included also such effects on kidneys and other organs. There is convincing evidence, from this symposium, as well as from data in the scientific literature, that human exposure to cadmium and mercury may give rise to adverse effects on the kidneys, even at relatively low-level exposures. There is also evidence that lead may give rise to such effects. It is indicated by the evidence presented, that adverse kidney effects may occur in sensitive subgroups of the general population, even at background exposures to cadmium and mercury.

Further studies on cadmium and mercury are needed in population groups in different countries on the occurrence of kidney dysfunction among persons with diabetes and/or autoantibodies against metallothionein. Dose–response relationships for each sensitive population subgroup and the possible reversibility after decreases in exposure should be delineated. The precise mechanistic and genetic background determining the development of antibodies against MT and subsequent increased sensitivity to metal toxicity should be identified.

The relationship between exposure to toxic metals, particularly cadmium, and the occurrence of low bone density and fractures should be further studied and the influence of dose, as well as possible reversibility subsequent to decreased exposures, delineated. Exposures to arsenic, copper, chromium, indium, tin, uranium and vanadium may give rise to adverse kidney effects, but present knowledge is limited. Well-designed experimental and epidemiological studies should be performed to further our understanding of when and how these metals may act as nephrotoxicants.

Acknowledgements

This symposium was organized by the Scientific Committee on the Toxicology of Metals (SCTM) of the International Commission on Occupational Health (ICOH), in collaboration with the Nordic Trace Element Society (NTES) and the International Society of Trace Element Research in Humans (ISTERH). The SCTM, ICOH Chair is Prof. Monica Nordberg (Karolinska Institutet, Stockholm, Sweden) and the Secretary is Prof. Ole Andersen (Roskilde University Center, Roskilde, Denmark). Gunnar Nordberg and Staffan Skerfving, as members of SCTM, ICOH, wrote the summary of the symposium based on discussions at the symposium and during a meeting of the SCTM the day after the Symposium.

This symposium was sponsored by FORMAS (FOrskningsRadet for Miljo, Areella naringar och Samhallsbyggande), NTES, and ICOH.

An invited paper presented in the symposium "Health effects of low dose exposure to toxic metals".

Proteomic and metabolomic biomarkers for assessing low dose toxic trace element interactions: an overview

Bruce A. Fowler[1], E. A. Conner[2], H. Yamauchi[3], G. Wang[4], M. H. Whittaker[5]
[1]Division of Toxicology and Environmental Medicine, ATSDR, Atlanta, GA, USA; [2]NCI, Bethesda, MD USA; [3]Kitasato University, Kanagawa, Japan; [4]Anderson Cancer Center, Houston, TX, USA; [5]ToxServices, Washington, DC, USA

Corresponding Author:
Email: bxf9@cdc.gov

Introduction

Humans are exposed to a number of toxic and essential trace elements from air, food, and water (Nordberg et al. 2007a) and there are major risk-assessment issues concerning to what extent these metallic mixture exposures produce toxic or beneficial public health outcomes. During recent decades, there has been growing interest in the development of sensitive, specific and rapid biological tests (biomarkers) capable of providing objective quantifiable data regarding cellular responses to low-dose trace element exposures either alone or as mixtures (Fowler 2005). In more recent years, the "omic" biomarkers (genomic, proteomic, and metabolomic) have been a major focus of biomarker development. This brief overview will focus on how metabolomic and proteomic biomarkers have provided useful quantifiable data of great value for interpreting the biological consequences of single or combined exposures to lead, cadmium, arsenic and the binary III–V semiconductors gallium arsenide and indium arsenide. Biomarker data will be correlated where possible with other quantitative morphological data and clinical outcomes. It is worth noting

that "omic" biomarkers will undoubtedly become of even greater importance for trace element risk-assessment purposes since all of the metals/metalloids, as well as others, are being utilized in the production of nanomaterials which will increase the probability of human exposures.

Metabolomic biomarkers and trace element exposures. The heme biosynthetic pathway

The heme biosynthetic pathway is essential for life and has a number of catalytic steps which are differentially sensitive to toxic trace elements. Specific disturbances in this pathway from low-dose exposures to lead (Fowler et al. 1980; Oskarsson and Fowler 1985; NAS/NRC 1993), methyl mercury (Woods and Fowler 1977), arsenic (Wood and Fowler 1978) or mixtures of lead, cadmium, and arsenic (Mahaffey et al. 1981), gallium arsenide (Goering et al. 1988) or indium arsenide (Conner et al. 1993, Fowler et al. 2005) have been shown to produce element or mixture-specific porphyrinuria patterns. A number of these exposures were also correlated with histological or ultrastructural morphometric findings in major target organ systems (Fowler et al. 1975; Fowler et al. 1979; Fowler and Woods 1979, Fowler et al. 1980; Fowler et al. 1983) thus providing supplemental data of value for interpretation of porphyrinuria patterns. These biomarker endpoints have proven useful for evaluating lead, cadmium, and arsenic interactions at even the lowest observed effect level (LOEL) dose levels (Fowler et al. 2004; Wang and Fowler 2008).

Proteinuria Patterns

Most of the major toxic trace elements are accumulated in the kidney where they may disrupt essential protein handling pathways leading to the production of element specific or characteristic proteinuria patterns. Excellent examples of these responses have been reported for cadmium (Nordberg et al. 2007b) and the III–V semiconductors gallium arsenide and indium arsenide (Fowler et al. 2005). It is likely that other specific proteinuria patterns exist for toxic trace elements alone or in combination and these may be resolved by increasingly sensitive and specific analytical methodologies.

Proteomic Biomarkers and Trace Element Exposures

Target cell proteomic responses following exposure to metals/ metalloids may occur as up and/or down regulation of a number of gene products (proteins). The constellation of changes in these protein expression patterns may be used to characterize exposures to trace elements on an individual (Aoki et al. 1990) or mixture basis (Conner et al. 1993; Fowler. 2005). The linkage of these changes in protein expression patterns to other biomarkers of cell injury such as metallic mixture-specific proteinuria patterns (Fowler et al. 2005) provides useful interpretive information regarding the potential clinical significance of the observed alterations in protein expression patterns in target cell populations such as renal tubule cells. Another advantage of proteomic analyses is the ability to delineate differences in proteomic responsiveness between genders (Fowler et al. 2008) as well as potentially sensitive subpopulations at special risk for toxicity. As with other classes of biomarkers, validation by correlations with other cellular, physiological or pathology endpoints is now a major focus of activity for investigators working in the area.

Summary and Conclusions

In conclusion, metabolomic and proteomic biomarkers show great promise for delineating early cellular responses following exposures to trace elements on an individual or mixture basis. The future value of these tests for improving risk assessments for exposures to toxic metals/metalloids alone or as mixture combinations now rests validation studies to provide ancillary data so that these classes of biomarkers may be correctly interpreted as biomarkers of exposure, biomarkers of response or harbingers of major long-term health effects such as chronic organ system disease or cancer. This information will be of particular importance for chronic low-dose metallic mixture situations.

References

Aoki Y, Lipsky MM, Fowler BA. Alteration of protein synthesis in primary cultures of rat kidney epithelial cells by exposure to gallium indium and arsenite. Toxicol Appl Pharmacol 1990; 106:462–8.

Conner EA, Yamauchi H, Fowler BA, Akkerman M. Biological indicators for monitoring exposure/ toxicity from III–V semiconductors. J Exposure Analysis and Environ Epidemiol 1993;3:431–40.

Conner EA, Yamauchi H, Fowler BA. Alterations in the heme biosynthetic pathway from III–V semiconductor metal indium arsenide (InAs). Chem Biol Interact 1995; 96:273–85.

Fowler BA. Molecular biomarkers: challenges and prospects for the future. Toxicol Appl Pharmacol 2005; 206(2):97.

Fowler BA, Brown HW, Lucier GW, Krigman MR. The effects of chronic oral methyl mercury exposure on the lysosome system of rat kidney morphometric and biochemical studies. Lab Invest 1975; 32:313–22.

Fowler BA, Conner EA, Yamauchi H. Metabolomic and proteomic biomarkers for III–V semiconductors: Chemical-specific porphyrinurias and proteinurias. Toxicol Appl Pharmacol 2005; 206(2):121–30.

Fowler BA, Conner EA, Yamauchi H. Proteomic and metabolomic biomarkers for III–V semiconductors: prospects for applications to nano-materials. Toxicol. Appl. Pharmacol. 2008; doi: 10.1016/j.taap.2008.01.014), in press.

Fowler BA, Kardish R, Woods JS. Alteration of hepatic microsomal structure and function by acute indium administration: Ultrastructural morphometric and biochemical studies. Lab Invest 1983; 48:471–8.

Fowler BA, Kimmel CA, Woods JS, McConnell EE, Grant LD. Chronic low level lead toxicity in the rat III. An integrated toxicological assessment with special reference to the kidney. Toxicol Appl Pharmacol 1980; 56:59–77.

Fowler BA, Whittaker MH, Lipsky M, Wang G, Chen XQ. Oxidative stress induced by lead, cadmium and arsenic mixtures: 30-day, 90-day, and 180-day drinking water studies in rats: an overview. Biometals 2004; 17(5): 567–8.

Fowler BA, Woods JS. The effects of prolonged oral arsenate exposure on liver mitochondria of mice: Morphometric and biochemical studies. Toxicol Appl Pharmacol 1079;50:177–87.

Fowler BA, Woods JS, Schiller CM. Studies of hepatic mitochondrial structure and function: morphometric and biochemical evaluation of in vivo perturbation by arsenate. Lab Invest 1979;41:313–20.

Goering PL, Maronpot RR, Fowler BA. Effect of intratracheal administration of gallium arsenide administration on δ-aminolevulinic acid dehydratase in rats: relationship to urinary excretion of aminolevu-linic acid. Toxicol Appl Pharmacol 1988;92:179–93.

Mahaffey KR, Capar SG, Gladen BC, Fowler BA. Concurrent exposure to lead cadmium and arsenic: effects on toxicity and tissue metal concentrations in the rat. J Lab Clin Med 1981; 98:463–81.

NAS/NRC: Report of the Committee on Measuring Lead Exposure in Infants, Children and Other Sensitive Populations. Washington, D.C., NAS/NRC, 1993, pp 337.

Nordberg GF, Gerhardsson L, Broberg K, Mumtaz M, Fowler BA. Interactions in metal toxicology. In: Nordberg GF, Fowler BA, Nordberg M, Friberg L. eds. Handbook of Toxicology of Metals, 3rd Edition. Elsevier, Amsterdam, 2007a. pp. 117–46.

Nordberg GF, Nogawa K, Nordberg M, Friberg L. Cadmium, In: Nordberg, GF, Fowler, BA, Nordberg, M, Friberg, L eds. Handbook on the Toxicology of Metals 3rd Edition, Elsevier, Amsterdam, 2007b. pp 445–86.

Oskarsson A, Fowler BA. Effects of lead on the heme biosynthetic pathway in rat kidney. Exper Molec Pathol 1985; 43:397–408.

Wang G, Fowler BA. Roles of biomarkers in evaluating interactions among mixtures of lead, cadmium and arsenic, toxicology and applied pharmacology (2008), doi: 10.1016/j.taap.2008.01.017, in press.

Woods JS, Fowler BA. Renal porphyrinuria during chronic methyl mercury exposure. J Lab Clin Med 1977;90:266–72.

Woods JS, Fowler BA. Altered regulation of mammalian hepatic heme biosynthesis and urinary porphyrin excretion during prolonged exposure to sodium arsenate. Toxicol Appl Pharmacol 1978; 43:361–71.

An invited paper presented in the symposium "Health effects of low dose exposure to toxic metals".

Neuropsychological and renal effects of low dose exposure to elemental mercury exposure from amalgam in children

Lars Barregard
Department of Occupational and Environmental Medicine, Sahlgrenska University Hospital and University of Gothenburg, Sweden

Corresponding Author:
lars.barregard@amm.gu.se

Introduction

Dental amalgam constitutes the most common source of exposure to elemental mercury in the general population and the possible health risks have been debated for a long time (WHO 2003; Clarkson and Magos 2006). Many studies have been performed in adults exposed to low levels of elemental mercury, but until recently few data were available on this topic in children, who might be more vulnerable.

In 2006, two large NIH-funded randomized controlled trials were published, comparing neuropsychological and renal outcomes between children treated with dental amalgam or composites over a 5-year trial period (Bellinger et al. 2006; DeRouen et al. 2006).

Neuropsychological effects: the children's amalgam trial studies

The NECAT study, performed in the North East USA, involved 534 children, 6 to 10 years of age, with no prior or existing amalgam restorations, but two or more occlusal dental caries lesions, recruited over a 2-year period in Boston and rural Maine (Bellinger et al. 2006). Baseline visits included a dental examination, blood and urine samples, anthropometric measurements, health interviews, and neuropsychological testing of the child. Exclusion criteria were clinical evidence of existing psychological, behavioral, neurologic, immunosuppressive, or renal disorders. These children were randomized to a study treatment group. Sample sizes were based on the requirement of an adequate power to detect a three-point difference between treatment groups in full scale IQ score.

A dispersed phase amalgam or a resin composite material (white filling) was used to restore all posterior teeth with caries at baseline and incident caries during the 5-year trial period, according to treatment group. Children in both groups had semi-annual dental examinations. At the annual visits, neuropsychological testing and anthropometric measurements were performed, and a urine sample collected. At baseline, also hair mercury levels and blood lead were measured, since methyl mercury and lead could affect neuropsychological performance and kidney function.

The number of dental restorations was highest early in the trial due to unmet treatment needs. The children had on average approximately one new surface filled per year, while decidual teeth (some with fillings) were shed. In year 5, the children had 0–36 surfaces filled, with a median of four surfaces (three amalgam) in the amalgam group and five in the composite group.

The key measure of mercury burden was mercury in urine, corrected for creatinine (U–Hg in microgram per gram creatinine; microgram per gramC). The U–Hg levels were only moderately increased in the children treated with dental amalgam (to about 0.9 μg/gC vs. 0.6 μg/gC in the composite group in year 5).

There were no significant differences in neuropsychological outcomes between treatment groups (Bellinger et al. 2006). In the primary outcome (WISC-III IQ score) there was a mean change (increase) of 3.1 IQ points in the amalgam group vs. 2.2 in the composite group. Further analyses of dose–response relations failed to show any associations with number of amalgam fillings or urinary Hg excretion (Bellinger et al. 2007).

Interestingly enough, the NECAT study was, however, powerful enough to detect highly significant negative associations between blood lead and IQ, as well as several other neuropsychological tests, also below blood lead of 100 μg/L (Surkan et al. 2007). This indicates that the NECAT study had a design, power, and confounder control good enough to detect also subtle effects.

The other large trial, the Casa Pia CAT study was similar in its design, although the urinary Hg levels of these Portuguese children were a little higher than in the US children (Woods et al. 2007). This trial, too, failed to demonstrate any statistically significant differences in neurobehavioral outcomes between treatment groups (DeRouen et al. 2006).

Renal effects: the Children's Amalgam Trial studies

In the NECAT study, there was no difference in mean albumin excretion between treatment groups, nor where there any associations with amalgam or U–Hg for the renal tubular markers γ-glutamyl transferase (γ-GT), alpha-1-microglobulin (A1M) or *N*-acetyl-glucose-aminidase (NAG) (Barregard et al. 2008).

However, the prevalence of urinary albumin >30 mg/g creatinine (microalbuminuria; MA) in year 3 or year 5 was higher in the amalgam group than in the composite group (repeated measures logistic regression, odds ratio=1.8; *P*=0.03). There were 48

occasions of MA in 38 children in the amalgam group at the 3-year and/or 5-year visits vs. 33 occasions in 31 children in the composite group. Ten children in the amalgam group had MA on both visits, but only two in the composite group (*P*=0.04).

There was no significant interaction between treatment group and gender (*P*=0.27), but the OR for MA was significantly increased only in boys. There was no significant increase in MA with increasing numbers of amalgam fillings or urinary mercury excretion. However, when an interaction term B-Pb×U-Hg was included in the model with urinary mercury as predictor, it was a statistically significant predictor of MA in year 5 (*P*=0.02) and nearly so in year 3–5 (*P*=0.07).

The Casa Pia CAT showed no difference between treatment groups in terms of albumin excretion, nor in excretion of urinary glutathione transferases (De Rouen et al. 2006).

Renal effects: a European cross-sectional study

In a large cross-sectional study, blood and urinary samples from more than 800 children in France, the Czech Republic, and Poland were examined. Concentrations of lead and cadmium in blood, and cadmium and mercury in urine, were determined as well as several markers of kidney function: Cystatin C in serum, and Clara cell protein, NAG, and retinol-binding protein in urine (de Burbure et al. 2006). Unexpectedly, there was a statistically significant positive association between the excretion of NAG and urinary mercury, although U-Hg levels were low, 0.1–1.0 μg/gC in the respective countries. This association was, however, only found in models including cadmium (in blood or urine) included, and the results indicated several complex metal interactions with respect to renal markers.

Discussion and conclusions

Regarding neuropsychological outcomes, the results from the CAT trials are reassuring regarding low-level mercury exposure from dental amalgam on a population scale. They do not, however, exclude effects in a small fraction of children, either due to variability in exposure (Barregard et al. 1995), or because some children may be especially sensitive to low doses of mercury (Needleman 2006). A differential sensitivity has been shown at high-dose mercury exposure, which may cause acrodynia (pink disease), not all children being affected (Counter and Buchanan 2004). It is unknown whether such differences occur also with respect to effects on the central nervous system at low-level exposure.

The European cross-sectional study indicated a possible effect of low-level mercury exposure on renal tubular biomarkers. This could not be reproduced in the randomized controlled NECAT study, but the latter study did not take into account cadmium or selenium status, factors which may influence the renal tubular toxicity of mercury (de Burbure et al. 2006; Ellingsen et al. 2000). The NECAT study unexpectedly found an association between microalbuminuria and dental amalgam. High exposure to inorganic mercury increases the prevalence of albuminuria in adults (Buchet et al. 1980), and in some cases causes clinical glomerulonephritis (Tubbs et al. 1982; Oliveira et al. 1987). Animal models indicate that the mechanisms behind mercury-induced autoimmunity are complex, and genetic factors, especially MHC genes, may be important (Enestrom and Hultman 1995; Nielsen and Hultman 2002; Pollard et al. 2005). In view of previous knowledge, our finding of microalbuminuria in children treated with dental amalgam may therefore represent a causal association. However, chance is clearly an alternative explanation for a higher occurrence of MA in the present study. A study specifically focussed on the possible association between dental amalgam and MA in children would be desirable, e.g., a case-referent or case cross-over studies in surroundings where substantial fractions of children have and have not had dental amalgam fillings.

References

Barregard L, Sällsten G, Järvholm B. People with high mercury uptake from their own dental amalgam fillings. Occup Environ Med. 1995;52:124–8.

Barregard L, Trachtenberg F, McKinlay S. Renal effects of dental amalgam in children: the New England Children's amalgam trial. Environ Health Perspect. 2008;116:394-9.

Bellinger D, Trachtenberg F, Barregard L, et al. Neuropsychological and renal effects of dental amal-gam in children. A randomized clinical trial. JAMA 2006;295:1775–83.

Bellinger DC, Trachtenberg F, Daniel D, et al. A dose–effect analysis of children's exposure to dental amalgam and neuropsychological function: the New England Children's Amalgam Trial. J Am Dent Assoc. 2007;138:1210–6.

Buchet JP, Roels H, Bernard A, Lauwerys R. Assessment of renal function of workers exposed to inorganic lead, cadmium or mercury vapour. J Occup Med. 1980;22:741–50.

Clarkson TW, Magos L. The toxicology of mercury and its chemical compounds. Crit Rev Toxicol. 2006;36:609–62.

Counter SA, Buchanan LH. Mercury exposure in children: a review. Toxicol Appl Pharmacol. 2004;198:209–30.

de Burbure C, Buchet J-P, Leroyer A, et al. Renal and neurologic effects of cadmium, lead, mercury, and arsenic in children: evidence of early effects and multiple interactions at environmental exposure levels. Environ Health Perspect. 2006;114:584–90.

DeRouen TA, Martin MA, Leroux BG, et al. Neurobehavioral effects of dental amalgam in children: a randomized clinical trial. JAMA. 2006; 295:1784–92.

Ellingsen DG, Efskind J, Berg KJ, et al. Renal and immunologic markers for chloralkali workers with low exposure to mercury vapor. Scand J Work Environ Health. 2000;26:427–35.

Enestrom S, Hultman P. Does amalgam affect the immune system? A controversial issue. Int Arch Allergy Immunol. 1995;106:180–203.

Needleman HL. Mercury in dental amalgam—a neurotoxic risk? JAMA 2006;295:1835–6.

Nielsen JB, Hultman P. Mercury-induced autoimmunity in mice. Environ Health Perspect. 2002;110 (suppl 5):877–81.

Oliveira DBG, Foster G, Savill J, et al. Membraneous nephropathy caused by mercury-containing skin lightening cream. Postgrad Med. 1987;63:303–4.

Pollard KM, Hultman P, Kono DH. Immunology and genetics of induced systemic autoimmunity. Autoimmunity reviews. 2005;4:282–8.

Surkan PJ, Zhang A, Trachtenberg F, et al. Neuropsychological function in children with blood lead levels <10 μg/dL. Neurotoxicology. 2007; 28:1170–7.

Tubbs RR, Gephardt GN, McMahon JT, et al. Membranous glomerulonephritis associated with industrial mercury exposure: Study of pathogenetic mechanisms. Am J Clin Pathol. 1982;77:409–13.

Woods JS, Martin MA, Leroux BG, et al. The contribution of dental amalgam to urinary mercury excretion in children. Environ Health Perspect. 2007;115:1527–31.

World Health Organization (WHO). Concise International Chemical Assessment Document 50. Elemental mercury and inorganic mercury compounds: human health aspects. Geneva, WHO, 2003.

An invited paper presented in the symposium "Health effects of low dose exposure to toxic metals".

Manganese exposure as a determinant of Parkinsonian damage

Roberto Lucchini[1], Rosanna Squitti[2], Elisa Albini[1], Laura Benedetti[1], Stefano Borghesi[1], Eleonora Nan[1], et al.

[1]Department of Applied and Experimental Medicine, Section of Occupational Health, University of Brescia, Italy; [2]AFaR, Department of Neuroscience, Hospital Fatebenefratelli, Rome, Italy

Corresponding Author:
Email address: lucchini@med.unibs.it

Introduction

Manganese (Mn) is an essential element for humans and animals and plays an important role in bone mineralization, protein and energy metabolism, metabolic regulation, cellular protection from damaging free radical species, and the formation of glycosaminoglycans (Roth and Garrick 2003). Homeostatic mechanisms regulate the absorption and excretion rates in order to keep manganese concentration within a strict range. Nevertheless, exposure to high doses determines a manganese overload in the central nervous system, given the slow elimination rate from this organ based on passive diffusion mechanism (Yokel 2006). In cases of overload, manganese accumulates in the globus pallidus of the basal ganglia where it causes cellular damage on the GABAergic (Gwiazda et al. 2007) and dopaminergic pathways. As a consequence, motor function and coordination of fine movements are affected, and mood regulation as well with marked aggressivity. Human exposure to air concentration higher then 1 mg/m^3 (WHO 1981) can determine the clinical picture of manganism, an atypical Parkinsonism that shows clinical differences from the typical features of Parkinson's Disease (Cersosimo and Koller 2006).

Parkinsonism after lifetime exposure to Mn

After prolonged exposure at much lower levels, manganese may act as an environmental trigger and favour the onset of Parkinsonian disturbances (Martin 2006). This can be determined by a damage of the dopaminergic neurons of the substantia nigra—pars compacta, which is located very closely to the globus pallidus and shares various interconnections within the basal ganglia (Weiss 2006). This hypothesis is based on epidemiological studies showing a higher frequency of Parkinsonian disease among Mn-exposed welders vs. age-standardized individuals in the general population (Racette et al. 2001; 2005a). Moreover, positron emission tomography (PET) has shown that the clinical features of Mn-induced Parkinsonism can overlap with those of Idiopathic Parkinson's Disease (IPD), characterized by prolonged L-dopa responsiveness and reduced [^{18}F] fluorodopa uptake (Racette et al. 2005b).

A recent epidemiological study investigated the risk of Parkinsonian disorders in the population of Toronto and Hamilton, Ontario, in relationship with industrial emissions of Mn and the use of methylcyclopentadienyl manganese tricarbonyl (MMT) as fuel additive. Results have pointed out that in Hamilton, the odds ratio for a physician's diagnosis was 1.034 (1.00–1.07) per 0.01 μg/m^3 increase in Mn in total suspended particles. Mn levels in Hamilton ranged from 0.050 to 0.092 μg/m^3 (Finkelstein and Jerrett 2007). This study is consistent with the theory that exposure to Mn may add to the natural loss of neurons attributable to the aging process.

Similar results were observed in Italy among the residents in the vicinities of ferroalloy plants located in Valcamonica, a valley in the pre-Alps located in the province of Brescia. Mn concentrations in settled dust were significantly higher in the surroundings and downwind from the industrial plants and airborne concentration in the city of Brescia averaged those reported in the Canadian study. Significantly higher SMRs (Kruskal–Wallis chi^2 1 df=17.55, P<0.001) were observed in 37 municipalities in the vicinities of ferromanganese plants (age- and sex-standardized prevalence 492/100,000), compared to the other 169 municipalities of the province (standardized prevalence 321/100,000). Row and Bayesian SMRs were associated with the concentrations of manganese in settled dust (Lucchini et al. 2007a).

Phenotype of Mn-related Parkinsonism

In a further cross sectional assessment, Parkinsonian patients, residents of Valcamonica were examined individually and compared with patients residents of the city of Brescia, and with age- and sex-matched healthy individuals. The protocol included information on clinical, occupational, residential history and life habits, neuro-psychological testing, and assessment of genetic polymorphism. A total number of 65 patients and 52 healthy controls residents in Valcamonica, and 28 patients and 14 controls from Brescia were examined. The age at onset was significantly lower among women (60.93±1.26) compared to men (65.96±1.77), independently from the residential area. After adjusting for age and sex, Parkinsonian patients from Valcamonica showed a more severe impairment of several neuropsychological tests exploring cognitive and motor functions. The Unified Parkinson's Disease Rating Scale (UPDRS) showed a significant contribution of the residential area in the model, with higher impairment of motor functions among the cases from Valcamonica. Parkinsonian patients from Valcamonica showed also lower cognitive performance at the Mini Mental State Examination (MMSE) and Token test. The prevalence of familiarity for Parkinsonian disturbances was more frequent among cases from Brescia, and the allelic distribution of gene DRD4 resulted significantly different between cases and controls in the area of Brescia (MonteCarlo test p=0.041-T1; p=0.012-T2) and not between cases and controls residents in Valcamonica (Lucchini et al. 2007b).

Low levels of occupational or environmental exposures, or clinical condition known to determine Mn overload, like chronic liver failure and total parenteral nutrition, can cause frontal and subcortical cognitive impairment (Klos et al. 2006; Bouchard et al. 2007; Bowler et al. 2007). An association between environmental exposure to Mn and deficits in measures of intellectual functioning has been described in children from France (Takser et al. 2003), Bangladesh (Wasserman et al. 2006) and the USA (Wright et al. 2006). Non-human primates have shown also subtle deficits in cognitive function, in addition to impaired fine motor control, after chronic exposure to Mn (Schneider et al. 2006). Therefore, differently from the classical features of manganism, caused by exposure to high levels of Mn, lifetime exposure to lower levels seems to determine a clinical picture that overlaps IPD but is characterized by more pronounced cognitive dysfunction.

Role of copper in Mn-related Parkinsonism

Biological levels of metals were assessed in the Mn-exposed area of Valcamonica, Italy. Parkinsonian patients resident in the exposed area showed significantly higher serum levels of Cu, Cu/Zn and AST/ALT ratios (p<0.0001) and lower serum Zn (p<0.0001) compared to Parkinsonian patients resident in other areas and to healthy controls from the same area. Within the Parkinsonian patients, Cu (rho=0.3, p<0.05), Cu/Zn ratio (rho=0.3, p<0.05), AST/ALT ratio (rho=0.4, p<0.05) and duration of illness (rho=0.5, p<0.05) correlated with UDPRS scores and Cu levels strongly correlated with peroxide levels (rho=0.7, p<0.01) in serum (Squitti et al. 2007).

Concentrations of Mn, copper, zinc and iron were measured also in the brain tissues of Mn-exposed non-human primates and control animals. Manganese and copper levels resulted significantly higher in Mn-exposed animals compared to controls both in the basal ganglia (Guilarte et al. 2006) and in frontal cortex tissues (Guilarte et al. 2008), whereas no changes were observed for zinc and iron. Immuno-histochemistry revealed also the presence of diffuse amyloid-β plaques in the frontal cortex of Mn exposed animals.

A recent study has also shown that saliva concentrations of Mn and Cu were significantly higher in welders compared to age and sex-matched controls and this variation was associated with airborne Mn levels. Saliva levels of Zn were significantly lower in the welders. Significant associations were observed between saliva and serum for Mn (r=0.575, p<0.05) and Cu (r=0.50, p<0.05; Wang et al. 2008).

In previous studies, Li et al. (2004) reported the same association between increased serum Mn, Cu and Fe and decreased serum Zn among welders. These Mn-induced changes of Cu and Zn corresponded to lipid peroxidative damage (Lu et al. 2005).

Taken all together, these observations point out the importance of Cu and Zn in Mn-induced toxicity. These metals are both important in cellular redox reactions, therefore, a dysregulation of their homeostasis may potentiate the cellular damage resulting from reactive oxygen species. Mn may induce changes in copper homeostasis also through liver damage. An increase in brain copper concentrations induced by Mn exposure may contribute to the neurodegenerative changes and formation of amyloid-β plaques as copper has been implicated in AD pathology (Bush 2003).

Conclusion

Chronic and lifetime exposure to low levels of Mn can increase the frequency of Parkinsonian disturbances. These do not reproduce the classical feature of clinical manganism that is caused by much higher exposure in shorter periods of time. In addition to extrapyramidal changes, Mn-induced parkinsonism is characterized by cognitive impairment. A dysregulation of copper and zinc homeostasis and a consequent oxidative-stress mechanism may ultimately contribute to Mn-induced neurotoxicity. The use of MMT in gasoline may increase environmental exposure to this metal on a world scale (Walsh 2007), with a possible increase of Parkinsonian disturbances in the population. This represents a new potential concern that must be addressed adequately by the scientific and public health community and the regulatory bodies at the international level.

References

Bouchard M, Mergler D, Baldwin M, Panisset M, Bowler R, Roels H. Neurobehavioral functioning after cessation of manganese exposure: a follow-up after 14 years. Am J Ind Med. 2007;50(11):831–40.

Bowler RM, Roels HA, Nakagawa S, Drezgic M, Diamond E, Park R, Koller W, Bowler RP, Mergler D, Bouchard M, Smith D, Gwiazda R, Doty RL. Dose–effect relationships between manganese exposure and neurological, neuropsychological and pulmonary function in confined space bridge welders. Occup Environ Med. 2007;64(3):167–77.

Bush AI. The metallobiology of Alzheimer's disease. Trends Neurosci. 2003; 26: 207–14.

Cersosimo MG, Koller WC. The diagnosis of manganese-induced parkinsonism. Neurotoxicology. 2006;27(3):340–6.

Finkelstein MM, Jerrett M. A study of the relationships between Parkinson's disease and markers of traffic-derived and environmental manganese air pollution in two Canadian cities. Environ Res. 2007;104:420–32.

Gwiazda R, Lucchini R, Smith D. adequacy and consistency of animal studies to evaluate the neurotoxicity of chronic low level manganese exposure in humans. J Toxicol Environ Health Part A. 2007; 70:594–605.

Guilarte TR, Chen MK, McGlothan JL, Verina T, Wong DF, Zhou Y, Alexander M, Rohde CA, Syversen T, Decamp E, Koser AJ, Fritz S, Gonczi H, Anderson DW, Schneider JS. Nigrostriatal dopamine system dysfunction and subtle motor deficits in manganese-exposed non-human primates. Exp Neurol 2006;202:381–90.

Guilarte TR, Burton NC, Verina T, Prabhu VV, Becker KG, Syversen T, Schneider JS. Increased APLP1 expression and neurodegeneration in the frontal cortex of manganese-exposed non-human primates. Journal of Neurochemistry. 2008;105(5):1948-59.

Klos KJ, Chandler M, Kumar N, Ahlskog JE, Josephs KA. Neuropsychological profiles of manganese neurotoxicity. Eur J Neurol. 2006;13(10):1139–41.

Li GJ, Zhang L, Lu L, Wu P, Zheng W. Occupational exposure to welding fume among welders: alterations of manganese, iron, zinc, copper, and lead in body fluids and the oxidative stress status. J. Occup. Environ. Med. 2004;46:241–8.

Lu L, Zhang LL, Li GJ, Guo W, Liang W, Zheng W. Serum concentrations of manganese and iron as the potential biomarkers for manganese exposure in welders. NeuroToxicology. 2005;26:257–65.

Lucchini R, Albini E, Benedetti L, Borghesi S, Coccaglio R, Malara E, Parrinello G, Garattini S, Resola S, Alessio L. High Prevalence of parkinsonian disorders associated to manganese exposure in the vicinities of ferroalloy industries. Am J Ind Med. 2007a;50(11):788–800.

Lucchini R, Albini E, Benedetti L, Zoni S, Caruso A, Nan E, Pasqualetti P, Rossigni PM, Binetti G, Benussi

L, Parrinello G, Gasparotti R, Padovani A, Draicchio F, Alessio L. Neurological and neuropsychological features in parkinsonian patients exposed to neurotoxic metals. G Ital Med Lav Ergon. 2007b;29(3):280–1.

Martin CJ. Manganese neurotoxicity: connecting the dots along the continuum of dysfunction. Neurotoxicology. 2006;27(3):347–9.

Racette BA, McGee-Minnich L, Moerlein SM, Mink JW, Videen TO, Perlmutter JS. Welding-related parkinsonism: clinical features, treatment, and pathophysiology. Neurology. 2001;56:8–13.

Racette, BA, Tabbal SD, Jennings D, Good L, Perlmutter JS, Evanoff B. Prevalence of Parkinsonism and relationship to exposure in a large sample of Alabama welders. Neurology. 2005a;64:230–5.

Racette BA, Antenor JA, McGee-Minnich L, Moerlein SM, Videen TO, Kotagal V, Perlmutter JS. [^{18}F]FDOPA PET and clinical features in Parkinsonism due to manganism. Mov Disord. 2005b;20:492–6.

Roth JA, Garrick MD. Iron interactions and other biological reactions mediating the physiological and toxic actions of manganese. Biochem Pharm. 2003;66:1–13.

Schneider JS, Decamp E, Koser AJ, Fritz S, Gonczi H, Syversen T, Guilarte TR. Effects of chronic manganese exposure on cognitive and motor functioning in non-human primates. Brain Res. 2006;1118 (1):222–31.

Squitti R, Gorgone G, Binetti G, Ghidoni R, Pasqualetti P, Draicchio F, Albini E, Benedetti L, Lucchini R, and Rossigni PM. [Metals and oxidative stress in Parkinson's Disease from industrial areas with exposure to environmental toxins or metal pollution]. G Ital Med Lav Ergon. 2007;29(3):294–6.

Takser L, Mergler D, Hellier G, Sahuquillo J, Huel G. Manganese, monoamine metabolite levels at birth, and child psychomotor development. Neurotoxicology 2003;24:667–74.

Yokel RA. Blood–brain barrier flux of aluminum, manganese, iron and other metals suspected to contribute to metal-induced neurodegeneration. J Alzheimers Dis. 2006;10:223–53.

Walsh MP. The global experience with lead in gasoline and the lessons we should apply to the use of MMT. Am J Ind Med. 2007;50(11):853–60.

Wang D, Du X, Zheng W. Alteration of saliva and serum concentrations of manganese, copper, zinc, cadmium and lead among career welders. Toxicol Lett. 2008;176:40–7.

Wasserman GA, Liu X, Parvez F, Ahsan H, Levy D, Factor-Litvak P, Kline J, van Geen A, Slavkovich V, LoIacono NJ, Cheng Z, Zheng Y, Graziano JH. Water manganese exposure and children's intellectual function in Araihazar, Bangladesh. Environ Health Perspect. 2006;114:124–9.

Weiss B. Economic implications of manganese neurotoxicity. Neurotoxicology. 2006;27(3):362–8.

WHO. Environmental Health Criteria 17. Manganese. World Health Organization, Geneva. 1981.

Wright RO, Amarasiriwardena C, Woolf AD, Jim R, Bellinger DC. Neuropsychological correlates of hair arsenic, manganese, and cadmium levels in school-age children residing near a hazardous waste site. Neurotoxicology. 2006;27(2):210–6.

An invited paper presented in the symposium "Health effects of low dose exposure to toxic metals".

Kidney and bone effects of low dose cadmium exposure in Sweden

Agneta Åkesson
Institute of Environmental Medicine, Karolinska Institutet, Stockholm, Sweden

Corresponding author
Institute of Environmental Medicine
Karolinska Institutet
Box 210
171 77 Stockholm, Sweden
Phone: +46-8-52487542
Fax: +46-8-304571

Cadmium is a toxic environmental pollutant (Järup et al. 1998; McMurray and Tainer 2003; Safe 2003) that we are exposed to via food and tobacco smoking. High concentrations of cadmium can be found in foods such as liver, kidneys, shellfish and mollusks and some seeds. The metal has been widely dispersed into the environment and contaminated agricultural soil even in industrially non-polluted areas. A high accumulation in agricultural crops results in the fact that plant foods generally contribute to more than 80% of the total cadmium intake (Olsson et al. 2002). The major contributors to the dietary cadmium intake are, thus, foods considered healthy such as cereals especially whole grains, vegetables and potatoes and roots.

In contrast to most other environmental pollutants, women have a higher body burden than men. This sex-difference is reflected as higher concentrations of cadmium in blood, urine and kidney cortex (Vahter et al. 2007). The main reason for the higher body burden in women is an increased intestinal absorption of dietary cadmium at low body iron stores. The duodenal metal transporter (DMT1) which is responsible for the uptake of iron into the mucosa cell and up-regulated by iron deficiency, has also a high affinity for cadmium (Gunshin et al. 1997; Tallkvist et al. 2001). Thus, at low iron stores, which are common in women at fertile age, especially during pregnancy (Berglund et al. 1994; Åkesson et al. 2002), the absorption of cadmium will be increased.

Cadmium exposure is monitored either in blood or urine. Despite a high correlation between these two parameters, cadmium in blood mainly reflects recent exposure. However, at long-term low-level exposure, blood cadmium also mirrors the body retention (Järup et al. 1998). Urinary cadmium, on the other hand, is considered to primarily reflect the accumulation of cadmium in the kidney cortex (Orlowski et al. 1998). Because the half-life of cadmium in the body is very long, in the order of 10–30 years, both measures of exposure are highly age-dependent. The age-related increase in blood and urinary cadmium is less evident, disappears or may even turns to a decrease at the age range of 50 to 70 years and older.

High cadmium exposure is well-known to cause kidney and bone damage (Järup et al. 1998). One of the first signs of the renal lesion is a tubular damage, characterized by increased excretion of low-molecular weight proteins (e.g. β_2-microglobulin, protein HC or retinol-binding protein) and tubular enzymes (e.g. *N*-acetyl-β-D-glucosaminidase; NAG). This increased excretion is caused by decreased tubular reabsorption of low-molecular weight proteins and by increased cell turnover in the tubuli. There is a general agreement that cadmium-induced tubular damage may occur at lower levels than previously anticipated. It has been suggested that the critical exposure of cadmium defined as 10 μg/g creatinine in urine, used by the WHO to estimate the provisional tolerable weekly intake of cadmium, is far too high. Thus, there is a need to define the critical exposure level in the general population, especially at long-term low-level exposure.

Within a population-based women's health survey in Southern Sweden (WHILA; 71% response rate; Åkesson t al. 2005; Åkesson et al. 2006), we investigated cadmium associated health effects among 820 women, aged 53 to 64 years. The area has no known historical cadmium contamination. Specifically, we assessed the associations between cadmium exposure and tubular and glomerular function, forearm bone mineral density and markers of bone metabolism. We also calculated the benchmark dose for kidney effects. Associations between exposure and effect markers were evaluated using multiple linear regression analysis including data on possible confounders and effect modifiers. The exposure levels were generally low; the median urinary cadmium concentration was 0.52 μg/L adjusted to the mean urinary density (1.015 g/mL), corresponding to approximately 0.67 μg cadmium/g creatinine ~ nanomole per millimole creatinine and blood cadmium was 0.38 μg/L (3.4 nmol cadmium/L).

Our results showed associations corresponding to negative effects of low-level cadmium exposure on tubuli, glumeruli and bone (Table 1). Cadmium seemed to potentiate diabetes-induced effects on kidney (Åkesson et al. 2005) as well as postmenopausal bone resorption (Åkesson et al. 2006).

It has been argued that the association between urinary cadmium and tubular effect markers may be the results of a parallel phenomenon and not an effect by cadmium. According to this argument, kidney deterioration, independent of cadmium, may result in increased excretion of both cadmium and the tubular effect markers. Although cross-sectional studies preclude conclusion to be drawn with respect to causality, several findings from this study support a causal relationship and also rules out that the associations merely are results of a parallel phenomenon. First, both blood and urinary cadmium were associated with the kidney effect markers (Table 1). Unless an extremely strong association is present between cadmium in blood and in urine, there is no reason to believe that blood cadmium can reflect tubular dysfunction. This implies that cumulative cadmium exposure—and not dysfunction related cadmium excretion—is associated with the tubular effects. As the associations between cadmium in urine and kidney effect markers were present also among those who reported to be never-smokers, it is also highly unlikely that the association were attributed solely to an effect by smoking. Second, cadmium in both blood and urine were also associated with decreasing glomerular function (estimated GFR; Table 1). The glomerular function was estimated via determination of serum cystatin C which is considered a very valid indirect marker of GFR. Because cystatin C is measured in serum, this measurement is not dependent on any excretion in urine. In addition, as cadmium in blood is mainly found in blood cells and in plasma Cd is bound to the small protein metallothionein, easily filtered through the glomerulus, a reverse causality, meaning that a low GFR increases the accumulation of cadmium in blood, can be ruled out.

Clear associations were also demonstrated between cadmium and bone. Cadmium body burden, on one hand, was associated with decreasing bone mineral density, increasing bone resorption (urinary excretion of deoxypyridinoline; U-DPD) and decreasing parathyroid hormone (PTH), on the other. There were, however, no associations between cadmium and markers of bone formation and excretion of calcium in urine. Because the skeleton contains only minor amount of cadmium (Petersson Grawe et al. 2000), it is unlikely that an increased bone turnover would release significant amounts of cadmium to the circulation. A direct effect of cadmium on bone, independent of the cadmium-induced kidney damage, is a more likely explanation. PTH is the main regulator of calcium metabolism and increased bone resorption would lead to a compensatory decrease in PTH, which is inline with the observed results. The fact that we observed no association between cadmium and bone formation, may reflect a cadmium-induced uncoupling between bone resorption and formation. Also for bone effects, the associations persisted among never-smokers with lower exposure, although smoking is an established risk factor for osteoporosis.

We estimated the concentration of urinary cadmium below which the probability of adverse health effects is low, using the benchmark dose (BMD) method (Suwazono et al. 2006). The BMD is the exposure that corresponds to a certain predefined increase in response compared to the background. We modified the method so that both the exposure and effects markers were kept as continuous variables. Because the changes occurring in this study are not at the level signifying clinical disease, dichotomization of the outcome is best avoided. Nevertheless, dichotomizing is often carried out, and the cutoff of the concentration of the effect markers is generally the 95th percentile in the study population or in a reference population. In the case of cadmium, when all people are "exposed", differences in exposure affect the level of the "cutoff", as will the choice of reference population. The chosen cutoff-value will then strongly affect the level of the estimated critical concentration. By using the hybrid approach, the concept of risk can be used for a continuous outcome without dichotomization, which gives a higher statistical validity and efficiency. The "cutoff" for adverse response was, thus, defined as the 95th percentile in the population under study, obtained by the model at "zero" cadmium exposure. By using this approach, the impact of the exposure in a reference group and problems related to compromised comparability between the study population and a reference group can be minimized.

For both the tubular effect markers, the BMDs at 5 to 10% additional risk and the corresponding 95% lower confidence bounds (BMDLs) of urinary cadmium ranged between 0.6 and 1.1 (0.5–0.8) μg/g creatinine (14). For estimated GFR, the BMDs (BMDLs) were 1.1–1.8 (0.7–1.2) μg cadmium/g creatinine. The obtained benchmark doses of urinary cadmium were substantially lower than the critical concentrations previously reported. Furthermore, the critical dose level for glomerular effects was only slightly higher than that for tubular effects.

Acknowledgement

Staffan Skerfving, Marie Vahter, Jonas Lidfelt, Thomas Lundh, Per Bjellerup, Yasushi, Suwazono, Salomon Sand, Agneta Falk-Filipsson, Ulf Strömberg, Göran Samsioe are acknowledged for all their important contributions. This study was supported by grants from The Swedish Research Council/Medicine.

References

Åkesson A, Berglund M, Schutz A, Bjellerup P, Bremme K, Vahter M. Cadmium exposure in pregnancy and lactation in relation to iron status. Am J Public Health. 2002;92(2):284–7.

Åkesson A, Lundh T, Vahter M, et al. Tubular and glomerular kidney effects in Swedish women with low environmental cadmium exposure. Environ Health Perspect. 2005;113(11):1627–31.

Åkesson A, Bjellerup P, Lundh T, et al. Cadmium-induced effects on bone in a population-based study of women. Environ Health Perspect. 2006;114(6):830–4.

Berglund M, Akesson A, Nermell B, Vahter M. Intestinal absorption of dietary cadmium in women depends on body iron stores and fiber intake. Environ Health Perspect. 1994;102(12):1058–66.

Gunshin H, Mackenzie B, Berger UV, et al. Cloning and characterization of a mammalian proton-coupled metal-ion transporter. Nature. 1997; 388 (6641):482–8.

Jarup L, Berglund M, Elinder CG, Nordberg G, Vahter M. Health effects of cadmium exposure—a review of the literature and a risk estimate. Scand J Work Environ Health. 1998;24 Suppl 1:1–51.

McMurray CT, Tainer JA. Cancer, cadmium and genome integrity. Nat Genet. 2003;34(3):239–41.

Olsson IM, Bensryd I, Lundh T, Ottosson H, Skerfving S, Oskarsson A. Cadmium in blood and urine—impact of sex, age, dietary intake, iron status, and former smoking—association of renal effects. Environ Health Perspect. 2002;110(12): 1185–90.

Orlowski C, Piotrowski JK, Subdys JK, Gross A. Urinary cadmium as indicator of renal cadmium in humans: an autopsy study. Hum Exp Toxicol. 1998; 17(6):302–6.

Petersson Grawe K, Oskarsson A. Cadmium in milk and mammary gland in rats and mice. Arch Toxicol. 2000;73(10–11):519–27.

Safe S. Cadmium's disguise dupes the estrogen receptor. Nat Med. 2003;9(8):1000–1.

Suwazono Y, Sand S, Vahter M, et al. Benchmark dose for cadmium-induced renal effects in humans. Environ Health Perspect. 2006;114(7):1072–6.

Tallkvist J, Bowlus CL, Lonnerdal B. DMT1 gene expression and cadmium absorption in human absorptive enterocytes. Toxicol Lett. 2001;122(2):171–7.

Vahter M, Akesson A, Liden C, Ceccatelli S, Berglund M. Gender differences in the disposition and toxicity of metals. Environ Res. 2007;104(1):85–95.

Table 1 The direction of the statistically significant multivariate-adjusted linear associations observed between cadmium exposure and markers of kidney and bone effects in women from a population-based study in Southern Sweden. Presented for all subjects and for urinary cadmium also for never-smokers (Åkesson et al. 2005, 2006)

	Cadmium exposure		
	Urine		Blood
	All	Never-smokers	All
Kidney			
Tubular effect markers			
U-NAG	Pos	Pos	Pos
U-HC	Pos	Pos	Pos
Glomerular effect marker			
Estimated GFR	Neg		Neg
Bone			
Bone mineral density	Neg	Neg	
Markers of bone remodeling			
PTH	Neg	Neg	Neg
Osteocalcin			
bALP			
U-DPD	Pos	Pos	
Urinary calcium			

Pos Significant positive associations, *Neg*, significant negative associations, *bALP* bone-specific alkaline phosphatase, *U-DPD* urinary deoxypyridinoline, *U-NAG* urinary N-acetyl-β-D-glucosaminidase

An invited paper presented in the symposium "Health effects of low dose exposure to toxic metals".

Factors influencing dose–response relationships of cadmium in humans—diabetes, metallothionein and metallothionein antibodies

Taiyi Jin[1,2,*] Liang Chen[1], Lijian Lei[1], Monica Nordberg[3], Gunnar F. Nordberg[2]
[1]Department of Occupational Health, School of Public Health, Fudan University, Shanghai, 200032, China; [2]Environmental Medicine; Department of Public Health and Clinical Medicine, Umeå University, S-90187 Umeå, Sweden; [3]Institute of Environmental Medicine, Karolinska Institutet, S-171 77, Stockholm, Sweden

*Corresponding Author:
E-mail: tyjin@shmu.edu.cn

Diabetes and cadmium nephrotoxicity

Currently, the susceptibility to toxic hazards in high risk population is of increasing concern. Diabetes mellitus is one condition in such high-risk groups which can be suspected of increasing the susceptibility to toxic hazards (Orth 2002). In diabetes, kidney disease is one of the dreaded complications. Diabetic renal damage is the leading cause of chronic kidney disease in patients starting renal replacement therapy (Hostetter 2001). A recent study in Swedish women also indicated that subjects with diabetes seem to be at an increased risk of renal damage, mainly tubular dysfunction (Åkesson, et al. 2005). Several experimental studies have shown increased susceptibility to cadmium nephrotoxicity (Jin et al. 1994; Jin and Frankel 1996a) in spontaneously diabetic mice and hamsters, when compared to normal animals of the same strain. Streptozotocin (STZ)-induced diabetic rats, subchronically exposed to cadmium chloride in drinking water, are more susceptible to cadmium nephrotoxicity than normal rats (Jin et al. 1999).

Metallothionein, antibody and cadmium nephrotoxicity

Metallothioneins (MTs) are a family of stress proteins containing a high content of cysteine and divalent metals. Several physiological roles have been proposed for MT, including detoxification of toxic metals, such as cadmium (Cd), and homeostasis of essential metals, such as zinc (Zn) and copper (Cu). MT is also a potent antioxidant, interacting with various reactive oxidative species (ROS) more efficiently than other antioxidants (Jin et al. 1998; Nordberg 1998; Nordberg and Nordberg 2000, Sato and Kondoh 2002). Elevated expression of MT in pancreatic beta cells has been shown to protect from STZ-induced beta cell damage and diabetes (Ohly et al. 2000; Yang and Cherian 1994; Chen et al. 2001). MT is significantly increased in the liver and kidney of diabetic animals (Cai et al. 2002; Jin et al. 1996b). The increased MT in the kidney may prevent cadmium nephrotoxicity in STZ induced diabetes in rats (Jin et al. 1996b). It has been reported that metallothionein antibody (MT-Ab) is present in the circulation of healthy subjects and in patients suffering from atopic dermatitis (Jin et al. 2003). The relationship between MT-Ab and renal dysfunction has firstly been studied within a cadmium exposed population in China (Chen et al.

2006a). It showed that the workers having high levels of MT-Ab display cadmium-induced tubular nephrotoxicity more frequently than those possessing low levels of MT-Ab, which suggests that subjects having higher MT-Ab levels more readily develop cadmium-induced renal dysfunction (Chen et al. 2006a). The relationship between MT-Ab and diabetic nephropathy, however, has yet to be studied. The aim of this study was to investigate the potential effect of MT-Ab on the renal dysfunction within a Chinese diabetic population. The levels of plasma MT-Ab, urinary cadmium (UCd) were measured and relationships between the levels of MT-Ab and UCd and renal dysfunction were explored.

Cadmium nephrotoxicity in a Chinese diabetic population

The major sources of cadmium exposure in the general population are cereals, vegetables, and shellfish. In this diabetic population, we found that UCd correlated with tubular biomarker UB2M. This result is in agreement with other studies in general populations (Åkesson et al. 2005; Buchet et al. 1990). However, we did not find any significant relationship between cadmium biomarkers and UALB in this study, although it is reported that cadmium can exacerbate glomerular damage in diabetes as well (Åkesson et al. 2005). It is noted that the UCd levels (average 0.38 µg/g Cr in all subjects), which is the main biomarker for cadmium body burden during chronic exposure, were relative lower compared with UCd (average 0.67 µg/g Cr in all subjects) in the study by Åkesson, et al. 2005. In another study with a low UCd level in studied subjects (0.26 nmol/mmol Cr≈ 0.26 µg/g Cr), there was no positive relationship between UCd and glomerular biomarkers (Olsson et al. 2002). It seems that the UCd level is not high enough to potentate glomerular dysfunction in this study. Despite the relative low UCd level in the present study, there still was a clear effect on tubular dysfunction. Those subjects with UCd ≥1 µg/g Cr are at 3.26 times higher risk to develop hyperB2Muria compared to those patients with UCd value below 1 µg/g Cr.

Numerous studies have confirmed the increased renal risk in smokers with type 1 and type 2 diabetes mellitus. Smoking can increase the risk to develop microalbuminuria and accelerates the rate of progression from microalbuminuria to manifest proteinuria (Orth 2002). In the present study, we have not found such an effect on UALB, but we found smoking could increase the risk to develop hyperB2Muria, and the OR is 1.84. Cigarettes smoking are significant way of cadmium exposure in generally population. In this study, the BCd levels (1.00 μg/L [range: 0.13–3.50]) in smokers statistically higher than that in previous smoker (0.50 μg/L [range: 0.03–1.41]) and never-smokers (0.51 μg/L [0.06–1.91]). In current smokers, MT-Ab showed good correlation with UB2M ($r=0.6$). It suggested that smoking had an interacted effect with MT-Ab on tubular function. During this study, only a few percent of the effects of smoking could be explained by cadmium because smoking had an independent effect on hyperUB2Mruia in the logistic regression. In fact, except increasing cadmium burden, the kidney injury effect of smoking could be indirect results of some other mechanisms, such as oxidative stress (Orth 2002, Righetti 2001). These mechanisms may play a role in smoking-related renal injury in this study.

Metallothionein, metallothionein antibody and cadmium nephrotoxicity in a Chinese diabetic population

Over the past several years, the concern has been raised that other factors such as oxidation and inflammatory factor play an essential role in the progress of diabetic complications, including renal damage (Yaqoob et al. 1994; Morcos et al. 2002, Rosen, et al. 2001). Metallothionein is a kind of multifunctional stress protein, and it also has a potent effect of scavenging free radicals because of its high thiol content (Sato and Kondoh 2002); the rate constant of MT for reaction with hydroxyl radical is 100-fold higher than that of glutathione. MT also could be easily induced by some chemicals that stimulate the production of reactive oxygen species (ROS; Bauman et al. 1991). It is reasonable to speculate that MT-Ab may interfere with such effect of metallothionein. This might be an alternative mechanism for its effect on diabetic tubular damage. However, we cannot rule out some other possibility. Additional mechanisms, such as secondary effect of MT-Ab on other tissues involved, might play a role, also.

In this study, MT-Ab showed positive correlation exclusively with UB2M, which is an important biomarker of tubular damage. Nevertheless, no statistically significant relationship between MT-Ab and ALB, one of the predominant biomarker of glomerular dysfunction, was found in this study. It

indicated that MT-Ab mainly interacted with tubular function in this diabetic population. This result was in accordance with our previous study within a cadmium-exposed population (Chen et al. 2006a). In that study, we found no significant correlations between the levels of MT-Ab and the cadmium exposure doses of cadmium, but the levels of MT-Ab did correlate positively with two biomarkers of renal tubular dysfunction—UB2M and *N*-acetyl-beta-D-glucosaminidase (UNAG), while UALB kept silent. We hypothesized that the interaction between circulating antibodies and glomeruli might be one reason for cadmium-induced nephrotoxicity, and if that is the case, MT-Ab should show positive relationship not only with tubular lesion but also glomerular damage (Chen et al. 2006a). However, we have not found any positive relationship between MT-Ab and UALB in this present study with a larger sample size. Thus, the discrepancies of MT-Ab on renal function implied that renal tubules might be one of the important target tissues of MT-Ab.

As the antibody against metallothionein, MT-Ab should interact with metallothionein. In the human body, metallothioneins are mainly stored in liver tissue and renal cortex, in general population and cadmium-exposed population. It is not strange that MT-Ab could enact its function at the place with higher concentrations of metallothionein, although relationship between MT-Ab and hepatic function has not been fully studied yet. Most of the evidence available at present indicates that the toxicity of cadmium to the kidneys is related to the balance between the levels of toxic "free" non-MT-bound Cd and CdMT in renal cells (Jin et al. 1998; Nordberg and Nordberg 2000). Even now, the definite mechanisms of MT-Ab on renal tubular dysfunction are still unclear. In our previous study, we hypothesize that the MT-Ab may interfere with the detoxification by MT in the renal tubular cells exposed to cadmium, in an occupational population (Chen et al. 2006b). It is reported that metallothionein immunization (induced MT-Ab) can impede the mercuric-chloride-induced increase of MT expression in the liver and lead to increases in the level of mercury in both the serum and liver while decreasing the level found in the kidneys (Jin et al. 2002a). MT is a low-molecular-weight protein, having a molecular weight of 6,600, which is even smaller than that of B2M (11,800). Urinary MT can be used as a sensitive biomarker of cadmium-induced tubular damage (Chen et al. 2006b). In this study, we found UMT increased significantly in the subjects with tubular dysfunction (hyperB2M) compared with those without renal dysfunction (non-hyperALBuria and non-hyperB2Muria). Relative to the group hyperALBuria(+) plus hyperB2M(−), UB2M and MT-Ab increased statistically in the group hyperALBuria(−) plus hyperB2M(+). As a biomarker of tubular toxicity, however, UMT did not show significant increase, even though it has been proved to be a sensitive urinary indicator within an occupational population. In those patients with only hyperB2Muria, UB2M was 3.7-fold higher than that in the subjects with only hyperALBuria, whereas UMT was only 0.5 times increased. We know that the elevation of urinary MT excretion is partly as a result of decreased reabsorption of low-molecular-weight proteins and partly because of a leakage of MT from tubular cells when renal tubular dysfunction occurs (Chen et al. 2006b). It is implied that urinary MT can partly reflect the change of MT within tubular cells. In this case, we thought inhibition of MT synthesis within tubular cells might be one reason for the effect of MT-Ab on renal dysfunction in this study of diabetics.

It is noted that MT-Ab also showed higher prevalence in some diabetic-related disease such as hyperlipidemia, coronary heart disease, and fat liver in male or female patients, although they are not statistically significant in this study. In addition, those subjects with paralysis showed higher MT-Ab levels compared with those without. It is suggested that MT-Ab should have an impact on other tissues and organs, except the kidney, to some extent. Further studies untangling the mechanism behind this intriguing side effect of MT-Ab may provide further clues as to the relationship between MT-Ab, cadmium toxicity, and diabetes that could have broader implications for our understanding of the pathogenesis of diabetic renal damage.

Acknowledgements

This study was funded by the National Key Basic Research and Development Program (No. 2002CB512905), the National Natural Science Foundation of China.

References

Akesson A, Lundh T, Vahter M, Bjellerup P, Lidfeldt J, Nerbrand C, Samsioe G, Stromberg U, Skerfving S. Tubular and glomerular kidney effects in Swedish women with low environmental cadmium exposure. Environ Health Perspect. 2005 Nov;113 (11):1627–31.

Bauman JW, Liu J, Liu YP, Klaassen CD. Increase in metallothionein produced by chemicals that induce oxidative stress. Toxicol Appl Pharmacol. 1991 Sep 1;110(2):347–54.

Buchet JP, Lauwerys R, Roels H, Bernard A, Bruaux P, Claeys F, Ducoffre G, de Plaen P, Staessen J, Amery A, et al. 1990. Renal effects of cadmium body burden of the general population. Lancet. 336 (8717), 699–702.

Cai L, Chen S, Evans T, Cherian MG, Chakrabarti S. Endothelin-1-mediated alteration of metallothionein and trace metals in the liver and kidneys of chronically diabetic rats. Int J Exp Diabetes Res. 2002 Jul–Sep;3(3):193–8.

Chen H, Carlson EC, Pellet L, Moritz JT, Epstein PN. Overexpression of metallothionein in pancreatic beta-cells reduces streptozotocin-induced DNA damage and diabetes. Diabetes. 2001 Sep;50(9):2040–6.

Chen, L, Jin, T, Huang, B, Chang X, Lei L, Nordberg, GF, Nordberg M, 2006a. Plasma metallothionein antibody and cadmium-induced renal dysfunction in an occupational population in China. Toxicol. Sci. 91(11)104–12.

Chen L, Jin T, Huang B, Nordberg G, Nordberg M. 2006b. Critical exposure level of cadmium for elevated urinary metallothionein—an occupational population study in China. Toxicology and Applied Pharmacology. 215:93–9.

Hostetter TH. Prevention of end-stage renal disease due to type 2 diabetes. N Engl J Med. 2001 Sep 20;345(12):910–2.

Jin GB, Inoue S, Urano T, Cho S, Ouchi Y, and Cyong JC. (2002a). Induction of anti-metallothionein antibody and mercury treatment decreases bone mineral density in mice. Toxicol. Appl. Pharmacol. 185, 98–110.

Jin GB, Nakayama H, Shmyhlo M, Inoue S, Kondo M, Ikezawa Z, Ouchi Y, Cyong JC. (2003). High positive frequency of antibodies to metallothionein and heat shock protein 70 in sera of patients with metal allergy. Clin. Exp. Immunol. 131, 275–9.

Jin T, Nordberg GF, Sehlin J, Leffler P, Wu J. The susceptibility of spontaneously diabetic mice to cadmium–metallothionein nephrotoxicity. Toxicology. 1994 Apr 18;89(2):81–90.

Jin T, Nordberg G, Sehlin J, Vesterberg O. Protection against cadmium–metallothionein nephrotoxicity in streptozotocin-induced diabetic rats: role of increased metallothionein synthesis induced by streptozotocin. Toxicology. 1996a Jan 8;106(1–3):55–63.

Jin T, Frankel BJ. Cadmium–metallothionein nephrotoxicity is increased in genetically diabetic as compared with normal Chinese hamsters. Pharmacol Toxicol. 1996 b Sep;79(3):105–8.

Jin T, Lu J, Nordberg M. (1998). Toxicokinetics and biochemistry of cadmium with special emphasis on the role of metallothionein. Neurotoxicology 19, 529–35.

Jin T, Nordberg G, Sehlin J, Wallin H, Sandberg S. The susceptibility to nephrotoxicity of streptozotocin-induced diabetic rats subchronically exposed to cadmium chloride in drinking water. Toxicology. 1999 Dec 20;142(1):69–75.

Morcos M, Sayed AA, Bierhaus A, Yard B, Waldherr R, Merz W, Kloeting I, Schleicher E, Mentz S, Abd el Baki RF, Tritschler H, Kasper M, Schwenger V, Hamann A, Dugi KA, Schmidt AM, Stern D, Ziegler R, Haering HU, Andrassy M, van der Woude F, Nawroth PP. Activation of tubular epithelial cells in diabetic nephropathy. Diabetes. 2002 Dec;51 (12):3532–44.

Nordberg M. (1998). Metallothioneins: historical review and state of knowledge. Talanta 46, 243–54.

Nordberg M, Nordberg GF. (2000). Toxicological aspects of metallothionein. Cell Mol Biol 46, 451–63.

Ohly P, Dohle C, Abel J, Seissler J, Gleichmann H. Zinc sulphate induces metallothionein in pancreatic islets of mice and protects against diabetes induced by multiple low doses of streptozotocin. Diabetologia. 2000 Aug;43(8):1020–30.

Olsson IM, Bensryd I, Lundh T, Ottosson H, Skerfving S, Oskarsson A. Cadmium in blood and urine—impact of sex, age, dietary intake, iron status, and former smoking—association of renal effects. Environ Health Perspect. 2002 Dec;110 (12):1185–90.

Orth SR. Smoking and the kidney. J Am Soc Nephrol. 2002 Jun;13(6):1663–72.

Righetti M, Sessa A. Cigarette smoking and kidney involvement. J Nephrol. 2001 Jan–Feb;14(1):3–6.

Rosen P, Nawroth PP, King G, Moller W, Tritschler HJ, Packer L. The role of oxidative stress in the onset and progression of diabetes and its complications: a summary of a Congress Series sponsored by UNESCO-MCBN, the American Diabetes Association and the German Diabetes Society. Diabetes Metab Res Rev. 2001 May–Jun;17(3):189–212.

Sato M, Kondoh M. Recent studies on metallothionein: protection against toxicity of heavy metals and oxygen free radicals. Tohoku J Exp Med. 2002 Jan;196(1):9–22.

Yang J, Cherian MG. Protective effects of metallothionein on streptozotocin-induced diabetes in rats. Life Sci. 1994;55(1):43–51.

Yaqoob M, McClelland P, Patrick AW, Stevenson A, Mason H, White MC, Bell GM. Evidence of oxidant injury and tubular damage in early diabetic nephropathy. QJM. 1994 Oct;87(10):601–7.

An invited paper presented in the symposium "Environmental stress and mineral homeostasis".

Overview of human physiological responses to environmental extremes

Andrew J. Young
Military Nutrition Division
USARIEM
Natick, MA 01760, USA

Corresponding Author:
Andrew.j.young@us.army.mil

INTRODUCTION

Millions of people live, work, and play in regions of the world where the weather is intemperate, or at terrestrial elevations where the ambient oxygen pressure is less than at sea level. Exposure to extreme environments can elicit physiological responses in humans, which assist the body in re-establishing and/or maintaining homeostasis. The environmental extremes that people usually experience do not elicit responses approaching physiological limits in sedentary people, and probably have little impact on nutritional requirements. However, stress of physical activity elicits responses approaching physiological limits, and that stress can be sufficiently exacerbated by exposure to extreme environments to have nutritional impact. Since exercise alone has a major influence on nutritional requirements, this chapter will examine environmental effects from the perspective of physically active persons.

HEAT EXCHANGE AND THERMAL BALANCE

Thermal stress arises from the combined effects of temperature, humidity, sun, wind, rain/water exposures, clothing worn, and body heat produced. Muscular contractions and other physiological processes produce metabolic heat that is transferred from the tissues to blood, and then distributed convectively throughout the body. The balance between internal heat production and its transfer to the environment determines body temperature. The heat balance equation (Gagge and Gonzalez 1996) summates the rates of body heat production and dissipation to calculate heat storage, which is positive when heat production is greatest or negative when heat dissipation is greatest. Body temperature increases when heat storage is positive, decreases when it is negative, and remains constant when it is zero.

The human thermoregulatory system normally compensates for altered heat storage and regulates core temperature within a narrow range (35° to 41°C) through behavioral and physiological responses to thermal stress. Behavioral responses operate to minimize or avoid thermal stress by modifying activity, changing clothes and seeking shade or shelter. When behavior cannot negate thermal stress, physiological responses are activated that, depending on whether the thermal stress is heat or cold, enhance dissipation or conservation of body heat stores through mechanisms to alter metabolic rate (shivering), blood flow between core to the skin (vasoconstriction or vasodilation), and sweating. Thermal receptors in the body core and skin send temperature information to a central integrator, and deviation between the controlled variable (body temperature) and a reference variable ("set-point") constitute a "load error" generating a "thermal command signal" that regulates sweating, vasodilation, vasoconstriction and shivering (Sawka et al. 1996). These responses, which operate until heat balance and body temperatures return to normal, produce physiological strain that can influence nutritional requirements.

HEAT STRESS

Exercise-induced thermogenesis tends to increase body temperature, eliciting increased skin blood flow and sweating, which work in tandem to dissipate heat (Sawka and Young 2006). Raising skin blood flow facilitates convective heat transfer from the deep body tissues to the skin surface, where it can be transferred to the environment via convective, conductive and evaporative transfer. An increase in sweating closely parallels increasing body temperature, and sweat evaporation cools the skin. Therefore, after sweating has begun, skin blood flow serves primarily to deliver to the skin the heat that is being removed by sweat evaporation.

Climatic conditions, clothing, and exercise intensity are the primary factors determining an individual's sweating rate. Sweating rates of 0.3 to 1.0 L/h are observed in persons engaged in routine occupational activities in hot-weather (Adolph et al. 1947), and 1.0 to perhaps as high as 2.5 L/h in athletes exercising in the heat (Sawka and Young 2006). However, people usually only sustain high sweating rates for several hours per day, and the remainder of time, when more sedentary, they will have lower sweating rates. Sweat losses must be replaced by fluid consumption, or else dehydration will ensue. For competitive athletes training in hot weather, daily fluid requirements might range from 4 to 12 L, whereas daily fluid requirements of less active or sedentary persons would fall nearer the bottom of that range (Sawka and Young 2006).

Sweating also results in electrolyte loss, primarily sodium chloride, but also measurable amounts of potassium, calcium, magnesium, and other trace minerals. Sweat sodium concentrations average 50 mEq/L, but vary widely over a range from 10–70 mEq/L (Sawka and Montain 2000). However, many factors influence sweat composition, including the specific sweating rate, diet, hydration, and heat acclimation status. Therefore, daily dietary electrolyte replacement requirements for hot climates are difficult to predict with precision. General guidance is that dietary sodium requirements in hot climates may be somewhat higher than the 4 g/d recommended for cool environments, ranging from 6 g/d for people engaged in light or sedentary activities, to as high as 12 g/d for persons performing extremely strenuous activities in very hot climates. Overall, when meals are consumed ad libitum, supplementation is not necessary because adjustments in an individual's salt appetite correct for changes in sodium stores (Convertino et al. 1996). Furthermore, when individuals increase their level of physical activity, ad libitum caloric intake usually increases, with a concomitant increment in sodium intake sufficient to compensate for increased losses due to exercise (Sawka and Montain 2000). Sweat potassium, calcium, and magnesium concentrations are typically 3–15 mmol/L, 0.3–2 mmol/L, and 0.2–1.5 mmol/L, respectively, but much less is known about sweating-associated losses of the other trace minerals. While sweat losses of those (minerals) are much lower than for sodium, the impact of hot weather on daily dietary trace element requirements should not be ignored.

COLD STRESS

When ambient temperature is colder than body temperature, the thermal gradient favors body heat loss, and wind exacerbates heat loss (i.e., windchill) by facilitating convection at the body surface (Sawka and Young 2006). Water has a heat transfer coefficient 25 times greater than air. Therefore, heat conduction away from the body is greater during cold air exposure when skin and/ or clothing are wet (e.g., from rain) than dry. That enhancement of conductive heat loss is more pronounced during water immersion, even in relatively mild water temperatures. Regardless of the severity of cold, body temperature changes will depend on the balance between heat loss and heat production. When behavioral thermoregulation provides inadequate protection, two physiological responses are exhibited: peripheral vasoconstriction and thermogenesis (Sawka and Young 2006). Peripheral vasoconstriction decreases peripheral blood flow, which reduces convective heat transfer between the body's core and shell (skin, subcutaneous fat, and skeletal muscle), thus retarding body heat loss at the expense of declining peripheral tissue temperature. In humans, cold-induced thermogenesis is attributable to skeletal muscle contractile activity. Humans initiate thermogenesis voluntarily by increasing activity (exercise, increased "fidgeting," etc.), or through involuntary shivering, which consists of repeated, rhythmic muscle contractions, the intensity of which varies according to the severity of cold. While certain animals exhibit a cold-induced, non-shivering thermogenesis by noncontracting tissues, humans lack this mechanism.

Physical activity during cold exposure elicits both thermogenesis and increased peripheral blood flow (Sawka and Young 2006), and, just as in hot conditions, the increased peripheral blood flow facilitates heat loss to the environment. The exercise-associated increase in heat loss during cold-water immersion can be so great that metabolic heat production during even intense exercise can be insufficient to maintain thermal balance, and body temperature falls. However, during cold-air exposure, exercise-induced thermogenesis usually increases metabolic heat production sufficiently to match or exceed heat loss, and sweating is often elicited. This is especially true when conditions do not allow individuals to adjust the amount of cold-weather protective clothing being worn. Therefore, even in cold climates, sweating may influence dietary trace mineral requirements.

Cold exposure increases urine flow. A cold-induced diuresis results from a blood-pressure mediated increase in filtration, and decreased reabsorption of water and solute by the kidney (Freund and Young 1996). Urine flow can increase by 50–100% (Lennquist 1972; Lennquist et al. 1974). Lennquist et al. (1974) have shown that cold-induced diuresis is accompanied by increases in daily urine solute losses, including sodium, potassium, chloride, calcium, and phosphate. Thus, cold-induced diuresis could, at least theoretically, influence daily dietary micronutrient requirements. Although there is insufficient rationale to recommend increased daily intakes of mineral micronutrients during cold exposure (Committee on Military Nutrition Research 1996), research is limited. Further, increased exercise/activity exacerbates oxidative stress, and optimal intakes of antioxidant minerals could be different in cold, as compared to temperate, climates (Reynolds 1996).

HIGH-ALTITUDE STRESS

The weight of the atmosphere causes air to be more dense at sea level than at higher elevations, and barometric pressure (P_B, mmHg) decreases from sea level (P_B=760 mmHg) to the summit of Mt. Everest (P_B=253 mmHg). Atmospheric gas concentrations are constant over the earth. Thus, ambient O_2 pressure (PO_2) falls with P_B as elevation increases. The atmospheric PO_2 (in dry air) is 159 mm Hg at sea level (760×0.2093) and 53 mmHg on the summit of Mt. Everest (253×0.2093). When the air is inspired, saturation with water vapor reduces inspired oxygen pressure (P_IO_2) below ambient PO_2. The P_IO_2 is 149 mmHg ($[760–47]\times0.2093$) at sea level and 43 mmHg ($[253–47]\times0.2093$) on the summit of Mt. Everest. Nevertheless, men have ascended Mt. Everest successfully without supplemental O_2. Clearly, humans have a great capacity for physiological compensation for hypoxia, and these compensations can influence nutrition.

The physiological responses to hypoxia at high altitude include increased pulmonary ventilation, although that response is insufficient to return alveolar oxygen pressure to sea level values. Therefore, the amount of O_2 in blood is less at high altitude than at sea level, necessitating a tachycardia-mediated elevation of cardiac output to meet metabolic demands (Stenberg et al. 1966). With long-term acclimatization to high altitude, expansion in red cell volume increase blood hemoglobin (Ward et al. 1989), facilitating oxygen transport with less cardiac strain.

High-altitude hypoxia exacerbates sweat losses during exercise compared to sea level (Young and Reeves 2002), but this effect is minimal for sedentary persons. Lowlanders also experience hormonally mediated diuresis at altitude (Hoyt and Honig 1995; Raff et al. 1996; Westerterp et al. 1996). Increased sweating and diuresis would be expected to impact mineral nutriture similarly at high altitude as described above. In addition, oxidative stress may be increased at high altitude, particularly for physically active persons, raising the possibility that dietary supplementation with antioxidant vitamins and minerals could have benefits. Increased erythropoietic activity stimulates increased red blood cell production and hemoglobin synthesis at high altitude (Young and Reeves 2002), but healthy, well-nourished lowlanders will not need to supplement iron intake (Reynolds 1996). Iron-deficient individuals, especially athletes, fail to demonstrate the erythropoietic response to altitude fully (Levine and Stray-Gundersen 1992), and, therefore, may need supplementation to achieve 15 (men) to 20 (women) mg/day (Reynolds 1996).

SUMMARY

Human trace mineral nutrition is influenced by exposure to extreme environments, especially in persons performing significant amounts of strenuous physical work or exercise. High sweating rates, elicited by exercise and/or environmental stress are probably the most significant mechanism accounting for increased mineral losses compared to losses of sedentary persons in temperate environments at sea level. In addition, diuresis may also contribute to accelerated mineral losses during cold exposure or sojourns at high altitude. If exercise or exposure to heat, cold, or altitude stress results in increased loss of trace minerals from the body stores, then the daily dietary intake requires compensatory adjustment. In addition, strenuous exercise, especially when performed under conditions of extreme environments, may contribute to oxidative stress sufficiently to merit increased consumption of dietary antioxidants, including antioxidant trace minerals.

DISCLAIMER

The opinions or assertions contained herein are the private views of the author and are not to be construed as official or as reflecting the views of the Army or the Department of Defense. Any citations of commercial organizations and trade names in this report do not constitute an official Department of the Army endorsement of approval of the products or services of these organizations.

REFERENCES

Adolph EF, et al. Physiology of Man in the Desert. New York: Intersciences, Inc.; 1947.

Committee on Military Nutrition Research. A Review of the Physiology and Nutrition in Cold and in High Altitude Environments. In: Marriot BM, Carlson SJ, editors. Nutritional Needs in Cold and in High-Altitude Environments. Washington, D.C.: National Academy Press; 1996:3–57.

Convertino VA, Armstrong LE, Coyle EF, Mack GW, Sawka MN, Senay LC, et al. Exercise and fluid replacement. Med Sci Sports Exerc. 1996;28:i–vii.

Freund B, Young AJ. Environmental influences on body fluid balance during exercise: cold exposure. In: Buskirk E, Puhl SM, editors. Body Fluid Balance. New York: CRC; 1996:159–81.

Gagge AP, Gonzalez RR. Mechanisms of heat exchange: biophysics and physiology. In: Fregly MJ, Blatteis CM, editors. Handbook of Physiology, Section 4, Environmental Physiology. New York: Oxford University Press; 1996:45–84.

Hoyt RW, Honig A. Body fluid and energy metabolism at high altitude. In: Fregley MJ, Blatteis

CM, editors. Handbook of Physiology: Section 4, Environmental Physiology, Volume II. New York: Oxford University Press; 1995:1277–89.

Lennquist S. Cold-induced diuresis. A study with special reference to electrolyte excretion, osmolal balance and hormonal changes. Scand J Urol Nephrol. 1972;9:Suppl 9:1–142.

Lennquist S, Granberg PO, Wedin B. Fluid balance and physical work capacity in humans exposed to cold. Arch Environ Health. 1974;29:241–9.

Levine BD, Stray-Gundersen J. A practical approach to altitude training: where to live and train for optimal performance enhancement. Int J Sports Med. 1992;13:S209–12.

Raff H, Janowski BM, Engel WC, Oaks MK. Hypoxia in vivo inhibits aldosterone synthesis and aldosterone synthase mRNA in rats. J Appl Physiol. 1996;81:604–10.

Reynolds RD. Effects of Cold and Altitude on Vitamin and Mineral Requirements. In: Marriot BM, Carlson LD, editors. Nutritional Needs in Cold and in High-Altitude Environments. Washington, D.C.: National Academy Press; 1996:215–44.

Sawka MN, Wenger CB, Pandolf KB. Thermoregulatory responses to acute exercise—heat stress and heat acclimation. In: Fregly MJ, Blatteis CM, editors. Handbook of Physiology, Section 4, Environmental Physiology. New York: Oxford University Press; 1996:157–85.

Sawka MN, Young AJ. Physiological Systems and Their Responses with Exposure to Heat and Cold. In: Tipton CM, Sawka, Tate CA, Terjung RL, editors. ACSM's Advanced Exercise Physiology Textbook. Baltimore: Lippincott, Williams & Wilkins; 2006: 535–80.

Sawka MN, Montain SJ. Fluid and electrolyte supplementation for exercise heat stress. Am J Clin Nutr. 2000;72:564–72.

Stenberg J, Ekblom B, Messin R. Hemodynamic response to work at simulated altitude, 4,000 m. J Appl Physiol. 1966;21:1589–94.

Ward MP, Milledge JS, West JB. Haematological changes and plasma volume. London: Chapman & Hall; 1989.

Westerterp KR, Robach P, Wouters L, Richalet JP. Water balance and acute mountain sickness before and after arrival at high altitude of 4,350 m. J Appl Physiol. 1996;80:1968–72.

Young AJ, Reeves JT. Human Adaptation to High Terrestrial Altitude. In: Pandolf KB, Burr RE, editors.

Medical Aspects of Harsh Environments, Volume 2. Washington, DC: Dept. of the Army, The Office of The Surgeon General; 2002:647–83.

An invited paper presented in the symposium "Environmental stress and mineral homeostasis".

Iron Homeostasis and Environmental Extremes: Focus on Physical Activity

James P. McClung, Ph.D.
Military Nutrition Division
US Army Research Institute of Environmental Medicine
Kansas St., Building 42
Natick, MA 01760, USA

Corresponding Author:
james.mcclung@na.amedd.army.mil

Introduction

Iron is a nutritionally essential trace element that functions primarily through incorporation into proteins and enzymes. Examples of these proteins and enzymes include hemoglobin and myoglobin for the transport and storage of oxygen, and cytochromes for the oxidative production of cellular energy. Iron deficiency is the most prevalent micronutrient deficiency disorder in the world. Recent estimates suggest that iron deficiency may affect up to 2 billion people globally (DeMaeyer and Adiels-Tegman 1985; Stoltzfus 2001), including up to 16% of premenopausal females in the United States (Looker et al. 2002). Iron deficiency has important public health implications, as changes in immune function, cognitive performance, and work capacity have been described in humans and animals with suboptimal iron status (Dallman 1986; Beard 2001; Haas and Brownlie 2001).

Iron status may be affected by a number of factors other than diet, including exposure to environmental extremes and engagement in heavy physical activity. A recent series of studies has explored the effects of combat training on iron status in female military personnel. Decrements in iron status indicators, including serum ferritin and transferrin saturation have been reported following 8 weeks of military training (McClung et al. 2006). This review will focus on the effects of environmental extremes on iron status, using training studies with female military personnel as an example of a population that may be sensitive to activity-induced decrements in iron status. Findings from studies with athletes will be reviewed as well, leading to a series of potential hypotheses explaining decrements in iron status in response to physical activity. Finally, nutritional strategies to mitigate the effects of environmental extremes and heavy physical activity on iron status will be described.

Iron Status in Female Military Personnel

Female military personnel are exposed to intense metabolic and cognitive demands during field training and operational deployment. Iron deficiency and iron deficiency anemia cause marked decrements in cognitive function and work capacity (Dallman 1986; Haas and Brownlie 2001). As female military personnel are typically premenopausal and at high risk of iron deficiency, and suboptimal iron intakes have been reported in this population (King et al. 1993), recent studies from our research group have focused on the effects of basic combat training (BCT) on iron status in female military personnel from the U.S. Army.

Army BCT consists of 8 to 9 weeks of activities, including aerobic and muscle strength training, tactical road marches, live fire training, and obstacle courses. Organized exercise generally occurs six times per week for an hour or more, and includes a variety of callisthenic exercises and running (Knapik et al. 2002). During BCT, trainees typically consume meals at a cafeteria-style dining facility with a wide variety of food choices. During field training, soldiers are provided military rations that contain all of the essential nutrients, including iron, and the energy required to maintain health and performance under all conditions. However, under-consumption of both calories and iron have been identified as a concern during military training (King et al. 1993; Baker-Fulco 1995).

A recent study from our laboratory determined the prevalence of iron deficiency and iron deficiency anemia among female soldiers immediately following entry to the Army, immediately following the BCT course, and following at least 6 months of permanent assignment to a regular duty station after BCT (McClung et al. 2006). Using a cross-sectional design and a series of iron status indicators, we found that the prevalence of iron deficiency and iron deficiency anemia in female soldiers upon initial entry to the Army was very similar to that of American women between the ages of 20–49. However, immediately following the completion of BCT, there was a striking increase in the prevalence of both iron deficiency and iron deficiency anemia. The prevalence of iron deficiency climbed from 13.4% upon initial entry to the Army to 32.8% following BCT. Likewise, the prevalence of iron deficiency anemia rose from 5.8% at the start of training to 20.9% following BCT. When iron status was determined at least 6 months beyond the completion of BCT, the prevalence of iron deficiency and iron deficiency anemia dropped to levels similar to initial entry to the Army. The prevalence of iron deficiency and iron deficiency anemia at each of the three timepoints appears in Figure 1.

The finding that iron status declines following military training may indicate a negative effect of sustained physical activity on iron homoeostasis. Although it is likely that suboptimal dietary iron intake is at least partially responsible for the decline in iron status, all soldiers in BCT have access to iron-containing foods, and their iron status returned to pre-training levels following permanent duty assignment. This suggests that the increased prevalence of iron deficiency observed in female soldiers during BCT might be prevented through improved iron nutrition in dining facilities, or by providing an iron supplement to maintain iron status during the training course.

Potential Causes of Diminished Iron Status Following Training

The decline in iron status observed in female soldiers during BCT is similar to that observed in college-age athletes during training periods (Beard and Tobin 2000), which may provide mechanistic evidence to determine the cause of activity-induced declines in iron status. "Sports anemia" was first described in 1970, and referred to diminished hemoglobin concentrations that occurred in response to physical activity (Yoshimura 1970). Diminished hemoglobin concentrations are typically attributed to the plasma volume expansion that occurs during training. More recent studies indicate that physical training affects not only hemoglobin, but other iron status indicators. In a retrospective review, Ashenden et al. (1998) described diminished serum ferritin levels during the training periods of female athletes participating in various sports. In another study, Magazanik et al. (1988) described reduced serum iron, total iron binding capacity, and serum ferritin in female athletes over a 7-week training period.

A number of hypotheses have been proposed to explain how physical activity could cause reduced iron status. For example, gastrointestinal bleeding may cause significant iron loss in athletes during training. Stewart et al. (1984) found elevated fecal hemoglobin levels in 20 of 24 runners following a long-distance race. Another possible mechanism for iron loss is increased whole body iron turnover during physical activity. Ehn et al. (1980) found that whole-body loss of isotopic iron occurred approximately 20% more quickly in female athletes as compared to non-athletes. Iron loss in athletes has also been attributed to hematuria, as one study found that up to 18% of marathon runners had blood in their urine following a race (Siegel et al. 1979).

A recent hypothesis that may explain reduced iron status in individuals exposed to heavy physical activity involves the function of hepcidin, a newly described protein that is synthesized and exported by the liver (Ganz and Nemeth 2006). The biological role of hepcidin has not been fully elucidated, although hepcidin is known to function in the regulation of cellular iron uptake, and its synthesis is directly affected by iron status (Pigeon et al. 2001) and inflammation (Nicolas et al. 2002a). Increased expression of hepcidin causes reduced iron status, as mice that overexpress hepcidin are born with severe iron deficiency and do not survive unless they are supplemented with parenteral iron (Nicolas et al. 2002b).

Pro-inflammatory cytokines, including IL-6, are major regulators of hepcidin synthesis (Ganz and Nemeth 2006). In fact, increased hepcidin expression in response to IL-6 infusion in humans leads to a significant reduction in indicators of iron status, including serum iron and transferrin saturation (Nemeth et al. 2004). At this point it is unclear as to whether inflammation caused by physical activity increases hepcidin expression. Current studies in our laboratory aim to determine whether military training elicits inflammatory responses and hepcidin release, which could explain the decrement in iron status observed in female military personnel during BCT, and perhaps athletes during training.

Conclusions

Iron status may be affected by factors other than diet, including exposure to harsh environments and heavy physical activity. Diminished iron status is associated with decrements in physical performance, including work capacity and cognitive function. The mechanism whereby heavy physical activity causes a reduction in iron status remains unknown, although changes in plasma volume, whole body iron turnover, and altered hepcidin expression may be contributing factors. In order to avoid the negative consequences of iron deficiency and iron deficiency anemia, individuals exposed to harsh environments and heavy physical activity should strive to consume the dietary reference intake (DRI) of iron. If iron deficiency or iron deficiency anemia has been diagnosed by a health care professional, supplementation with low doses of iron under the supervision of appropriately trained medical or dietary personnel should be considered.

Acknowledgements

The author acknowledges Nancy Andersen, Stephen Hennigar, and Tyson Tarr for their technical assistance in the preparation of this manuscript. The opinions or assertions contained herein are the private views of the authors and are not to be construed as official or as reflecting the views of the Army or the Department of Defense. Any citations of commercial organizations and trade names in this report do not constitute an official Department of the Army endorsement of approval of the products or services of these organizations.

References

Ashenden MJ, Martin DT, Dobson GP, Mackintosh C, Hahn AG. Serum ferritin and anemia in trained female athletes. Int J Sport Nut Ex Metab. 1998; 8:223–9.

Baker-Fulco CJ. An overview of dietary intakes during military exercises. In: Marriott BM, ed. Not eating enough. Washington, DC: National Academy Press; 1995:121–49.

Beard J, Tobin B. Iron status and exercise. Am J Clin Nutr. 2000; 72: 594S–7S.

Beard JL. Iron biology in immune function, muscle metabolism, and neuronal functioning. J Nutr. 2001;131:568S–80S.

Dallman PR. Biochemical basis for the manifestations of iron deficiency. Annu Rev Nutr. 1986;6:13–40.

DeMaeyer E, Adiels-Tegman, M. The prevalence of anemia in the world. World Health Stat Q. 1985; 38:302–16.

Ehn L, Carlmark B, Hoglund S. Iron status in athletes involved in intense physical activity. Med Sci Sports Exerc. 1980;12:61–4.

Ganz T, Nemeth E. Hepcidin and regulation of body iron metabolism. Am J Physiol Gastrointest Liver Physiol. 2006;290:G199–203.

Haas JD, Brownlie T. Iron deficiency and reduced work capacity: A critical review of the research to determine a causal relationship. J Nutr. 2001;131:676S–90S.

King N, Fridlund KE, Askew EW. Nutrition issues of military women. J Am Coll Nutr. 1993;12:344–8.

Knapik JJ, Canham-Chervak M, Hauret K, Laurin M, Hoedebecke E, Craig S, Montain SJ. Seasonal variations in injury rates during US Army basic combat training. Ann Occup Hyg. 2002;46:15–23.

Looker AC, Cogswell ME, Gunter MW. Iron deficiency—United States, 1999–2000. MMWR Morb Mortal Wkly Rep. 2002;51:897–9.

Magazanik A, Weinstein Y, Dlin RA, Derin M, Schwartzman S, Allalouf D. Iron deficiency caused by 7 weeks of intensive physical exercise. Eur J Appl Physiol Occup Physiol. 1988;57:198–202.

McClung JP, Marchitelli LJ, Friedl KE, Young AJ. Prevalence of iron deficiency and iron deficiency anemia among three populations of female military personnel in the US Army. J Am Coll Nutr. 2006;25:64–9.

Nemeth E, Tuttle MS, Powelson J, Vaughn MB, Donovan A, Ward DM, Ganz T, Kaplan J. Hepcidin regulates cellular iron efflux by binding to ferroportin and inducing its internalization. Science. 2004;306:2090–3.

Nicolas G, Chauvet C, Viatte L, Danan JL, Bigard X, Devaux I, Beaumont C, Kahn A, Vaulont S. The gene encoding the iron regulatory peptide hepcidin is regulated by anemia, hypoxia, and inflammation. J Clin Invest. 2002a;110:1037–44.

Nicolas G, Bennoun M, Porteu A, Mativet S, Beaumont C, Grandchamp B, Sirito M, Sawadogo M, Kahn A, Vaulont S. Severe iron deficiency anemia in transgenic mice expressing liver hepcidin. Proc Natl Acad Sci USA. 2002b;99:4596–601.

Pigeon C, Ilyin G, Courselaud B, Leroyer P, Turlin B, Brissot P, Loreal O. A new mouse liver-specific gene, encoding a protein homologous to human antimicrobial peptide hepcidin, is overexpressed during iron overload. J Biol Chem. 2001;276:7811–9.

Siegel AJ, Hennekens CH, Solomon HS, Van Boeckel BV. Exercise-related hematuria: findings in a group of marathon runners. JAMA. 1979; 241: 391–2.

Stewart JG, Ahlquist DA, McGill DB, Ilstrup DM, Schwartz S, Owen RA. Gastrointestinal blood loss and anemia in runners. Ann Intern Med. 1984;100:843–5.

Stoltzfus RJ. Defining iron-deficiency anemia in public health terms: time for reflection. J Nutr. 2001;131:565S–7S.

Yoshimura H. Anemia during physical training (sports anemia). Nutr Rev. 1970;28:251–3.

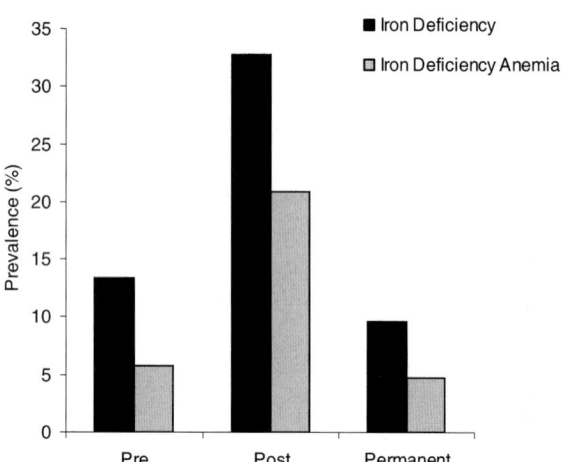

Fig. 1 Prevalence of Iron Deficiency and Iron Deficiency Anemia in Female Military Personnel. Iron status was determined before BCT (*Pre*), immediately following BCT (*Post*), and after 6 months of permanent duty assignment (*Permanent*). The definition of iron deficiency was an abnormal value for at least two of the following three indicators of iron status: serum ferritin, transferrin saturation, and red cell distribution width. Iron deficiency anemia was defined as iron deficiency as well as a low hemoglobin value (adapted from McClung et al. 2006)

An invited paper presented in the symposium "Environmental stress and mineral homeostasis".

Calcium Metabolism during Space Flight

Scott M. Smith[1] and Sara R. Zwart[2]
[1]Nutritional Biochemistry Laboratory, Human Adaptation and Countermeasures Office, NASA Johnson Space Center, Houston, TX 77058, USA; [2]Universities Space Research Association, Houston, TX 77058, USA

Corresponding Author:
Email address: scott.m.smith@nasa.gov

Calcium

Calcium is critical for maintaining the body's structural and mechanical functions, and it makes up 37% to 40% of the bone mineral hydroxyapatite in the body (Heaney et al. 1999). Total skeletal calcium is on average 1,100 to 1,500 g, and inadequate calcium intake has significant impact on adult bone (Institute of Medicine 1997). About 1% of the body's calcium stores reside in the intracellular structures, cell membranes, and extracellular fluids (Sauberlich 1999). In addition to its obvious role in the musculoskeletal system, calcium has a critical role in modulating the function of important proteins and regulating metabolic processes. Calcium binding activates proteins involved in a wide range of cell functions (Sauberlich 1999; Weaver and Heaney 1999). Circulating calcium levels are under tight control and are maintained within a narrow range (Nordin 1990).

Calcium Metabolism during Space Flight

As a result of skeletal unloading during space flight (Smith et al. 1977; Whedon 1984; Rambaut and Goode 1985; LeBlanc et al. 1996), bone mineral is lost, leading to increased urinary excretion of calcium (Smith et al. 1977; Whedon et al. 1977; Whedon 1984). Bone loss is a significant health concern for long-duration space flight (Holick 2000; Carmeliet et al. 2001; LeBlanc et al. 2007). It is estimated that the rate of bone mineral loss during space flight is about 0.5% to 1% per month (LeBlanc et al. 2000; Vico et al. 2000; Weaver et al. 2000). The bone loss, increased calcium excretion, and subsequent increased risk of renal stone formation during and after flight (Whitson et al. 1993; Whitson et al. 1997) are significant.

Data from the space station Skylab demonstrate that during space flight, bone mineral is not uniformly lost from all parts of the skeleton. Loss of bone tissue is most profound in weight-bearing bones such as the os calcis. Of the three men aboard the 59-day Skylab 3 mission, one lost a significant amount of os calcis bone mineral (−7.4%) but the other two did not (+2.3% and +1.4%). Calcium excretion in the urine was 200% of the preflight value for the man who lost os calcis mineral and 50% of the preflight values for the other two men (Smith et al. 1977).

Negative calcium balance was observed during both the Skylab (Whedon et al. 1974; Whedon et al. 1976; Smith et al. 1977; Whedon et al. 1977; Whedon 1984) and Mir (Smith et al. 1999; Smith et al. 2005) missions. During the 84-day Skylab 4 mission, calcium balance was −200 mg/day (Whedon et al. 1977; Rambaut and Johnston 1979), but no significant calcium losses occurred during the 28-day Skylab 2 mission (Smith et al. 1977; Weaver et al. 2000). Increased urinary and fecal calcium excretion accounted for most of the deficit in calcium (Whedon et al. 1976; Smith et al. 1977; Whitson et al. 1997; Smith et al. 1999; Smith et al. 2005). During the Skylab 4 mission, calcium losses correlated roughly with mineral losses in the os calcis (Whedon and Heaney 1993) and increases in the excretion of hydroxyproline.

Bone resorption increases during space flight, as shown by the concentrations of bone markers (Collet et al. 1997; Caillot-Augusseau et al. 1998; Smith et al. 1998) and by the results of calcium tracer kinetic studies (Smith et al. 1999; Smith et al. 2005). Urinary hydroxyproline was elevated 33% after 84 days of flight (Whedon et al. 1977; Leach et al. 1979). Urinary collagen crosslinks, also markers of bone resorption, were elevated >100% during space flight compared to preflight levels (Smith et al. 1998; Smith et al. 1999). Calcium tracer kinetic data indicated that bone resorption increased about 50% during flight (Smith et al. 1999).

Bone formation either remains unchanged or decreases during space flight (Smith et al. 1999; Weaver et al. 2000; Smith et al. 2005). As indicated by serum concentrations of bone-specific alkaline phosphatase and osteocalcin, bone formation was unchanged during Mir flights, but increased 2 to 3 months after landing (Smith et al. 1999; Smith et al. 2005). Trends toward decreased levels of bone formation markers were noted in two Mir studies with one subject each (Collet et al. 1997; Caillot-Augusseau et al. 1998). Studies, using calcium tracer techniques, of bone formation in three Mir crew members (Smith et al. 1999; Smith et al. 2005) were equivocal (formation unchanged or decreased). Together, increased resorption and decreased or unchanged formation yield an overall negative calcium balance (Smith et al. 1999; Smith et al. 2005).

A number of related factors likely contribute to the loss of bone mineral during weightlessness. Decreased calcium absorption by Mir astronauts has been observed (Smith et al. 1999; Smith et al. 2005) and likely resulted from the decreased concentration of circulating 1,25-

dihydroxyvitamin D that was also observed in these crew members (Smith et al. 1999; Smith et al. 2005). It is important to maintain calcium intake during flight, but the lower absorption during flight suggests that this is not a viable countermeasure for weightlessness-induced bone loss, a fact documented in bed rest studies (Baecker et al. unpublished observations).

Space flight analog studies (such as bed rest) with humans have shown qualitative effects on bone and calcium homeostasis similar to those shown in flight studies, with quantitative effects generally being of smaller magnitude. Effects include loss of bone mass (Vico et al. 1987; LeBlanc et al. 1990; Zerwekh et al. 1998), decreased calcium absorption (LeBlanc et al. 1995), increased urinary calcium and biochemical markers of resorption (Donaldson et al. 1970; LeBlanc et al. 1995; Heer et al. 2005), increased risk of renal stone formation (Dietrick et al. 1948; Hwang et al. 1988), and decreased serum concentrations of parathyroid hormone (Arnaud et al. 1992; Smith et al. 2003) and 1,25-dihydroxyvitamin D (LeBlanc et al. 1995; Smith et al. 2003).

If the rate of bone calcium loss is constant throughout a flight (a reasonable assumption judging by collagen crosslink excretion data (Smith et al. 1998; Smith et al. 1999; Smith et al. 2005), then about 250 mg of bone calcium are lost per day (Whedon et al. 1977; Grigoriev et al. 1998; Smith et al. 1999; Smith et al. 2005). The nature and degree of bone mineral loss over time varies between subjects (LeBlanc et al. 1990; LeBlanc et al. 1996).

Long-term follow-up data on bone recovery are lacking (Tilton et al. 1980). However, if the rate of postflight recovery is also assumed to be constant [reasonable according to ground-based (LeBlanc et al. 1990) and flight (Smith et al. 1999; Smith et al. 2005) data], then the rate of recovery is about +100 mg/day (Smith et al. 1999; Smith et al. 2005). By these estimates, on flights up to about 6 months, it takes 2 to 3 times the mission duration to recover the lost bone. For longer flights, however, the usefulness of these assumptions comes into question, as space flight data are not available. Although more data clearly are required to validate this hypothesis, it nevertheless has significant implications as mission durations increase.

Risks of Bone Mineral Loss during Exploration Missions

The ability to understand and counteract weightlessness-induced bone mineral loss will be critical for crew health and safety during and after extended-duration space station and exploration missions (Schneider and McDonald 1984; Heer et al. 1999). Changes in the endocrine regulation of bone metabolism seem to reflect adaptation to the weightless environment. Decreases in calcium absorption and plasma levels of parathyroid hormone and 1,25-dihydroxyvitamin D are expected physiological responses to increased resorption of bone that may occur as the body adapts to an environment in which bones bear less weight. This evidence, and the lack of improvement provided by earlier dietary countermeasures, indicate that supplementation of the diet with nutrients such as calcium and vitamin D will not correct this problem (Heer et al. 2003). Adequate nutrition will, however, be a required component in the success of whatever countermeasures are identified and implemented (Heer et al. 1995; Heer et al. 1999).

Summary

The effect of near-weightlessness on the human skeletal system is one of the greatest concerns in safely extending space missions (Holick 2000). Adequate intake of dietary calcium will be critical for maintaining skeletal health. Many other dietary factors, including dietary protein (amount and type) and dietary sodium affect calcium metabolism (Zwart and Smith 2005; Frings-Meuthen et al. 2008). Although it is unlikely that diet is solely responsible for the bone mineral loss associated with space flight, even modest protective effects from a balanced diet would benefit crew health.

References

Arnaud SB, Sherrard DJ, Maloney N, Whalen RT, Fung P. Effects of 1-week head-down tilt bed rest on bone formation and the calcium endocrine system. Aviat Space Environ Med 1992;63:14–20.

Caillot-Augusseau A, Lafage-Proust MH, Soler C, Pernod J, Dubois F, Alexandre C. Bone formation and resorption biological markers in cosmonauts during and after a 180-day space flight (Euromir 95). Clin Chem 1998;44(3):578–85.

Carmeliet G, Vico L, Bouillon R. Space flight: a challenge for normal bone homeostasis. Crit Rev Eukaryot Gene Expr 2001;11(1–3):131–44.

Collet P, Uebelhart D, Vico L et al. Effects of 1- and 6-month spaceflight on bone mass and biochemistry in two humans. Bone 1997;20:547–51.

Dietrick JE, Whedon GD, Shorr E. Effects of immobilization upon various metabolic and physiologic functions of normal men. Am J Med 1948;4:3–36.

Donaldson C, Hulley S, Vogel J, Hattner R, Bayers J, McMillan D. Effect of prolonged bed rest on bone mineral. Metabolism 1970;19:1071–84.

Frings-Meuthen P, Baecker N, Heer M. Low grade metabolic acidosis may be the cause of sodium chloride induced exaggerated bone resorption. J Bone Miner Res 2008;23:517–24.

Grigoriev AI, Oganov VS, Bakulin AV et al. [Clinical and physiological evaluation of bone changes among astronauts after long-term space flights]. Aviakosm Ekolog Med 1998;32:21–5.

Heaney RP, McCarron DA, Dawson-Hughes B et al. Dietary changes favorably affect bone remodeling in older adults. J Am Diet Assoc 1999;99(10):1228–33.

Heer M, Baecker N, Mika C, Boese A, Gerzer R. Immobilization induces a very rapid increase in osteoclast activity. Acta Astronaut 2005;57(1):31–6.

Heer M, Boese A, Baecker N, Smith SM. High calcium intake does not prevent disuse-induced bone loss. 24th Annual International Gravitational Physiology Meeting, Santa Monica, CA; 2003.

Heer M, Kamps N, Biener C et al. Calcium metabolism in microgravity. Eur J Med Res 1999; 4:357–60.

Heer M, Zittermann A, Hoetzel D. Role of nutrition during long-term spaceflight. Acta Astronaut 1995;35(4–5):297–311.

Holick MF. Microgravity-induced bone loss—will it limit human space exploration? Lancet 2000;355:1569–70.

Hwang TIS, Hill K, Schneider V, Pak CYC. Effect of prolonged bedrest on the propensity for renal stone formation. J Clin Endocrinol Metab 1988;66:109–12.

Institute of Medicine. Dietary reference intakes for calcium, phosphorus, magnesium, vitamin D, and fluoride. Washington, DC: National Academy Press; 1997.

Leach C, Rambaut P, Di Ferrante N. Amino aciduria in weightlessness. Acta Astronaut 1979;6:1323–33.

LeBlanc A, Schneider V, Shackelford L et al. Bone mineral and lean tissue loss after long duration space flight. J Bone Miner Res 1996;11 Suppl 1:S323.

LeBlanc A, Schneider V, Shackelford L et al. Bone mineral and lean tissue loss after long duration space flight. J Musculoskelet Neuronal Interact 2000;1:157–60.

LeBlanc A, Schneider V, Spector E et al. Calcium absorption, endogenous excretion, and endocrine changes during and after long-term bed rest. Bone 1995;16(4 Suppl):301S–4S.

LeBlanc AD, Schneider VS, Evans HJ, Engelbretson DA, Krebs JM. Bone mineral loss and recovery after 17 weeks of bed rest. J Bone Miner Res 1990;5:843–50.

LeBlanc AD, Spector ER, Evans HJ, Sibonga JD. Skeletal responses to space flight and the bed rest analog: a review. J Musculoskelet Neuronal Interact 2007;7(1):33–47.

Nordin BE. Calcium homeostasis. Clin Biochem 1990;23(1):3–10.

Rambaut P, Johnston R. Prolonged weightlessness and calcium loss in man. Acta Astronaut 1979;6:1113–22.

Rambaut PC, Goode AW. Skeletal changes during space flight. Lancet 1985;2(8463):1050–2.

Sauberlich H. Laboratory tests for the assessment of nutritional status. Boca Raton: CRC; 1999.

Schneider VS, McDonald J. Skeletal calcium homeostasis and countermeasures to prevent disuse osteoporosis. Calcif Tissue Int 1984;36(1 Suppl):S151–44.

Smith MC, Jr, Rambaut PC, Vogel JM, Whittle MW. Bone mineral measurement—experiment M078. In: Johnston RS, LF Dietlein, eds. Biomedical results from Skylab (NASA SP-377). Washington, DC: National Aeronautics and Space Administration; 1977:183–90.

Smith SM, Davis-Street JE, Fesperman JV et al. Evaluation of treadmill exercise in a lower body negative pressure chamber as a countermeasure for weightlessness-induced bone loss: a bed rest study with identical twins. J Bone Miner Res 2003;18:2223–30.

Smith SM, Nillen JL, Leblanc A et al. Collagen cross-link excretion during space flight and bed rest. J Clin Endocrinol Metab 1998; 83(10): 3584–91.

Smith SM, Wastney ME, Morukov BV et al. Calcium metabolism before, during, and after a 3-mo spaceflight: kinetic and biochemical changes. Am J Physiol 1999; 277(1 Pt 2): R1–10.

Smith SM, Wastney ME, O'Brien KO et al. Bone markers, calcium metabolism, and calcium kinetics during extended-duration space flight on the Mir space station. J Bone Miner Res 2005;20(2):208–18.

Tilton FE, Degioanni JJC, Schneider VS. Long-term follow-up of Skylab bone demineralization. Aviat Space Environ Med 1980;51:1209–13.

Vico L, Chappard D, Alexandre C et al. Effects of a 120 day period of bed-rest on bone mass and bone cell activities in man: attempts at countermeasure. Bone Miner 1987;2:383–94.

Vico L, Collet P, Guignandon A et al. Effects of long-term microgravity exposure on cancellous and cortical weight-bearing bones of cosmonauts. Lancet 2000;355(9215):1607–11.

Weaver CM, Heaney RP. Calcium. In: Shils ME, JA Olson, M Shike, AC Ross, eds. Modern nutrition in health and disease. Baltimore, MD: Lippincott Williams & Wilkins; 1999: 141–55.

Weaver CM, LeBlanc A, Smith SM. Calcium and related nutrients in bone metabolism. In: Lane HW, DA Schoeller, eds. Nutrition in spaceflight and weightlessness models. Boca Raton, FL: CRC; 2000:179–201.

Whedon G, Heaney R. Effects of physical inactivity, paralysis and weightlessness on bone growth. In: Hall B, ed. Bone. Boca Raton: CRC; 1993;7:57–77.

Whedon G, Lutwak L, Rambaut P et al. Mineral and nitrogen balance study observations: the second manned Skylab mission. Aviat Space Environ Med 1976;47:391–6.

Whedon GD. Disuse osteoporosis: physiological aspects. Calcif Tissue Int 1984;36:S146–50.

Whedon GD, Lutwak L, Rambaut PC et al. Mineral and nitrogen metabolic studies, experiment M071. In: Johnston RS, LF Dietlein, eds. Biomedical results from Skylab (NASA SP-377). Washington, DC: National Aeronautics and Space Administration; 1977: 164–74.

Whedon GD, Lutwak L, Reid J et al. Mineral and nitrogen metabolic studies on Skylab orbital space flights. Trans Assoc Am Physicians 1974;87:95–110.

Whitson P, Pietrzyk R, Pak C. Renal stone risk assessment during Space Shuttle flights. J Urol 1997;158:2305–10.

Whitson P, Pietrzyk R, Pak C, Cintron N. Alterations in renal stone risk factors after space flight. J Urol 1993;150:803–7.

Zerwekh JE, Ruml LA, Gottschalk F, Pak CY. The effects of twelve weeks of bed rest on bone histology, biochemical markers of bone turnover, and calcium homeostasis in eleven normal subjects. J Bone Miner Res 1998;13:1594–601.

Zwart SR, Smith SM. The impact of space flight on the human skeletal system and potential nutritional countermeasures. International SportMed Journal 2005;6(4):199–214.

An invited paper presented in the symposium "Environmental stress and mineral homeostasis".

Mineral Losses During Extreme Environmental Conditions

Henry C. Lukaski
USDA, ARS
Grand Forks Human Nutrition Research Center
Grand Forks, ND 58202

Corresponding Author:
Email: henry.lukaski@ars.usda.gov

Introduction

Broad interest in the effects of the loss of minerals in sweat during physical activity persists because of its potentially adverse impact on nutrient requirements. Advisory groups that make recommendations for mineral intakes seek reliable information on the effects of usual activity patterns at work and recreation on mineral losses of children, adolescents and adults (Food and Nutrition Board 2001). Similarly, there is renewed attention on mineral needs associated with strenuous physical activity, stress and other conditions encountered during military life (Committee on Military Nutrition 2006). The public also seeks substantiation of claims in advertisements that mineral and other nutrient needs increase when people participate in regular physical activity as recommended to achieve and maintain healthy body weight (Dietary Guidelines for Americans 2005). Thus, there is a need to ascertain whether conditions that promote surface loss of minerals affect the mineral needs of people.

Factors affecting sweat mineral concentrations

For nearly 50 years, investigators have reported highly variable data describing the concentrations of calcium, iron, and zinc in sweat at rest and during exercise in the heat. Several factors contribute to the diversity in the reported sweat mineral concentrations including the methods and sites selected for sweat collection, possible sources of sample contamination, analytical methods, environmental conditions used to stimulate sweating, and type and duration of exercise.

One confounding issue is the use of regional sites to estimate whole body mineral losses in sweat. Costa et al. (1969) reported that mineral concentrations obtained with patches from regional collection sites were greater than whole-body (shorts, shorts, socks, lower arm, and bath) determinations of men undergoing moderate amounts of work. Palacios et al. (2003) found that losses of calcium and magnesium using whole body wash-down procedures were $103\pm$ 13 and 35 ± 13 mg/day, respectively. However, projection of the whole body losses based on electrolyte concentrations determined with patches at eight sites and extrapolated to body surface area yielded values more than three times greater than the measured losses. Other investigators showed a similar magnitude of underestimation of whole body sweat mineral concentrations compared to arm sweat (Cohn and Emmett 1978; Jacob et al. 1981; Hoshi et al. 2001). Thus, use of regional measurements to estimate whole body loss overestimates total body mineral losses.

Sweat concentrations of minerals vary among collection sites. Aruoma et al. (1988) found that iron concentrations were greater on the abdomen and chest ($\sim$0.5 mg/dL) compared to the arm and back ($\sim$0.2 mg/dL); zinc concentration also was greater on the abdomen ($\sim$0.8 mg/dL) compared to the arm, chest and back ($\sim$0.4 mg/dL) in response to acute exercise in the heat. Palacios et al. (2003) reported similarity in calcium (1.0–1.45 mg/d) and magnesium (0.43–0.49 mg/day) losses estimated by collections at sites on the arms, legs and back.

Environmental temperature and humidity affect mineral concentrations. Sweat concentrations of zinc and iron were lower in warm than in cool environments (Tipton et al. 1993; Waller and Haymes 1996). Sweat rates increased in the warm environments resulting in dilute sweat mineral concentrations. However, the amounts of zinc and iron lost (concentration multiplied by volume) were the same in these environments.

Physiological adaptations to environmental conditions impact sweat mineral concentrations. Repeated exposures over 1–2 weeks reduced sweat calcium, magnesium, iron, and zinc (Consolazio et al. 1964; Chinevere et al. 2008). Mineral concentrations also decrease during a bout of prolonged exercise in the heat. Serial measurements revealed that iron and zinc concentrations decreased during a 2–7-h exercise in a hot environment (DeRuisseau et al. 2002; Montain et al. 2007). These changes are the result of increased rates of sweating during prolonged exercise and exfoliation of cells and cellular debris from sweat glands during the initial period of sweating.

Effects of sweat mineral losses on nutritional requirements

Assessment of whole body surface loss of minerals has been restricted to non-exercise states. Jacob et al. (1981) reported that mean losses of copper, iron and zinc of 13 men were 0.34, 0.33, and 0.50 mg/day that represented 26, 2 and 4% of daily intakes, respectively. Attempts to determine the impact of minerals lost in the sweat on mineral needs are hampered by a paucity of reports that describe both mineral concentrations and sweat losses. Thus, the following estimates should be considered as preliminary.

Calcium

Whole body sweat calcium concentrations were measured during exercise in a few studies. Among 12 men who exercised for 40 min at variable total work outputs, calcium loss in sweat was measured to be between 72 ± 10 and 74 ± 17 μg (Costa et al. 1969). Palacios et al. (2003) reported calcium losses of $103\pm$ 22 mg/day among six women who performed uncontrolled exercise during a 24-h period. Based on the adequate intake of 1,000 mg/d for calcium as a reference (Food and Nutrition Board 1997), mild exercise was associated with a $\sim$10% calcium loss.

Iron

Determination of iron concentrations in sweat has been studied extensively. Initial reports of whole body surface iron losses ranged from 0.24 to 0.33 mg/day under non-exercise conditions (Green et al. 1968; Jacob et al. 1981). Vellar (1968) found iron losses of 0.38 mg/h during a 1-h heat exposure. Lamanaca et al. (1988) reported iron losses ranging from 0.21 to 0.28 mg/h among trained runners during 30–60 min of exercise in the heat. In contrast, a 30-min heat exposure in a sauna resulted in 0.02-mg iron loss in sweat (Brune et al. 1986).

The duration of physical activity affects sweat iron losses. DeRuisseau et al. (2002) reported that sweat iron concentrations decreased significantly from 0.20 mg/L at 30 min to 0.10 mg/L at 120 min whereas sweat rate increased progressively. Sweat iron losses were estimated to be 3% of the recommended dietary allowance or RDA (Food and Nutrition Board 2001).

The interaction of dietary iron and exercise on iron metabolism has been reported (Table 1). Heat-acclimatized men consumed diets containing two levels of iron for 3-day periods, performed their habitual activities and exercised 2 h once during each diet period; and whole body sweat was collected with a wash-down technique (Wheeler et al. 1973). When iron intake was high, iron balance was positive (e.g., iron retention). However, when iron intake was reduced to 17.5 mg/d, iron balance was negative (e.g., iron loss exceeded intake). Sweat iron loss apparently did not respond to the change in iron intake, but was greater (2 vs 1%) when dietary iron was reduced.

Table 1 Effects of Exercise and Iron (Fe) Intake on Iron Losses and Balance[a]

Condition	Fe Intake (mg/day)	Urinary Fe (mg/day)	Fecal Fe (mg/day)	Sweat Fe (mg/day)	Balance (mg/day)
UA	34.8	0.22	22.0	0.38	+12.2
UA+ST	36.8	0.23	26.0	0.32	+10.3
UA+ST	17.5	0.19	25.2	0.34	−8.2

Adapted from Wheeler et al. (1973)

UA usual activity pattern, *ST* 2 h of step exercise

[a]Balance = intake − [urinary + fecal + sweat losses]

Zinc

Interest in the contribution of sweat zinc to daily zinc needs began with the finding that almost 5% of the daily intake (11 mg) of young men was lost under thermoneutral conditions (Jacob et al. 1981). Al-though data from 2-h periods of exercise in the heat indicated a reduction in the concentrations of zinc (0.9 to 0.6 mg/L), the calculated loss of zinc was 8–9% of the RDA (DeRuisseau et al. 2002). The combination of exercise and heat acclimation resulted in marked decreases in zinc losses, estimated from arm sweat, from 13.7 to 2.41 mg/day (Consolazio et al. 1964). Whereas the initial estimate of sweat zinc loss is very large, the sweat losses during the subsequent 11 d of heat and exercise exposure ranged from 2.18 to 2.41 mg/day, which represent 20–21% of the RDA for zinc (Food and Nutrition Board 2001).

Table 2 shows an example of the potentially adverse effect of different estimates of sweat zinc loss on zinc balance of young men fed different amounts of zinc while engaged in regular physical activity. Use of a conservative estimate of surface zinc loss, derived without an exercise or temperature stressor, shows a negative zinc balance with limited zinc intake. When the experimentally-derived estimate of exercise-heat induced sweat zinc loss is included in the calculation, both estimates of zinc balance reveal net loss of zinc. Thus, under conditions of regular physical activity, sweat zinc losses may be detrimental to maintenance of body zinc stores.

Table 2 Impact of Sweat Zinc (Zn) on Zinc Retention in Physically Active Men

	Zn supplement	Low Zn
Intake, mg/day[a]	18.7	3.6
Losses, mg/day		
Urine	0.5	0.4*
Feces	16.8	3.1*
Sweat, mg		
Basal	0.8[b]	0.8[b]
Exercise	2.4[c]	2.4[c]
Balance, mg/day		
Basal	+0.6	−0.8
Exercise	−1.0	−2.4

*$p<0.05$

[a]Lukaski et al. (2005)

[b]Jacob et al. (1981)

[c]Consolazio et al. (1964)

Other Considerations

Collection of sweat from various sites on the body during exercise may result in a heterogeneous solution containing aqueous and cellular components. Prasad et al. (1963)

found that zinc concentrations were similar in whole compared to cell-free sweat (115±30 vs 93±26 µg/dL). However, iron concentrations were greater in whole than cell-free sweat (120±36 vs 46±11 µg/dL). Confirmation of these differences is needed to develop a uniform preparatory method for analysis of sweat samples.

Mineral deficiency affects sweat mineral concentrations. Prasad et al. (1963) found that zinc-deficient, compared to zinc-adequate, men had significantly reduced concentrations of zinc and iron in both whole and cell-free sweat collected from their arms while performing exercise in a hot environment. Milne et al. (1983) reported that whole body zinc losses decreased when men were fed diets low in zinc (~4 mg/day) compared to higher zinc intakes (~33 mg/day). The decreases in sweat zinc losses paralleled the observed reductions in zinc status indicators. Thus, changes in zinc nutrition affect sweat zinc concentrations.

Summary and conclusions

Accurate assessment of mineral losses in sweat during exposure to extreme environmental conditions is a challenge because of the need to minimize contamination while requiring a practical collection method. Mineral losses can be appreciable regardless of collection site or method used. Based on empirical data, losses in sweat can adversely affect body mineral retention. Key issues to resolve include the determination of practical sites for sweat collection during physical activity and establishment of valid estimates of regional sweat loss for use in calculation of total mineral losses during exercise in various environmental conditions.

Acknowledgements

Mention of a trademark or proprietary product does not constitute a guarantee of the product by the United States Department of Agriculture and does not imply its approval to the exclusion of other products that may also be suitable. U.S. Department of Agriculture, Agricultural Research, Northern Plains Area is an equal opportunity/affirmative action employer and all agency services are available without discrimination.

References

Aruoma OI, Reilly T, MacLaren D, Halliwell B. Iron, copper and zinc concentrations in human sweat and plasma: the effect of exercise. Clin Chim Acta 1988;177:81–8.

Brune M, Magnusson B, Perrson H, Hallberg L. Iron losses in sweat. Am J Clin Nutr 1986;43:438–43.

Chinevere TD, Kenefick RW, Cheuvront SN, Lukaski HC, Sawka MN. Effect of heat acclimation on sweat minerals. Med Sci Exerc Sport 2008;40:886–91.

Cohn JR, Emmett EA. The excretion of trace metals in human sweat. Ann Clin Lab Sci 1978;8:270–5.

Committee on Military Nutrition, Food and Nutrition Board, Institute of Medicine. Mineral Requirements for Military Personnel. Levels Needed for Cognitive and Physical Performance During Garrison Training. Washington, DC: National Academy of Sciences, 2006.

Consolazio CF, Nelson RA, Matoush LO, Hughes RC. The trace mineral losses in sweat. Denver, CO: US Army Medical Research and Nutrition Laboratory. 1964. Report No. 284.

Costa F, Calloway DH, Margen S. Regional and total body sweat composition of men fed controlled diets. Am J Clin Nutr 1969;22:52–8.

DeRuisseau KC, Cheuvront SN, Haymes EM, Sharp RG. Sweat iron and zinc losses during prolonged exercise. Int J Sport Nutr Exerc Metabol 2002;12:428–37.

Dietary Guidelines for Americans 2005. U.S. Department of Health and Human Services and U.S. Department of Agriculture (www.healthierus.gov/dietaryguidelines).

Food and Nutrition Board, Institute of Medicine. Dietary reference intakes for vitamin A, arsenic, boron, chromium, copper, iodine, iron, manganese, molybdenum, nickel, silicon, vanadium, and zinc. Washington, DC: National Academy of Sciences, 2001.

Food and Nutrition Board, Institute of Medicine. Dietary reference intakes for calcium, phosphorus, magnesium, vitamin D, and fluorine. Washington, DC: National Academy of Sciences, 1997.

Green R, Charlton R, Seftel H, Bothwell T, Mayet F, Finch C, Layrisse M. Body iron excretion in man. Am J Med 1968; 45: 336–53.

Hoshi A, Watanabe H, Kobayashi M, Chiba M, Inaba Y, Kimura N, Ito T. Concentrations of trace elements in sweat during sauna bathing. Tohoku J Exp Med 2001;195:163–69.

Jacob RA, Sandstead HH, Munoz JM, Klevay LM, Milne DB. Whole body surface loss of trace elements in normal males. Am J Clin Nutr 1981;34:1379–83.

Lamanaca JJ, Haymes EM, Daly JA, Moffatt RJ, Waller MF. Sweat iron losses of male and female runners during exercise. Int J Sports Med 1988; 9: 52–5.

Lukaski, H.C. Low dietary zinc decreases erythrocyte carbonic anhydrase activities and impairs cardiorespiratory function in men during exercise. Am. J. Clin. Nutr. 2005;81:1045–51.

Milne DB, Canfield WK, Mahalko JR, Sandstead HH. Effect of dietary zinc on whole body surface loss of zinc: impact on estimation of zinc retention by balance method. Am J Clin Nutr 1983;38:181–86.

Montain SJ, Cheuvront SN, Lukaski HC. Sweat mineral-element responses during 7 hour of exercise-heat stress. Int J Sport Nutr Exerc Metabol 2007;17: 574–82.

Palacios C, Wigertz K, Weaver CM. Comparison of 24-hour whole body versus patch tests for estimating body surface electrolyte losses. Int J Sport Nutr Exerc Metabol 2003;13:479–88.

Prasad AS, Schulert AR, Sandstead HH, Miale A, Farid Z. Zinc, iron and nitrogen content of sweat of normal and deficient subjects. J Lab Clin Med 1963;62:84–9.

Tipton K, Green NR, Haymes EM, Waller M. Zinc loss in sweat of athletes exercising in hot and neutral temperatures. Int J Sport Nutr 1993;3:261–71.

Vellar OD. Studies on sweat losses of nutrients I: iron content of whole body sweat and its association with other sweat constituents, serum iron levels, hematological indices, body surface area, and sweat rate. Scand J Clin Lab Med 1968;21:157–67.

Waller MF, Haymes EM. The effects of heat and exercise on sweat iron loss. Med Sci Exerc Sport 1996;28:197–03.

Wheeler EF, El-Neil H, Willson JOC, Weiner JS. The effect of work level and dietary intake on water balance and the excretion of sodium, potassium and iron in a hot environment. Br J Nutr 1973;30:127–37.